Application of Electrophysical Agents in Physiotherapy

Dimitrios Stasinopoulos
Editor

Application of Electrophysical Agents in Physiotherapy

Springer

Editor
Dimitrios Stasinopoulos
University of West Attica
Athens, Greece

ISBN 978-3-032-32143-5 ISBN 978-3-032-32144-2 (eBook)
https://doi.org/10.1007/978-3-032-32144-2

This Springer imprint is published by the registered company Springer Nature Switzerland AG
The registered company address is: Gewerbestrasse 11, 6330 Cham, Switzerland

Acknowledgments

The writing of this book is the culmination of many years of academic teaching, clinical practice, research activity, and collaboration with remarkable individuals, to whom I owe my sincere gratitude.

First and foremost, I would like to express my deepest gratitude to my PhD supervisor, Professor Mark I. Johnson. He has been far more than an academic mentor to me. He taught me how to approach scientific research with critical thinking, how to write scientific papers, and how to communicate scientific knowledge with clarity and rigor. Above all, he instilled in me the academic values that continue to guide every aspect of my scientific work. His contribution to my academic and professional development has been invaluable.

I would also like to express my sincere appreciation to all my undergraduate, postgraduate, doctoral, and PhD candidate students. Through our interactions in teaching, research, and clinical practice, they have continuously challenged my thinking, broadened my knowledge, and contributed significantly to my scientific development.

My heartfelt thanks also go to my publisher and friend, **Giannis Konstantaras**, who first inspired me to write a book of this kind. I am equally grateful to my dear friend **Angelos Prasas**, whose dedication, hard work, and unwavering commitment throughout the preparation of this book were invaluable.

I would also like to thank all my patients. Every patient has represented a unique opportunity to learn, reflect, and grow as both a clinician and an academic. My daily clinical practice has been the greatest source of inspiration for many of the ideas, observations, and clinical approaches presented in this book.

I would also like to express my sincere appreciation to everyone at **Springer** who contributed to the development and publication of this book. My special thanks go to the editorial and production teams for their professionalism, guidance, and continuous support throughout the publishing process. Their dedication, efficiency, and attention to detail have played an essential role in transforming this project into a finished book.

Finally, I would like to express my deepest gratitude to my wife, **Eirini**, and to our children, **Argyri** and **Ioannis**, for their love, patience, understanding, and unwavering support throughout these years. Their presence has been a constant source of strength and inspiration at every stage of my academic career and throughout the writing of this book.

I dedicate this book to my parents, **Argyri** and **Ioannis**, and to my beloved sister, **Kelly**, whose love, encouragement, and unwavering belief in me have supported me throughout every stage of my life and academic journey.

Most importantly, I dedicate this book to the memory of my father. From the very beginning of my academic career, he continually encouraged me to write scientific papers and books, believing in my abilities long before I believed in them myself. Sadly, he did not live to see the publication of this book or the fulfillment of a dream that we shared. Nevertheless, his faith in me, his perseverance, and his wisdom continue to accompany me in every new scientific endeavor.

This book is dedicated to his memory, with profound love, gratitude, and respect.

Contents

About the Editor

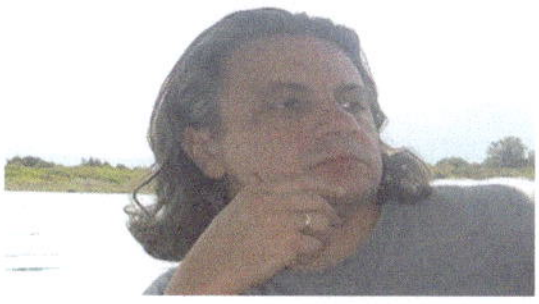

Dimitrios Stasinopoulos, PT, MSc, PhD is Associate Professor of Physiotherapy in the Department of Physiotherapy, School of Health and Caring Sciences, University of West Attica, Greece. His academic position is in **Electrotherapy and Electrophysical Agents in Physiotherapy**.

He graduated from the Department of Physiotherapy at the Technological Educational Institute (TEI) of Athens, Greece, in 1998. He obtained his **MSc in Physiotherapy** from the **University of Manchester**, UK, in 2001 and completed his **PhD** at **Leeds Metropolitan University**, UK, in 2006. His doctoral thesis, entitled "Cyriax Physiotherapy, a Supervised Exercise Program and Bioptron Light for the Treatment of Lateral Epicondylitis," focused on the conservative management of lateral elbow tendinopathy using Cyriax physiotherapy, therapeutic exercise, and Bioptron light therapy.

During his academic career, he served as an Academic Associate at the Department of Physiotherapy, TEI of Lamia (2007–2011), and subsequently joined the **European University Cyprus** (2010–2012), where he was promoted to Assistant Professor and later Associate Professor of Physiotherapy. At the same institution, he taught courses in electrophysical agents, clinical electrotherapy, musculoskeletal physiotherapy, sports physiotherapy, and soft tissue techniques. He also served as Coordinator of the MSc Program in Sports Physiotherapy, Coordinator of the PhD Program in Physiotherapy, Vice Chair and Chair of the Department of Health Sciences, and Coordinator of the Cyprus Musculoskeletal and Sports Trauma Research Center **(CYMUSTREC)**.

He currently serves as Associate Professor at the **University of West Attica**, where he teaches undergraduate and postgraduate courses in **Electrophysical Agents** and **Clinical Electrotherapy**. During previous academic years, he also taught **Soft Tissue Techniques**. In addition, he is Director of the **Musculoskeletal Physiotherapy Research Laboratory** at the University of West Attica.

His research and clinical interests focus on the conservative management of tendinopathies, the application of electrotherapy and electrophysical agents in neuromusculoskeletal disorders and injuries, soft tissue techniques, and evidence-based physiotherapy practice. He has participated in numerous research projects related to musculoskeletal rehabilitation and the clinical application of electrophysical agents.

He has authored more than **225** scientific publications in international and national peer-reviewed journals, contributed chapters to academic books, edited scholarly volumes, and supervised numerous MSc and PhD theses. His published work has received more than **3500 citations** according to Google Scholar. In 2026, he served as Editor of the international textbook *Application of Electrophysical Agents in Physiotherapy*, published by **Springer**.

He has presented his research extensively at national and international scientific conferences, seminars, and symposia. He has served as **Editor-in-Chief** of the international scientific journal *Biology of Exercise* and as **Managing Editor** of *Physiotherapy*, the official scientific journal of the Hellenic Physiotherapists' Association, until January 2025. He has also served as a member of the editorial boards of several international scientific journals, including the *British Journal of Sports Medicine*. He regularly acts as a reviewer for numerous international journals in the fields of physiotherapy, rehabilitation, and sports medicine. He is also a member of the **International Society for Electrophysical Agents in Physical Therapy (ISEAPT)**.

He is internationally recognized for his contributions to the conservative management of tendinopathies, clinical electrotherapy, and the application of electrophysical agents in physiotherapy. His scientific, research, and educational work has made a significant contribution to the advancement of evidence-based physiotherapy practice and the international dissemination of knowledge in musculoskeletal rehabilitation, clinical electrotherapy, and electrophysical agents.

1 Introduction to Electrophysical Agents (EPAs)

Dimitrios Stasinopoulos

1.1 Introduction

Electrophysical agents (EPAs) constitute a foundational component of contemporary physiotherapy practice and education. Their application spans a wide range of clinical settings, from musculoskeletal and sports rehabilitation to neurological, cardiopulmonary, and integumentary care. Despite their long-standing presence in physiotherapy, EPAs remain an area of ongoing scientific development, clinical debate, and educational challenge. This introductory chapter aims to establish the conceptual, terminological, and clinical foundations necessary for the systematic study of EPAs in subsequent chapters.

1.2 Definitions of EPAs

According to the International Society for Electrophysical Agents in Physiotherapy (ISEAP), EPAs are defined as the application of electrophysical or biophysical ener gies to evaluate, treat, and prevent impairments, activity limitations, and participation restrictions [6]. Evaluation procedures involving EPAs include (but are not limited to) ultrasound imaging and electro-neurophysiological testing to assist with physical therapy diagnosis, guide treatment procedures, and evaluate treatment outcomes [6]. Ultrasound imaging and electro-neurophysiological testing are outside the scope of the present book and will not be covered. Treatment procedures involving EPAs include (but are not limited to) the use of thermal, electromagnetic, acoustic, and mechanical energies to produce biophysical effects at the cellular, tissue,

D. Stasinopoulos (✉)
University of West Attica, Athens, Greece
e-mail: dstasinopoulos@uniwa.gr

D. Stasinopoulos (ed.), *Application of Electrophysical Agents in Physiotherapy*,
https://doi.org/10.1007/978-3-032-32144-2_1

organ, and whole-body levels, thereby achieving physiological and clinical effects that maintain and optimize health [6].

This textbook focuses specifically on the therapeutic application of electrophysical agents and their role in contemporary physiotherapy practice. While the ISEAP provides a comprehensive global framework, translating these standards into local clinical practice often requires a nuanced understanding of regional educational traditions. In the Greek healthcare and education system, specific terminological distinctions have been established that influence how clinicians categorize and prioritize these interventions. Having established a working definition of EPAs and clarified the scope of this textbook, it is necessary to examine how these agents are categorized. Classification systems are not merely semantic; they shape educational structure, clinical reasoning, and research interpretation.

1.3 Types/Categories of EPAs

EPAs are core therapeutic interventions in academic physical therapy curricula worldwide. The term "EPAs" refers to the electrical and physical forms of energy delivered by these agents to soft tissues [1]. Many other terms are used instead of EPAs. The term "physical agents" refers to physical energies but excludes the purpose or intention behind their use [3]. The term "therapeutic modalities" better reflects the ability of these interventions to confer therapeutic benefits [3]. The term "biophysical agents" refers to physical agents and modalities [3]. The term "biophysical energies" refers to electromagnetic, acoustic, light, and mechanical energies that produce biophysical effects [3]. The term "electrotherapy" relates to the delivery of electrical energy [11].

Although these terms are often used interchangeably in the international literature, their application varies across countries, professional organizations, and educational systems. Understanding this variability is essential for both academic clarity and clinical communication.

The term "electrotherapy" in Greece refers to modalities that deliver electrical energy to tissues, including electrical stimulation for muscle dysfunction, pain, and wound healing, as well as iontophoresis. All other modalities that deliver thermal, electromagnetic, and acoustic energy to tissues are referred to as EPAs in Greece. The modalities that deliver mechanical energy to tissues, such as spinal traction therapy, intermittent pneumatic compression therapy, and continuous passive motion therapy, are not included in EPAs in Greece. Therefore, this book will cover EPAs in accordance with the Greek protocol. EPAs are classified into three categories—thermal, electromagnetic, and acoustic—based on the type of energy they deliver to the body. The thermal category includes thermotherapy and cryotherapy. The electromagnetic category includes diathermy (shortwave and microwave), phototherapy (low-level laser therapy [LLLT] or photobiomodulation, high-intensity laser therapy [HILT], and polarized polychromatic noncoherent light therapy [PPCCLT]), and magnetic field therapy (magnetotherapy). The acoustic category includes therapeutic ultrasound (ultrasound therapy [US]), low-intensity pulsed ultrasound (LIPUS), and extracorporeal shockwave therapy (ESWT).

This classification system provides the organizational framework of this textbook and will be used consistently throughout subsequent chapters.

While such classifications are useful for organizing content and understanding biophysical principles, they do not, in themselves, determine how EPAs are applied in clinical practice. To fully appreciate their role in physiotherapy, it is necessary to consider how EPAs are used therapeutically and their position within broader rehabilitation strategies.

1.4 Application of EPAs

One of the most persistent conceptual issues surrounding EPAs concerns their classification as "passive" interventions. This characterization has important implications for clinical reasoning, professional identity, and the interpretation of research evidence.

It is important to note that the absence of robust clinical evidence for certain modalities does not necessarily imply a lack of efficacy; rather, it often reflects methodological weaknesses in existing research. This reality underscores why a deep understanding of biophysical principles and physiological rationale is essential for clinical reasoning.

EPAs are called passive physical therapy modalities. The terms "passive modality" and "passive intervention" have gained popularity in recent years. Several published papers from North America (Canada and the United States), Australia, the United Kingdom, and other regions have used this term extensively, often in a negative way. A passive physical modality, or passive intervention, is defined as a physical treatment that uses a device and requires no active patient participation [5]. More specifically, the therapist administers the treatment directly, and the patient does not actively participate in exercise or movement.

However, EPAs are not the only passive physical therapy modalities. Passive physical therapy modalities also include the following:

- Joint mobilizations and manipulations
- Soft-tissue mobilizations
- Electrotherapy modalities
- Acupuncture/dry needling
- Mechanical energy modalities
- Passive exercise therapy
- Orthotics (bracing) and taping

The above-mentioned approaches are typically aimed at reducing pain, improving circulation, increasing flexibility, and/or promoting tissue healing. It is worth mentioning two examples from the literature. Firstly, Wong et al. [12] examined the effectiveness of manual therapies, passive physical modalities, and acupuncture in managing whiplash-associated disorders (WAD) or neck pain–associated disorders (NAD). Passive physical modalities were divided into two categories: physicochemical (thermal or electromagnetic modalities) and structural (nonfunctional assistive devices). However, all of the above treatments are passive physical therapy. Manual therapies and acupuncture should be included among passive physical therapy modalities.

Secondly, Dion et al. [5] evaluated the effectiveness of passive physical modalities for managing common soft-tissue injuries of the elbow in their systematic review (SR). Manual therapies, such as manipulation, mobilization, and soft-tissue therapy, were excluded from this SR. They did not refer to acupuncture. The authors did not explain why manual therapies were not included in the SR when the title of the SR is "Are Passive Physical Modalities Effective? A Systematic Review by the Ontario Protocol for Traffic Injury Management (OPTIMa) Collaboration." Based on the SR title, the reader would expect all passive physical modalities to be included. Therefore, this SR did not evaluate the effectiveness of all passive physical modalities; only some were evaluated, and the conclusions should be read with great caution.

These two examples from the literature support the conclusion that not only EPAs but also electrotherapy, taping, and bracing are considered passive physical therapy modalities. On the other hand, there seems to be a trend in which manual mobilization, manipulation, soft-tissue mobilization, and acupuncture are not considered passive physical therapy modalities, even though these treatments meet the definition of passive physical therapy modalities outlined in the first paragraph of this section.

Beyond methodological inconsistencies in the literature, the passive–active dichotomy has also shaped professional attitudes toward EPAs.

It appears that academics and practitioners do not want to include manual mobilization, manipulation, soft-tissue mobilization, and acupuncture as passive physical therapy modalities because passive modalities have been portrayed negatively (in simple terms, no patient-active involvement = bad) [9]. This issue has been the subject of extensive, detailed professional debate. EPAs are often described as part of a treatment package and are frequently used alongside active interventions, such as exercise programs, to achieve optimal outcomes in rehabilitation and pain management [9]. However, reliance solely on passive treatments may not address the underlying causes of musculoskeletal problems or promote long-term functional movement. Therefore, a comprehensive physiotherapy approach typically combines passive and active treatments tailored to the patient's individual needs.

Crucially, the clinical utility of EPAs often lies in their ability to create a "therapeutic window." By modulating pain or reducing inflammatory responses in the early stages of rehabilitation, these agents can lower the physiological and psychological barriers to movement. This temporary symptomatic relief allows patients to engage in active exercise programs that might otherwise be intolerable, effectively bridging the gap between acute impairment and functional recovery.

EPAs are not the only passive physical therapy modalities. EPAs are not the sole intervention a patient should receive, but adding EPAs alongside an active treatment program provides evidence-based added value; the patient benefits from this addition. EPAs and other passive physical therapy modalities are not necessarily "bad" because they are passive [9]. Finally, it is overly simplistic to dichotomize interventions as passive and active [9].

Another prejudice put forward to single out and undermine the practice of EPAs is that these agents, because they are passively delivered, may be harmful to patients [2]. To claim that EPAs may be harmful to patients simply because they are passively delivered is prejudicial and, as such, must be dismissed from the conversation [2]. The bottom line is that the question of harm and benefit to the patient has little to do with the way a therapeutic intervention is delivered (i.e., passively or actively) and much to do with the clinician's responsibility to provide proper instructions aimed at maximizing the efficacy of the therapeutic intervention received by the patient [2].

An important conceptual question arises regarding the therapeutic classification of electrophysical agents (EPAs): should EPAs themselves be considered active treatment modalities? From the perspective of energy-based classification frameworks, EPAs are formally categorized as active interventions because their devices generate and deliver energy to biological tissues. For example, therapeutic ultrasound and extracorporeal shockwave therapy transmit acoustic energy, whereas diathermy and phototherapy deliver electromagnetic energy. Similarly, electrotherapeutic modalities introduce electrical currents directly into the tissues.

When the EPA application is combined with therapeutic exercise, the overall intervention assumes a clearly active clinical character, as the patient becomes directly engaged in the therapeutic process. In this context, EPAs may be conceptualized as facilitating modalities that optimize the biological and neuromuscular environment in preparation for, or in conjunction with, active rehabilitation. Nevertheless, the device itself continues to function as the primary source of externally applied energy. Empirical evidence indicates that combining therapeutic ultrasound with passive stretching produces significantly greater improvements in joint range of motion than either intervention applied in isolation [8, 10].

These observations support reconsidering conventional EPA application protocols, with greater emphasis on integrating active patient participation into treatment delivery. Comparable integrative approaches have already been successfully implemented using neuromuscular electrical stimulation and biofeedback-based interventions, in which externally applied energy is combined with voluntary motor activity to enhance neuromuscular adaptation and functional recovery. However, further rigorously designed clinical studies are required to establish standardized application frameworks, clarify optimal combinations with active rehabilitation strategies, and strengthen the evidence base supporting this integrative model.

These conceptual biases have contributed to more extreme positions regarding the clinical legitimacy of EPAs.

Many physical therapists around the world argue that the application of EPAs constitutes fraud and therefore do not recommend them for managing conditions and disorders. However, EPAs, when used based on the best available evidence and concomitantly with other therapeutic interventions, are efficacious in that they provide symptom management and positively affect soft-tissue healing, commonly without side effects, in comparison with medications and surgical techniques, which carry their own burden of potential side effects and severe health risks [2]. Recommendations regarding EPAs should reflect current evidence and guidelines based on systematic reviews and meta-analyses.

Finally, it is essential to remember that EPAs are part of a comprehensive treatment approach, used as an adjunct within a broader program rather than as a standalone treatment for a clinical case. They are dose–response modalities. The optimal treatment dose varies across the stages of patient recovery (acute, subacute, and chronic conditions), with distinct tissue problems and corresponding treatment goals, leading to different EPA dosages for these conditions [11]. The topic of dosology will be covered in Chaps. 2, 3, 4, 5, 6, 7, and 8.

Within contemporary rehabilitation, EPAs should be understood as components of a broader biopsychosocial approach to patient care. Their effects are not limited to local biophysical interactions at the tissue level; they may also influence pain modulation, sensorimotor processing, patient expectations, and engagement in movement-based rehabilitation. As such, EPAs are not isolated technical procedures but interventions embedded within therapeutic relationships and clinical contexts.

From a biopsychosocial perspective, EPAs may contribute to symptom modulation, facilitate movement initiation, reduce fear-related responses, and support participation in active rehabilitation. Their clinical value, therefore, lies not only in their direct physiological effects but also in their capacity to create conditions that enable functional restoration, motor learning, and behavioral change.

Consequently, the appropriate use of EPAs requires integration with exercise therapy, patient education, and psychosocially informed clinical reasoning. When applied within such frameworks, EPAs can support goal-directed rehabilitation strategies rather than function as standalone symptomatic treatments.

If EPAs are to be integrated responsibly within comprehensive rehabilitation programs, their clinical use must ultimately be grounded in scientific evidence. This necessitates an examination of the research base supporting their effectiveness.

The clinical application of EPAs should be guided by structured clinical reasoning rather than routine or protocol-driven use. Decision-making must be informed by a comprehensive assessment of the patient's condition, functional limitations, goals, and stage of tissue healing.

Key considerations include identifying treatment objectives (e.g., pain modulation, movement facilitation, tissue healing, neuromuscular activation), selecting the most appropriate modality, and determining treatment parameters based on available evidence and physiological rationale. The patient's stage of recovery (acute, subacute, or chronic), comorbidities, psychosocial factors, and treatment tolerance should further inform the choice of modality and dosage.

EPAs should be integrated within broader care pathways that include active rehabilitation, education, and functional training. Continuous reassessment of patient response is essential to determine effectiveness, guide progression, and decide whether to continue, modify, or discontinue an EPA.

1.5 Clinical Effectiveness of Electrophysical Modalities

Clinical physiotherapy practice is increasingly guided by evidence-based healthcare principles, requiring clinicians to integrate the best available research evidence with clinical expertise and patient values.

This paradigm shift toward a biopsychosocial perspective also requires a more sophisticated interpretation of the "placebo effect" in EPA research. Rather than dismissing nonspecific effects as clinical failures, contemporary practice recognizes that the context of EPA application—including the therapeutic alliance and patient expectations—interacts with biophysical mechanisms to shape the overall clinical outcome.

There is a belief that the body of research-based evidence on EPAs is of poor scientific quality compared with other physiotherapy interventions and disciplines, and therefore not credible enough to establish a scientific foundation for the field of EPAs [2]. However, in the peer-reviewed scientific literature, one can find articles demonstrating that the quality of research in EPAs is higher than that in other physical therapy disciplines [2]. Studies examining the effectiveness of EPAs are often plagued by heterogeneity in design, outcomes, chronic pain conditions, and methodological quality [3]. Therefore, it is time to dismiss such beliefs.

There is substantial research-based evidence supporting the practice of EPAs. Databases such as PubMed and PEDro list tens of thousands of peer-reviewed articles in the field of EPAs, including randomized controlled trials, systematic reviews with meta-analyses, and reviews of reviews that clinicians and scientists can consult for clinical and research purposes [2]. Research-based evidence can also be found in several academic textbooks on EPAs [1, 3, 4, 7, 11].

When reading the literature on EPAs, practitioners should carefully consider how EPAs were used. EPAs can be efficacious therapeutic interventions. Search results from databases reveal many randomized controlled trials, systematic reviews, and meta-analyses demonstrating the efficacy of EPAs for a wide range of disorders [2]. Some studies evaluate the effectiveness of EPAs as monotherapies; however, in clinical practice, they are most often used to complement other therapeutic approaches. This topic will be covered in detail in Chaps. 2, 3, 4, 5, 6, 7, and 8. It is important to remember that EPAs are seldom used as monotherapy. They are used alongside a broad range of other medical and/or physiotherapeutic interventions to manage a wide array of disorders. The research evidence suggests that EPAs can be effective as elements of treatment. Future research is needed to evaluate the most effective treatment approaches for combinations of therapies. Moreover, EPAs are effective when used appropriately; when used inappropriately, they may achieve nothing [11]. If they are omitted from a therapist's practice, a patient may not, in fact, be receiving the best evidence-based treatment [11]. The evidence suggests that when the appropriate modality is applied at the right dose for the presenting problem, it can significantly contribute to patient improvement and well-being.

It is unproductive to read only abstracts of systematic reviews. Practitioners should evaluate the details of every included study. Just because a conclusion appears in a systematic review does not mean it is sufficient evidence to underpin practice [11]. Often, conclusions are based on a homogeneous patient group but a heterogeneous intervention. Ideally, readers should return to the original studies and critically appraise them.

Despite the extensive volume of literature on EPAs, several methodological challenges complicate the interpretation of research findings. These include variability in treatment parameters, inadequate reporting of dosage, heterogeneity of patient populations, and inconsistencies in outcome measures. Such factors limit comparability across studies and contribute to conflicting conclusions within systematic reviews.

The design of credible placebo or sham interventions presents an additional challenge, particularly for modalities that produce perceptible sensory experiences. Therapist dependence, difficulties with blinding, and technological variability further affect study quality and reproducibility.

Moreover, translational gaps often exist between controlled experimental settings and real-world clinical practice. These limitations underscore the need for cautious interpretation of findings, adherence to detailed reporting standards, and continued high-quality research focused on clinically meaningful outcomes and treatment fidelity.

Demonstrating effectiveness, however, is only one component of responsible clinical application. Equally important is an understanding of when and how EPAs can be applied safely.

1.6 Overview of Indications, Contraindications, and Precautions

However, the clinical efficacy of an intervention cannot be dissociated from its safety profile. A rigorous, evidence-based approach requires that an EPA be selected not only for its potential to achieve physiological goals but also through a meticulous screening process to mitigate inherent risks.

Sound clinical decision-making requires not only knowledge of potential benefits but also a clear understanding of indications, contraindications, and precautions associated with therapeutic interventions.

Indications, contraindications, and precautions for EPAs will be covered in detail in Chaps. 2, 3, 4, 5, 6, 7, and 8. Appropriately applied EPAs may (1) relieve pain, (2) alter collagen extensibility, (3) increase range of motion, and (4) support tissue healing. EPAs may influence these outcomes when they are applied appropriately as part of a comprehensive plan of care during specific phases of rehabilitation or throughout the entire rehabilitation program.

Restrictions on the use of specific treatment interventions are referred to as contraindications or precautions. Contraindications are defined as conditions or factors in which the application of a modality over a specific location or region of the body could be harmful. They should therefore not be used in that location or region [3]. Precautions apply when a patient is at risk of adverse effects [3]. In such cases, treatment may proceed with special care, limitations, and proactive measures, such as adjusting the treatment dose and/or closely monitoring the patient's response, to reduce the risk of potential harm [3]. The terms "absolute contraindications" and "relative contraindications" may be used in place of "contraindications" and "precautions," respectively [4].

Although contraindications and precautions for the application of EPAs vary, several conditions are contraindications or precautions for most EPAs. Therefore, caution should be exercised when applying EPAs to patients with the following conditions:

- Malignancy
- Hemorrhagic conditions
- Impaired sensation
- Thrombophlebitis
- Impaired or diminished cognition or communication
- Pregnancy
- Pacemakers or other implanted electronic devices

It is important to note that many of these conditions, such as pregnancy, are often classified as relative contraindications depending on the specific modality and the anatomical site of application. For instance, while most EPAs are strictly avoided over the gravid uterus due to potential risks to fetal development, some may be applied with caution to peripheral joints, provided there is no risk of systemic energy transfer. This underscores the necessity for clinicians to move beyond a binary "yes/no" approach and instead employ a risk-benefit analysis based on biophysical principles and the latest safety guidelines.

The clinician should determine whether the patient's history and current status present any factors or risks that may render a specific therapeutic modality harmful or disadvantageous to the patient's health [3].

This introductory chapter has outlined the conceptual foundations, classifications, applications, and evidence base of EPAs. The chapters that follow will build on this framework by examining each category of electrophysical agent in detail, with emphasis on biophysical mechanisms, physiological effects, clinical indications, treatment parameters, safety considerations, and evidence-informed application. Understanding fundamental physical principles such as energy transfer, dose–response relationships, and tissue interaction is essential for the safe and effective clinical application of electrophysical agents. Therefore, each subsequent chapter will integrate biophysical foundations with clinical reasoning and evidence-informed practice.

Key Concepts

- Electrophysical agents are therapeutic applications of biophysical energies used to support rehabilitation and health optimization.
- EPAs are categorized according to the type of energy delivered, providing an organizational framework for education and clinical reasoning.

- Classifying EPAs as passive modalities is conceptually limited and should not determine their clinical value.
- EPAs are most appropriately used as components of comprehensive, goal-directed rehabilitation programs.
- Evidence supports the clinical effectiveness of EPAs when appropriately selected and dosed.
- Safe application requires an understanding of indications, contraindications, and precautions.

Reflective and Critical Questions

In what ways can EPAs support, rather than replace, active rehabilitation strategies?

How does the passive–active dichotomy influence clinical decision-making and professional attitudes toward EPAs?

What challenges arise when interpreting research on EPAs, and how should clinicians address them?

How can EPAs be integrated within a biopsychosocial model of rehabilitation?

What ethical and professional responsibilities accompany the clinical use of electrophysical agents?

Clinical Relevance

Understanding the conceptual foundations, evidence base, and safety principles of EPAs enables clinicians to integrate these interventions responsibly into patient-centered rehabilitation programs. Appropriate use of EPAs can enhance symptom management, support functional restoration, and facilitate engagement in active therapy when guided by structured clinical reasoning and evidence-informed practice.

Declarations

Competing Interests The author(s) have no competing interests to declare that are relevant to the content of this manuscript.

References

1. Belanger AY. Therapeutic electrophysical agents: an evidenced-based handbook. 4th ed. Philadelphia: Wolters Kluwer; 2023.
2. Belanger AY, Selkowitz DM, Lawson D. On putting an end to the backlash against electrophysical agents. Int J Sports Phys Ther. 2023;18:1230–7.
3. Bellew J, Nolan T. Michlovitz's modalities for therapeutic intervention. 7th ed. Philadelphia: FA Davis; 2022.
4. Cameron M. Physical agents in rehabilitation. An evidence – based approach to practice. 6th ed. St. Louis: Elsevier; 2023.
5. Dion S, Wong JJ, Côté P, Yu H, Sutton D, et al. Are passive physical modalities effective for the management of common soft tissue injuries of the elbow? A systematic review by the Ontario Protocol for Traffic Injury Management (OPTIMa) collaboration. Clin J Pain. 2017;33:71–86.
6. ISEAP. https://iseapt.wixsite.com/home. Accessed 17 Oct 2025.

7. Prentice WE. Therapeutic modalities in rehabilitation. 6th ed. New York: McGraw-Hill Medical; 2021.
8. Reda F, Eman E. Effectiveness of two combined techniques of ultrasound therapy and stretching in the treatment of mechanical neck pain: a randomized controlled trial. Int J Ther Rehabil Res. 2016;5:7–15.
9. Stasinopoulos D. Are electrophysical agents the only passive physical therapy modalities? J Orthop Res Ther. 2024;9:1351.
10. Stasinopoulos D, Constantinou A, Cheimozidou AZ, Lamnisos D. The best arm position for therapeutic ultrasound application in lateral elbow tendinopathy patients. Ann Physiother Occup Ther. 2023;6:000247.
11. Watson T, Nussbaum EL. Electrophysical agents: evidence-based practice. 13th ed. Edinburgh: Elsevier; 2021.
12. Wong JJ, Shearer HM, Mior S, Jacobs C, Côté P, et al. Are manual therapies, passive physical modalities, or acupuncture effective for the management of patients with whiplash-associated disorders or neck pain and associated disorders? An update of the bone and joint decade task force on neck pain and its associated disorders by the OPTIMa collaboration. Spine J. 2016;16:1598–630.

Cryotherapy-Thermotherapy

2

Konstantinos Fousekis

2.1 Fundamental Thermodynamic Principles in Thermotherapy and Cryotherapy

The clinical application of thermotherapy and cryotherapy is grounded in basic principles of thermodynamics and heat transfer. Understanding these principles is essential for rational selection of modality, appropriate dosing, and accurate prediction of tissue responses.

According to the fundamental laws of thermodynamics, energy is conserved and transferred between systems that are at different temperatures. In physiotherapy, the human body may also be regarded as a thermodynamic system that exchanges heat with its surrounding environment and therapeutic agents. Thermal equilibrium is a state in which the flow of heat between two objects ceases, and no change occurs.

It is important to clarify the distinction between heat and temperature, as these terms are often used interchangeably in clinical practice, even though they are conceptually distinct. Temperature, on the other hand, is simply a measure of how "hot" or "cold" something is, i.e., the average kinetic energy of the molecules in a material. Heat is the transfer of energy between two bodies, whereas temperature indicates the sensible heat within a system. Therefore, a 0 °C ice pack may deliver different amounts of heat to different patients due to tissue properties, blood perfusion, and contact conditions.

Heat is transferred in biological tissues primarily by conduction, convection (perfusion), radiation, and evaporation. Conduction is the primary mechanism of heat transfer when ice packs, hot packs, or paraffin baths are applied in clinical practice. At the same time, convection, driven by blood flow, plays a significant role in transporting heat to deeper tissues.

K. Fousekis (✉)
Department of Physical Therapy, University of Patras, Patras, Greece
e-mail: kfousekis@upatras.gr

D. Stasinopoulos (ed.), *Application of Electrophysical Agents in Physiotherapy*,
https://doi.org/10.1007/978-3-032-32144-2_2

Heat capacity is the heat required to increase a material's temperature by 1 °C. Tissues containing high water content, such as muscle and blood, have a higher specific heat capacity and therefore take longer to both heat up and cool down than fatty tissue, which has a lower specific heat capacity. This is why fat acts as an insulator, protecting deeper structures from extreme temperatures, both warm and cold.

Thermal capacity is the ability of a tissue or system to store heat. The greater the thermal capacity, the more energy is required to change its temperature. Clinically, this means that large muscle masses or highly perfused areas are more resistant to rapid temperature changes during cryotherapy or thermotherapy.

Thermal conductivity is the property of a material to conduct heat. High-conductivity tissues, such as muscle, facilitate heat transfer, while low-conductivity fat impedes it. This feature accounts for the fact that identical treatment (e.g., 15 min of ice application) can result in different depths and degrees of cooling or warming in individual patients.

In general, thermodynamics and tissue properties would decide the spatial and temporal distribution of temperature in cryotherapy or thermotherapy. The clinical efficacy and safety of these methods also depend on knowledge of the concepts and on treatment parameters adjusted to each patient's individual traits.

2.2 Cryotherapy

Cryotherapy is the use of cold as a treatment modality to minimize secondary tissue damage and pain and promote recovery through various physiological and biochemical responses. Cryotherapy reduces skin and tissue temperature, local metabolic rate, blood flow through vasoconstriction, and nerve conduction velocity (NCV), all of which contribute to analgesia while modulating inflammatory activity and reducing secondary damage (postinjury or overuse) to tissues. In the clinical and sports medicine settings, cryotherapy is often used as an adjunctive therapy to treat acute musculoskeletal conditions, postoperative pain, and exercise-induced muscle soreness [51].

Cryotherapy is applied both locally and systemically. Local cryotherapy treatments, including cold packs, gel packs, ice massage, and cold compression therapy, can be used to cool limited anatomic sites [14]. These techniques help with localized symptoms of pain, tenderness, swelling, or inflammatory irritation in soft-tissue structures. Since local cooling predominantly influences surface tissue through to subcutaneous tissue, treatment can be localized to the injured area while reducing whole-body systemic exposure. Such a localized treatment has favorable implications for rehabilitation delivery, as it may enable greater comfort, reduce pain levels, facilitate earlier mobilization, and increase tolerance to therapeutic exercise [90].

Cold water immersion (CWI) is another popular local-to-regional treatment that involves immersing a limb or the body (in whole or in part) in cold water for a predetermined period. Compared with a standard ice pack, CWI can provide more consistent cooling of submerged tissues and enhance vascular responses, particularly during postexercise recovery after high-intensity exercise. CWI is most commonly used in athletic populations to reduce delayed onset muscle soreness (DOMS), subjective fatigue, and short-term recovery needs following training or competition [33]. Importantly, although CWI is thermogenically capable of inducing mild systemic responses (specific to the temperature and depth of immersion), it may be considered a practical intermediate strategy between LC and WBC for stimulating recovery benefits without the same extent of neuroendocrine activation [55].

Overall, techniques employing local cryotherapy are popular due to their availability, low cost, and ease of application. The main clinical effects are to reduce immediate pain, moderate inflammatory signs, and restore some functional capacity by improving tolerance to mobility and rehabilitation exercises. Nevertheless, the effectiveness of cryotherapy in acute and chronic sports injuries depends on protocol specifics (i.e., temperature, duration, frequency), the type/stage of injury, and patient-level moderators such as adipose tissue thickness and sensitivity to thermal stimuli. For these reasons, cryotherapy is most effective as a structured, goal-oriented therapy component of an overall rehabilitation or recovery plan rather than as an isolated modality.

2.2.1 Biophysics of Cryotherapy

Depending on the context, cryotherapy can be applied systemically or topically for recovery, pain/edema, and/or inflammation-modulating purposes. Despite its widespread use in rehabilitation, sports medicine, and postoperative care, the effects of cryotherapy are largely based on biophysical principles [17]. The clinical response to cryotherapy is based on the physics of heat transfer from body tissues to a colder medium, the ability of human tissues to conduct and store heat, and the physiologic mechanisms (such as vascular responses) that respond during these physical processes [17]. It is important to understand the biophysics of cryotherapy to make appropriate choices of modality and dosing parameters, and to avoid adverse effects.

At the heart of cryotherapy is a basic thermodynamic principle: heat tends to flow from a warmer object to a cooler one [49]. The tissues are cooled with ice bags, cold-water immersion, or cooler air surrounding the body. This irreversibility of heat flow is consistent with the second law of thermodynamics, which states that energy transfer occurs from higher- to lower-temperature bodies. Thus, the efficacy of cryotherapy depends on the temperature difference (ΔT) between the skin surface and the cooling medium. A greater ΔT leads to faster heat loss and cooling than when ΔT is smaller [49]. It is also important to note that tissue cooling does not depend solely on the temperature gradient. The magnitude and intensity of cooling are also affected by contact time, quality of skin-cooling source contact, area treated, and whether the mechanism for heat flow is primarily one of exchange by conduction or convective transport between tissues beneath the skin (most notably the proportionate amounts of fat and muscle) [32].

Conduction and convection are the predominant modes of heat exchange underpinning cryotherapy, whereas evaporation and radiation make less significant contributions in most clinical settings [16]. Conduction is the process of thermal energy transfer through direct contact between two materials of differing temperatures. Conduction is the primary mechanism of action for ice packs, gel packs, ice massage, and cold compression wraps [26]. Here, contact quality is the decisive factor: The greater the skin area in contact with the cooling medium—and the closer these two points are to each other—the higher the conductive heat loss. Compression wraps are effective in reducing insulating air pockets, decreasing the surface contact area, and increasing the rate of heat extraction from superficial tissues.

Convection is typically a more effective means of cooling, as it extracts heat by moving fluid that replaces the warm boundary layer at the skin with cooler fluid. CWI, circulating cold-water devices, and forced cold-air systems rely heavily on convection. This results in faster, more uniform cooling (than by conduction) since cooling occurs through a continuously renewed coolant. Thus, water movement prevents the formation of a warm, insulating layer at the skin, resulting in a strong temperature gradient that supports ongoing heat exchange with and from core tissue. For these reasons, convection-based cryotherapy is often associated with deeper or more uniform cooling than the traditional application of ice pack(s), a distinction that is accentuated when treating larger portions of the body [48].

In cryotherapy, evaporation is especially important in applications where energy absorption is highly localized (e.g., vapocoolant sprays or wet towel cooling in moving air). Evaporation absorbs heat: To turn liquid water into water vapor, energy is required, and that energy comes from your skin's surface. Radiation (heat dissipated in the infrared spectrum) is also present but is negligible under normal therapy conditions and can generally be ignored relative to conduction and convection [93].

The rate of heat removal is determined by the cooling medium, not by how deeply or for how long it penetrates, based on the physical properties of biological tissues. Heterogeneity in tissue cooling is further exacerbated by variations in thermal conductivity, specific heat capacity, and blood perfusion across tissues. Thermal conductivity (k) is a measure of how well heat travels through materials. The thermal conductivity of muscle tissue is higher than that of adipose tissue, thus enabling better heat transfer; as a result, muscle can cool more effectively than adipose under similar exposure [31, 62]. Adipose tissue, on the other hand, has low thermal conductance and serves as a good insulator. This is one reason why superficial skin cooling becomes more intense in some subjects with a thick subcutaneous fat layer. At the same time, the temperature change in the underlying muscles and connective tissues remains small [62]. Clinically, this is of paramount importance: the same cryotherapy protocol could yield different deep-tissue effects when tested on subjects with different body compositions, and, consequently, different analgesic effects and recovery responses.

Tissue cooling dynamics are also dependent on the specific heat capacity. Specific heat is a measure of the amount of energy necessary to change the temperature of a unit mass of tissue by one degree. Tissues having high water content (i.e., muscle) store and transfer heat differently than those that have higher lipid contents.

Thus, the "cooling profile" is determined not only by exposure time but also by the energy required to cool the tissue to the desired temperature. These differences are particularly important when the intent is to modify deeper structures (muscle and tendon insertions) rather than superficial ones.

Another major influencer is blood perfusion, a "reheating" factor. The cooled periphery is opposed by the warm heart—it circulates blood from the body's core, thereby minimizing cooling [95]. With high perfusion, internal cooler tissues resist cooling and then reheat very quickly. Perfusion is also directly disrupted by cryotherapy-induced vasoconstriction, which reduces blood flow in the cooled area. This reduces the supply of warm blood, and Tissue temperature at the local level can then drop further. Thus, tissue cooling is not merely a passive physical event, but rather may be actively influenced by physiological thermoregulation. The combination of reduced perfusion and thermal conduction can affect the magnitude and duration of cooling, thereby modulating the therapeutic window for analgesia and inflammation [95].

As tissue cooling proceeds, it creates a thermal gradient across tissue layers. The skin is the coolest region, and temperatures increase with depth during cryotherapy. This gradient is responsible for the rapid decline in skin temperature during cold, while a slower, less severe cooling occurs in deeper muscles. Cooling depth can increase over time, but only up to a point of diminishing returns, because the temperature gradient progressively steepens as the tissue cools. A 10-min application could obviously decrease skin temperature, have some superficial analgesic effects, and have no thermal effect on deep tissue. Extending exposure allows greater tissue-depth cooling (20–30 min), although in both cases, fat thickness and modality type are the predominant factors influencing deep-tissue cooling. This has implications for clinical protocols: superficial tissues may be treated more effectively with shorter exposures, while deeper and/or larger tissues benefit from longer exposures [94].

Water (in case of CWI) has a high heat capacity—that is, it can absorb a lot of thermal energy without warming much. This is advantageous because water can absorb heat from the body more effectively than most solid-based cooling apparatuses. CWI also adds a mechanical component: hydrostatic pressure, which aids in venous return and affects hemodynamics. While hydrostatic effects are not strictly thermal biophysics, they provide a counterpoint to the clinical consequences observed during immersion-based recovery interventions.

Analgesia is commonly elicited at skin temperatures below 10–15 °C (though this depends on how we measure it). With decreasing temperature, there is a gradual attenuation of nerve conduction velocity and inhibition of pain transmission [72]. Metabolic processes are also temperature-dependent. Cooling decreases enzymatic activity and cellular metabolism, a reduction generally described by Q10 [Q10 = (reaction rate at T + 10 °C) ÷ (reaction rate at T)], where biochemical reaction rates decrease as temperature decreases. Vasoconstriction usually appears after the temperature drops from mild to moderate. This causes poor tissue perfusion, thereby increasing the local cooling effect. When cold exposure is long-term, an oscillatory vascular pattern termed the "hunting responses" has been reported, with alternating periods of vasoconstriction and vasodilation that might help protect tissues against excessive cold damage [14]. Previous theories have proposed that reactive vasodilation develops during sustained cryotherapy to prevent ischemia. Still, recent evidence indicates that the response is inconsistent and primarily confined to the distal extremities, such as the fingers and toes. In the usual clinical musculoskeletal applications over larger body areas, meaningful vasodilation is unlikely to occur; physiologically, vasoconstriction predominates. Therefore, therapists should not rely on the presumed hunting response to increase blood flow with cryotherapy.

Cryotherapy can be safe when used correctly, but it is not free of biophysical risks at higher intensities or longer durations. Freezing damage develops when tissues are ischemic due to excessive reduction in blood flow, when membranes become less flexible or stiff, and, finally, during severe exposures, when ice crystals form in or rupture cells. Excessive cooling for an extended period, particularly under constriction or compression, may also induce irritation or trauma to peripheral nerves. These hypothermia-related risks can present in the clinic as superficial cold burns resembling frostbite, nerve irritation (most commonly of the superficial nerves), and prolonged numbness or sensory changes. These negative results stress the need for customized settings when working with cold, poor-circulation patients, cold-sensitive patients, and those with limited thermal sensitivity.

In summary, the biophysics of cryotherapy is founded on basic heat-transfer mechanisms that drive cooling-induced changes in tissue temperature and biological responses. Convection and conduction are the primary heat-transfer mechanisms in clinical cryotherapy, with convective modes of administration, such as cold-water immersion, typically providing more rapid, homogeneous cooling. Depth and duration of cooling are predominantly influenced by thermal properties of tissue, specifically subcutaneous adipose insulation, muscle conductivity, and blood perfusion. Temperature gradients and thresholds: due to predictable cue-response relationships, clinical effects are highly dependent on modality selection and dosing. Above all, optimizing cryotherapy's therapeutic benefits involves integrating biophysical effects with treatment considerations to avoid excessive cooling and cold-induced damage.

2.2.2 Methods and Techniques of Cryotherapy

The numerous forms of cryotherapy are distinguished by the medium of cold, method of application, and depth of tissue effect (Table 2.1). In the sports injury rehabilitation practice, the most frequently used cooling techniques are: use of solid or crushed ice, standard gel packs, cold water immersion; reliefs also provided by application of cold sprays including ethyl chloride spray or device for generation of a cold air flow (cold-air devices) for certain treatments where muscle relaxation is required in addition to pain relief/limiting inflammation of injured tissues (with subsequent swelling) [11, 59]. More recently, therapeutic compression has been combined with cold modalities (e.g., chilled water or gel) for active cooling and

Table 2.1 Classification of cryotherapy methods in sports injury rehabilitation

Cryotherapy modalityl	Application type	Therapeutic characteristics	Indicated phase
Solid or crushed ice	Static	Ice cubes or ice in a bag	Acute
Gel packs	Static	Standardized cold packs	Acute—Subacute
Cold whirlpool bath-Ψ	Dynamic	Limb immersion in a cold-water whirlpool	Subacute—Chronic
Ice massage	Dynamic	Local circular ice application over a small area	Subacute—Chronic
Cold sprays (ethyl chloride)	Static	Superficial analgesia	Acute (analgesic use)
Cold air (air-cooling devices/cold rooms)	Dynamic	Controlled cold exposure via a device	All stages
Cold water immersion (ice immersion)	Dynamic	Immersion in a basin or bathtub for recovery	Recovery—Chronic
Compression cryotherapy	Combined	Specialized equipment (e.g., game ready) combining compression and cooling	Acute—Subacute—Recovery

therapeutic compression during the acute phase, when edema and inflammation are present [23].

Cryotherapy techniques are further classified as static or dynamic based on the mode of application, offering clinicians options tailored to different therapeutic needs. In static use, the cold medium is applied to the treated area for a specific period, such as with an ice or gel pack. Alternatively, dynamic applications comprise a flowing cold medium applied to the treatment area (e.g., ice massage), or a flow environment in which the affected limb is moved (e.g., cold whirlpool baths or cryokinetics). By understanding these categories, practitioners can more effectively match treatment type to injury stage and desired effect.

Simultaneous application of compressive treatment and cryotherapy is performed using specific devices (e.g., Game Ready, ZAMAR), which deliver cyclic compression combined with controlled cooling via water or air [23]. This approach is especially recommended for treating acute edema and promoting venous and lymphatic return, thereby accelerating the reabsorption of posttraumatic fluid accumulation and providing analgesia.

2.2.2.1 Static Cryotherapy Application: Cold Packs

The most popular cryotherapy for sports injuries is the static use of cold packs, which can be either solid ice or crushed ice or gel-based cold packs (Fig. 2.1). This method allows for the application of compression with an elastic bandage, and, when combined with limb elevation, has been reported to be more effective in improving treatment outcomes and promoting venous return. Understanding the popularity and mechanism of this technique provides important practical context for its widespread clinical adoption, as outlined in the classifications described above.

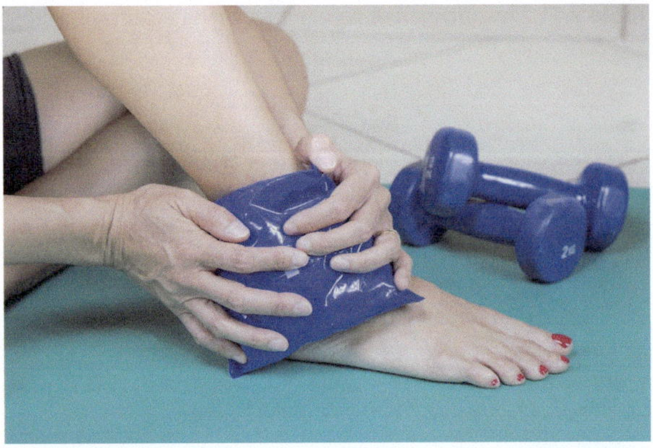

Fig. 2.1 Standardized gel packs. (© Stedata/Dreamstime.com)

Ice is ordinarily placed in a plastic bag, and the air is evacuated from the bag before application, so that the cold pack fits more closely to the part being treated and increases cooling. The pliable gel packs will continue to optimize cryotherapy of one or more anatomical areas requiring cooling, as they retain their flexibility after chilling. Cold packs can retain their chill longer when wrapped in a moist towel. This mode of operation insulates the cold medium and minimizes heat transfer between the cold pack and its surroundings.

Studies have found significantly lower skin temperatures with various forms of cryotherapy, a therapeutic technique that uses cold to treat injuries. The application modalities can be broadly classified as wet (i.e., ice applied directly to the skin, usually with a damp towel), dry (i.e., placed in a bag or towel to prevent them from becoming wet during use), and custom cold packs (i.e., commercially available gel packs). In particular, the lowest skin temperature is with wet ice at 12 °C below baseline, whereas with dry ice and gel packs it is 9.9 and 7.3 °C below baseline, respectively [9]. This "cooling" effect is also key for treating acute injuries and reducing edema (swelling due to fluid buildup).

Cryotherapy's efficacy depends on the amount of ice and the area of skin contact. Research shows that 0.3 kg is as effective as 0.6 kg. Another study finds ice weight above 0.5 kg is effective.

In summary, research shows that, for optimal effect with cold packs, using more ice yields better outcomes [36]. Skin temperature at the ice–skin interface drops substantially during a 20-min application, with most of the drop occurring during the initial 8–9 min [36]. In addition, using compression during ice application decreases skin temperature compared with applying ice without compression. These results reinforce the importance of both method selection and parameter adjustment, as discussed in relation to technique classifications, for achieving optimal therapeutic effects.

Findings from various studies demonstrate how different cryotherapy methods reduce temperature. For example, the mean cooling amplitude was 10.4 °C (range: 19.7 °C) when crushed ice with synthetic braces was applied to the limbs [60]. Likewise, cold packs with compression had a mean surface temperature of 6.1°, which was significantly lower than that of the group without compression [28]. In comparison with other methods, ice and water–alcohol mixtures significantly lowered skin temperature to 10.2 and 10.0 °C, respectively, compared with gel packs or frozen vegetables (mean skin temperatures after 20 min of application) [41]. Altogether, these results underscore the need to link the choice of cryotherapy modality and parameters to the specific therapeutic goal, building on the principles outlined previously.

2.2.2.2 Ice Massage

Ice massage is a common clinical modality used to produce analgesia in human skin and to provide cooling. During ice massage, a piece of ice (usually in a paper cup) is applied directly to the desired skin area without any intervening material [15] (Fig. 2.2). The motion is an uninterrupted, slow, circular, or linear stroke applied over the entire treatment area. The application time is 5–10 min, or until the patient develops local numbness, without producing features of cold-induced skin damage. In an ice massage, the pressure and treatment duration may be adjusted based on patient tolerance and therapeutic goals for pain relief, edema, and muscle tone. This is especially useful in the subacute stage of musculotendinous injuries to deliver analgesia for active and exercise programs, while allowing monitoring of skin response and patient sensation.

Ice massage can lower skin temperature to 13.6 °C, which is sufficient for analgesia. This cooling relieves pain and inflammation, making ice massage a popular choice in sports medicine and physiotherapy. The rapid temperature drop supports rehabilitation routines by providing rapid relief and broader benefits than standard ice therapy.

Ice massage cools the skin more effectively than other forms of cryotherapy, such as cold packs. The nadir temperature is achieved at 17.9 min with ice massage and at 28.2 min with packs [94]. The rapid cooling is attributed to the intimate contact and sliding of ice. Compression also accelerates early cooling, but eventually

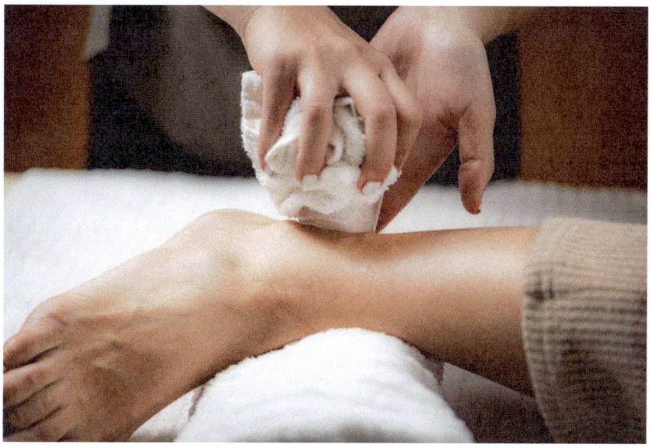

Fig. 2.2 Ice massage. (© Microgen/Dreamstime.com)

tissue temperature stabilizes as the body adjusts. So while compression does seem to control early pain and inflammation, it does not alter the overall cooling effect of extended treatment.

Several studies report skin temperature falls of 5.8–6.8 °C in the first few minutes of ice massage, and up to 12 °C after 15 min. This suggests that ice massage is an effective modality for therapeutic cooling. Its ability to lower skin temperature makes it a useful clinical and athletic tool [2].

2.2.2.3 Cold Air Therapy

Cold air therapy notably changes tissue temperatures at both the surface and deeper levels.

Cold air is a treatment modality that significantly affects tissue temperature and is effective at both superficial and deeper depths. In one study, a 5-min cold-air application caused a rapid decrease in skin temperature of 22.1 °C and a fall in intra-articular temperature of 3.9 °C, with intra-articular temperatures not returning to baseline levels even 2 h after application, suggesting that cooling was maintained for an extended period [2, 36].

Endurance and performance could also be influenced by cold-air exposure. In another investigation, endurance decreased by 71.6% following exposure to cold air (0 °C), and mild hypothermia was accompanied by a 1.0 °C decrease in core temperature. This observation indicates that skin cooling and incomplete protection can largely reduce endurance [89].

Furthermore, tissue oxygenation and perception may also be affected by CAT. Professional athletes were exposed to cold air at −135 °C for 2 min, and significant decreases in oxyhemoglobin and tissue oxygenation were observed, but not in core body temperature. Sensory and subjective comfort perception scores also reduced markedly.

In conclusion, cold-air therapy can significantly lower cutaneous and subcutaneous tissue temperatures, likely influencing endurance performance and thermal perception. These reactions might be therapeutic in both clinical and athletic applications, but care should be taken not to overcool and cause hypothermia.

Cold Sprays (Ethyl Chloride)

Cold sprays (ethyl chloride) are also used as a form of superficial cryotherapy, primarily for short-term analgesia. They produce rapid skin cooling through evaporation, leading to a temporary reduction in pain and muscle spasm. Refrigerant sprays are commonly used in combination with stretching techniques (e.g., spray-and-stretch) to manage myofascial pain. However, their effects are transient and limited to superficial tissues, and they should be used with caution to avoid skin irritation or frostbite.

Cold Water Immersion (CWI)

Cold water immersion (CWI) is one common method in cryotherapy, involving lowering a limb or full body into cold water, usually at a temperature between 10 and 15 °C (Fig. 2.3). The method mainly relies on heat transfer by conduction and

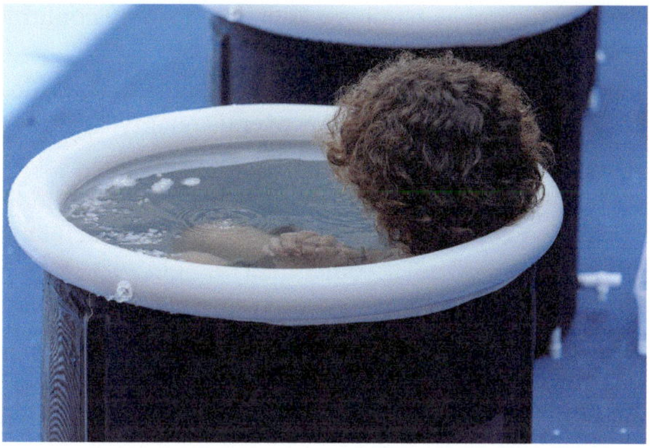

Fig. 2.3 Cold water immersion. (© Giorgio Rossi/Dreamstime.com)

convection, so cooling of tissue happens faster yet more uniformly than traditional ice packs. Tissue temperature decreases below normal, triggering vasoconstriction. Circulation drops significantly as local blood flow diminishes, and edema is also limited; in addition, significant analgesic effects result from slower nerve conduction. This may be clinically useful in both rehabilitation and postexercise recovery contexts. For example, when muscle fatigue is reduced in circulating cold water, metabolic by-products can be removed more rapidly, and the inflammatory response in muscles is checked to some extent. These factors combine to give earlier recovery and better function, whether patients are performing exercises or simply walking. Application time is generally 10–15 min, and care must be taken to identify contraindications, such as cold hypersensitivity or circulatory disorders, to ensure safe and effective use of this technique.

2.2.2.4 Cold Air Cryotherapy Modality and Devices

Cold air cryotherapy involves brief exposure of the whole body to extremely low temperatures (e.g., below −100 °C) for 2–4 min in special chambers. Athletes strip down and stand in the cold, dry air to minimize soft-tissue pain and swelling after strenuous workouts or injuries. The temperature, time, and frequency parameters for these technologies differ, and the exposure protocols used with them are not homogeneous in the literature.

Cryo-induced exposure to cold air might be an effective stimulus for beneficial modulation of biochemical and inflammatory variables. Research in athletes shows that muscle enzymes (e.g., creatine kinase and lactate dehydrogenase) decrease, indicating rapid recovery from muscle strain. Moreover, the downregulation of pain and inflammation, and cold air cryotherapy, whether administered via cold air devices or cold chambers, seems to have beneficial effects on the immune response. Anti-inflammatory cytokines such as IL-10 are upregulated, whereas proinflammatory mediators IL-2 and IL-8 are downregulated, without compromising immune defense. Exposure to cold may also help stabilize the cell membrane and diminish the deleterious effects of enzymes released during injury or inflammation. Finally, the available literature suggests that cryotherapy does not appear to adversely affect cardiologic and hematologic function, thereby confirming overall safety as a therapeutic measure [7, 21].

However, despite encouraging biochemical evidence and reports of reduced muscle pain and fatigue, the overall quality of the evidence remains low due to small sample sizes and variability in study designs. Most studies have shown that cold-air cryotherapy is safe for otherwise healthy athletes and does not elicit adverse events; however, insufficient data are available to interpret its long-term effects or to directly compare it with other interventions (e.g., topical ice water immersion) [36]. Overall, this technique may improve short-term recovery, but more work is needed to establish its effectiveness and safety [4].

2.2.2.5 Applications of Compression Cryotherapy

Compression cryotherapy, provided by devices such as Game Ready, consists of cold, intermittent, or continuous pneumatic compression applied to the injured or overloaded site. This treatment involves sleeves (hoses) applied around a limb or joint to circulate chilled water under pressure. The synergistic action of cold and compression leads to accelerated reduction in tissue temperature, reduced edema by increasing venous and lymphatic return, and analgesia. Customizable pressure and temperature settings allow personalized therapy to meet the athlete's needs during the onset of injury (acute phase) or during posttraining and postcompetition recovery.

Cryotherapy with compression in sports has been successful for conditions such as sprains, strains, and postsurgical conditions (e.g., arthroscopic procedures), as well as for situations requiring rapid reduction of inflammation and pain relief. One such study, which was conducted on patients after anterior cruciate ligament reconstruction, found that a compressive cryotherapy device produced superior objective functional outcomes (i.e., range of motion and isokinetic strength) compared to controls receiving standard cryotherapy—though differences in subjective pain scores or quality-of-life metrics were not significant [3]. The application of controlled pressure, in conjunction with conventional cryotherapy, significantly enhances reabsorption at sites of edema and bleeding. With these advantages comes the need for proper training and monitoring during use, as complications can occur, especially in patients with a sensation of vascular or nerve involvement. In high-performance sport, compression cryotherapy is now recognized as a potent and essential treatment for injury prevention and recovery [3].

Cryokinetics

Cryokinetics is a clinical approach that combines cryotherapy with active exercise. Cooling is applied to reduce pain and allow the patient to perform movements that would otherwise be limited. Once analgesia is achieved, the patient engages in controlled exercises to restore range of motion and function. This approach is commonly used in the management of acute musculoskeletal injuries and reflects the integration of electrophysical agents with active rehabilitation strategies.

General Principles of Cryotherapy Application

The duration of cryotherapy application should not be determined solely by time but by the patient's sensory response. Typically, patients experience a sequence of sensations described as cold, burning, aching, and finally numbness. The onset of numbness is commonly used as a clinical indicator for achieving analgesia and may guide the appropriate duration of treatment.

Several factors, including the thickness of subcutaneous adipose tissue, influence treatment duration. Areas with higher fat content require longer application times to achieve the desired cooling effect, whereas superficial regions or areas with minimal soft-tissue coverage require shorter application times.

Clinicians should continuously monitor patient response and adjust application time accordingly to ensure therapeutic effectiveness while minimizing the risk of cold-related injury.

2.2.3 Physiological Mechanisms of Cryotherapy

Cryotherapy is a commonly used therapeutic intervention in rehabilitation and sports medicine that is applied to minimize pain, inflammation, and secondary injury mechanisms after trauma or overuse-related injuries. Local tissue cooling and, in some modalities (e.g., whole-body cryotherapy [WBC]), systemic neuroendocrine responses are also responsible for its physiological effects. In conclusion, cryotherapy affects vascular dynamics, nerve conduction, metabolic rates, inflammatory cascades, and the immune system, providing lasting and clinically relevant benefits in pain control, edema reduction, and enhanced recovery (Table 2.2).

2.2.3.1 Decrease in Tissue Temperature and Its Major Effects

The primary action of cryotherapy is to reduce tissue temperature, which, in turn, induces a series of closely related physiological responses. Lower tissue temperature is associated with reduced local metabolic rate, with implications for the management of acute trauma. Cryotherapy might reduce cellular metabolism, thereby

Table 2.2 Physiological mechanisms of cryotherapy

Physiological mechanism	Primary biological effect	Clinical implication
Tissue temperature reduction	Analgesia, reduced metabolism, decreased edema	Pain relief, limitation of acute inflammatory response
Vasoconstriction	Reduced local blood flow	Limitations of swelling and secondary tissue injury
Decreased nerve conduction velocity	Attenuation of nociceptive transmission	Analgesic effect
Cytokine modulation	↓ IL-1β, IL-2, IL-6, PGE2	Anti-inflammatory response
Reduced immune cell activation	↓ T-cell and monocyte activity	Modulation of postinjury inflammation
Systemic neuroendocrine effects	Altered autonomic and hormonal responses	Improved mood, anxiety reduction, perceived well-being

decreasing oxygen requirements in injured tissues, and inhibit free radical formation and secondary injury mechanisms [51]. This reduction in metabolic demand is particularly relevant in an acutely injured state, where inflammation and hypoxia can promote tissue damage and impede repair.

Tissue cooling also reduces local tissue blood flow. There is diminished perfusion predominantly due to cold-induced vasoconstriction, which plays a significant role in preventing fluid extravasation into the interstitium and thus limiting swelling. As edema may lead to tissue pressure and mobility limitations, further pain, decreased blood flow, and, in sum, metabolic changes were addressed through symptom control and preservation-of-function goals from early on [1].

In addition, a significant effect of the temperature decline on nerve conduction velocity (NCV) is evident. Sensory nerve fibers become less sensitive to cold, ultimately leading to slower, less effective transmission of pain signals. This information is one reason cryotherapy exhibits strong short-term analgesic properties, enabling earlier movement, more tolerable rehabilitation exercises, and improved patient comfort [50].

2.2.3.2 Vasoconstriction and Edema Control

Vasoconstriction is an essential hemodynamic response to cold exposure. Constricting the superficial blood vessels saves fuel and retains core temperature, but it has its own issues. In vivo, this response reduces blood and plasma inflow to damaged tissues, thereby preventing edema formation and minimizing tissue impairment from excessive fluid accumulation [1, 50].

This would help to justify the traditional use of cryotherapy as an adjunct therapy for early-phase injury management when swelling and pain are predominant. By reducing edema, cryotherapy could also help increase the range of motion and decrease mechanical inhibition caused by joint swelling. In fact, this ability is of particular clinical benefit in musculoskeletal applications, where irritation causes local inflammatory exudate and functional impairment.

The vasoconstrictor effect would not only limit blood flow but also reduce the formation of inflammatory exudate and diminish capillary permeability during the acute phase. When not accompanied by subsequent vasoactive effects, vasoconstriction helps create a microenvironment less conducive to undue swelling and prolonged irritation without control [1, 50].

2.2.3.3 Inhibition of Pain Signal Transduction and Analgesia

Analgesia is one of the most consistent and clinically recognized effects of cryotherapy. The analgesic action is mainly produced by alterations in nerve conduction and decreased sensitivity of peripheral nociceptors. Cold, as such, decreases nerve conduction velocity, slowing pain transmission and raising the pain threshold. Therefore, patients commonly perceive an immediate decrease in pain after using cryotherapy [50] (Kaya Mumcu et al. 2025).

This has practical therapeutic implications. Decreased pain may also enable more efficient early mobilization and rehabilitation exercise, thereby minimizing potential inactivity and functional decline. Furthermore, attenuated pain perception may reduce some guarding and allow for higher-quality movement patterns as well as greater tolerance to stretching or strengthening measures.

It is also worth noting that the analgesia induced by cryotherapy is not solely sensory but rather a combined, integrated effect involving reduced activity of inflammatory mediators and modulation of central pain pathways. Consequently, cryotherapy does not function merely as an attenuator of symptoms, but works in a similar way to modulate biological elements that support the chronicity of pain.

2.2.3.4 Cellular and Molecular Changes: Inflammatory and Immune-Associated Responses

In addition to vascular and neural effects, cryotherapy affects inflammation at the cellular and molecular levels. There is cumulative evidence suggesting that cooling can influence inflammatory cytokine production and immune signaling pathways. A few studies highlight alterations in Cytokine profiles with cryotherapy exposure, affecting important mediators, including IL-1β, IL-2, and IL-6 [43, 54, 69]. Because these cytokines are important in the initiation and propagation of the inflammatory response, their modulation could partly explain decreases in swelling, soreness, and perceived fatigue.

In addition, cryotherapy has also been associated with decreases in some biochemical pain mediators such as prostaglandin E2 (PGE2), which is responsible for making the nerve endings more sensitive to pain and causing an increase in painful and inflammatory perception [43, 54, 69]. By attenuating PGE2 action, cryotherapy might provide an additional analgesic effect and reduce the endurance of inflammatory pain.

The activation of immune cells could also be modulated by cryotherapy. Leukocyte function, including inflammatory cell recruitment and activation, which can alter tissue recovery and adaptation, may also be influenced by cold exposure. Acute inhibition of inflammation may be advantageous for restricting excessive irritation, whereas the role of cryotherapy in long-term tissue remodeling is complex. Once more, in some situations, blunting of inflammatory signaling may theoretically interfere with a normal reparative or training strategy. Therefore, the timing and application procedure (modality) of cryotherapy should be tailored to clinical requirements.

2.2.3.5 Systemic Neuroendocrine Activation: Whole Body Cryotherapy (WBC)

In contrast to localized cold application, whole-body cryotherapy induces systemic physiological responses outside the treated area. WBC modulates neuroendocrine pathway activation, leading to global effects on the regulation of inflammation, autonomic balance, and psychological well-being [67]. This whole-system "shift" may involve stress hormones and other signaling molecules known to cross regulatory boundaries between the immune and nervous systems.

One of these WBC-specific concepts in the scientific literature is "pleiotropy", which refers to multiple downstream effects on diverse systems following a treatment. These probably involve reductions in systemic inflammation [67], potentially increased perceived recovery or improved mental well-being/mood states [68]. Also in applied settings and athletic scenarios, these broader effects could explain why WBCs sometimes not only reduce soreness but also improve subjective recovery quality and perceived readiness.

In addition, systemic activation of the nervous system has been associated with central modulation of pain processing; thus, it may provide an alternative mechanism for pain reduction beyond the peripheral nerve conduction changes caused by cryotherapy. As the body of literature grows, so does the understanding that WBC may influence neurophysiological mechanisms beyond those that directly regulate tissue cooling.

In conclusion, the mechanism of cryotherapy is multifactorial and involves integrated physiological responses. Metabolic activity, blood flow, and nerve conduction velocity are reduced by local tissue cooling, leading to analgesic and anti-inflammatory effects [1, 50] (Kaya Mumcu et al. 2025). Cold-induced vasoconstriction can reduce edema formation, which may decrease the susceptibility to further tissue damage [1, 50]. The analgesic effects are primarily mediated by altered pain signal conduction due to decreased nerve conduction velocity [50] (Kaya Mumcu et al. 2025). At the cellular and molecular levels, cryotherapy modulates inflammatory cytokines (e.g., IL-1β) and pain mediators (e.g., PGE2), and activates immune cells [43, 54]. In the last place, methods like WBC provoke systemic neuroendocrine stimulation associated with pleiotropic impact on inflammation and psychological condition [67, 68]. Taken together, these mechanisms support cryotherapy as the primary interventional tool in sports recovery programs and clinical rehabilitation settings.

2.2.4 Clinical Indications of Cryotherapy

Cryotherapy has a well-established role in clinical/cognitive and performance applications due to its analgesic, anti-inflammatory, and recovery benefits. Its uses are broad and include pain after injury, as an adjunct in postoperative care, for chronic disease management, for symptom control during cancer treatment, and recovery strategies for athletes (Table 2.3). Cryotherapy mechanisms of action at the level of biological tissue include decreasing tissue temperature, vasoconstriction, slowing nerve conduction velocity, and modulating local inflammatory mediators. During application, patients typically experience a predictable sequence of cold-related sensations—cold/freezing, burning, pain, and eventually numbness—reflecting

Table 2.3 Clinical indications and reported effects of cryotherapy

Clinical context	Primary effects of cryotherapy
Acute soft-tissue injury	Pain/edema ↓, possible function ↑
Postoperative pain (various surgeries)	Pain ↓, opioid use ↓
Chronic inflammatory diseases (RA, MS)	Inflammation ↓, pain ↓, well-being ↑
Sports recovery	Soreness ↓, subjective recovery ↑

progressive neural and vascular responses; notably, reduced subcutaneous fat thickness is associated with a faster onset of the freezing sensation. However, its clinical significance lies in its ability to reduce pain perception, limit swelling, improve patient movement sensitivity, and accelerate perceived recovery as part of a pain management protocol.

2.2.5 Acute Soft Tissue Injuries

Cryotherapy is widely used after acute soft-tissue injury to relieve pain and swelling during the initial recovery stage. Its clinical impact is primarily due to cold-induced vasoconstriction and decreased nerve conduction velocity, which together reduce edema formation and nociceptive signaling. In acutely injured subjects, cryotherapy is used to reduce inflammation and relieve symptoms, thereby facilitating a faster return to mobility and function by limiting the spread of inflammation at the site of injury [20, 70]. There is also evidence that cryotherapy may improve functional outcomes, depending on injury type and severity and exposure parameters; however, findings may vary about timing and clinical setting [61]. In sports and musculoskeletal rehabilitation, it is still a common nonpharmacological adjunct for pain and edema control in the early stages [40].

The acute treatment of soft-tissue injuries has historically been guided by acronyms to aid clinical assessment (Table 2.4). In recent years, these models have progressed from ICE to RICE, PRICE, POLICE, PEACE, LOVE, and CARE [13, 25, 29, 34, 80]. Each subsequent model was developed in response to the shortcomings of previous constructs, and both scientific understanding and rehabilitation philosophy evolved during that period. However, although they are of educational value, most acronyms focus more on the early temporal phase of injury, and they tend to overlook the severity of trauma, the extent of damage, and the functional effect in terms of swelling.

The role of cryotherapy is among the most contentious issues in current acute injury management. In this context, avoiding ice use in the acute phase is a recommendation within the PEACE framework and appears to be based on the idea that excessive modulation of the proinflammatory response could impair tissue repair, as observed in animal models [25]. However, it does not differentiate well between minor injuries with minimal swelling and moderate-to-severe injuries, which may involve considerable edema, hematoma formation, and limited function. In the clinical setting, soft-tissue injuries are highly heterogeneous, and across all injury severities, a one-size-fits-all approach might lead to less favorable outcomes [25].

Patients with soft-tissue injuries of moderate to severe degree frequently present with swelling and pain that reduce joint mobility, impair neuromuscular function, and delay rehabilitation. Early therapeutics that reduce edema and pain may make movement safer and enable earlier recovery without attenuating the necessary inflammation.

In this setting, acute cases should be managed by severity. We capture the key acronyms for common acute injury presentations and appraise them using the

Table 2.4 Summary of acute soft-tissue injury acronyms and clinical emphasis

Protocol	Core components	Primary aim	Main limitation/ criticism	Recommended clinical phase
ICE	Ice, compression, elevation	Symptom control, swelling	No guidance on loading or rehab	Very early symptomatic management
RICE	Rest, ice, compression, elevation	Protection and symptom relief	Overemphasis on rest	Acute phase, short-term use
PRICE	Protection, rest, ice, compression, elevation	Injury protection	Risk of prolonged immobilization	Acute injuries requiring protection
POLICE	Protection, optimal loading, ice, compression, elevation	Early safe loading	Limited severity differentiation	Broad acute injury management
PEACE	Protect, elevate, avoid anti-inflammatories, compression, educate	Education and inflammation modulation	Avoids cryotherapy regardless of severity	Minor injuries with minimal swelling
LOVE	Load, optimism, vascularization, exercise	Subacute rehabilitation	Not designed for acute swelling control	Subacute to chronic phases
CARE	Cryotherapy and compression, avoid harmful loading, rehabilitation, elevation	Severity-based acute management	Requires clinical justification	Moderate—severe injuries with significant edema

modified CARE framework (Cryotherapy and compression, Avoid harmful loading, Rehabilitation, Elevation)—a shift away from "acutist" based approach. CARE does not contradict modern rehabilitation theories but rather adds to them, specifically addressing swelling and pain in patients with moderate-to-severe injuries, while also promoting early, evidence-based rehabilitation and load management [29].

2.2.5.1 Evolution of Acute Injury Acronyms

One of the first organized approaches to soft-tissue injury management was proposed as the ICE acronym (Ice, Compression, Elevation), in which cryotherapy was strongly recommended for its effects on pain and swelling. While ICE remains effective for short-term analgesia, it offers little guidance on activity modification, progressive loading, or long-term rehabilitation planning [42].

Both the RICE (Rest, Ice, Compression, Elevation) and its extended version, PRICE (Protection, Rest, Ice, Compression, Elevation), have been designed to protect tissue during the acute phase [34]. Nevertheless, evidence indicates that severe rest- or immobilization-induced healing delay is due to muscle atrophy, joint stiffness, neuromuscular inhibition, and changes in limb biomechanics. As such, these models have been challenged for promoting atrophy following the acute phase of injury.

POLICE (Protection, Optimal Loading, Ice, Compression, Elevation) marked a notable conceptual leap by introducing optimal loading. It acknowledged the early use of controlled mechanical stimuli for healing and recovery, while preserving cryotherapy and compression to modulate symptoms and control edema. POLICE was a move from protective to re-educational models [13].

More recently, the PEACE and LOVE taxonomy was proposed to further extend the management of acute and subacute injuries. PEACE (Protect, Elevate, Avoid anti-inflammatory medications, Compression, Education) targets the acute phase, and LOVE (Load, Optimism, Vascularization, Exercise) targets the subacute stage, using an active rehabilitation-based approach that focuses on psychosocial elements as well as cardiovascular loading. The model aligns with the current concept of rehabilitation, but the recommendation against using cryotherapy in the acute phase for moderate and severe injuries is controversial because it is based on theoretical considerations of inflammation regulation, and no clear differences across levels of severity have yet been defined [25].

In an effort to address this clinical challenge, the management of acute soft-tissue injury has now been clearly refined on a severity-based basis (i.e., the CARE approach: Cryotherapy and compression; Avoidance of harmful loading; Rehabilitation; Elevation). CARE does not dispute the importance of optimal loading or education, nor does it support the indiscriminate use of cryotherapy. It rather recognizes from research both clinical trials and meta-analysis, that moderate to severe injuries (substantial edema, delayed resolution of hematoma, and functional limitation generated by pain) are types of injury that benefit mostly from early combined cryotherapy as well as compression in preventing excessive swelling, reduction in severity of symptoms, and speeding up recovery [29].

On this spectrum, CARE represents a progressive, dynamic development beyond POLICE and serves as a reciprocal balance to PEACE. PEACE is appropriate for mild injuries with limited swelling, whereas CARE provides a more evidence-based approach to managing acute-phase injuries with moderate-to-severe swelling and significant functional impairment [29].

2.2.5.2 Injury Severity as the "Missing" Clinical Variable

The limitation of acronyms is that most do not confine the extent of injury. Two patients labeled alike may present with a range of differences in the clinic. A mild internet injury will be defined by low levels of swelling or edema and little loss of function. Higher-grade injuries may have significant edema or hematoma, severe pain, decreased ROM, and impaired neuromuscular control.

Swelling from injury not only affects the injured area but also increases pain, reduces range of motion, inhibits surrounding muscles, and may lead to secondary hypoxic damage in nearby tissues. In these cases, interventions that reduce pain and swelling prior to movement may facilitate earlier and more effective rehabilitation.

Accordingly, decisions regarding acute intervention should be based on the time elapsed since injury, the severity of tissue injury, and the functional consequences of edema.

2.2.5.3 The Care Algorithm: An Acute Strategy Based on Severity [29]

CARE (Cryotherapy and compression, Avoidance of harmful loading, Rehabilitation, Elevation) is introduced as an acute treatment strategy for managing moderate-to-severe soft-tissue injuries with substantial swelling and dysfunction. This combination of cryotherapy and compression is intended to reduce pain and limit swelling in the early postinjury period. The intent is not to remove all inflammation, since inflammation is needed for healing, but to control the extent of the inflammatory response and minimize its harmful mechanical and neuro-motor consequences. There is strong evidence that cryotherapy provides pain relief, and moderate evidence that, when combined with compression and used early, it can also reduce swelling and improve joint range of motion [29].

Avoiding harmful loading does not mean total rest—it means avoiding any activity that worsens pain or swelling. Expedient offloading techniques, such as the use of braces or crutches when appropriate, along with patient education, may be employed. Rehabilitation should be initiated as soon as clinically feasible, based on the nature and severity of the injury, and should employ evidence-based therapies. Early mobilization, muscle recruitment, and graded loading are required to maintain condition and promote functional recovery.

Cryotherapy and compression, aided by elevation to improve venous and lymphatic fluid return, help reduce edema.

2.2.5.4 Clinical Bottom Line

Acronyms are useful educational tools, but should not replace clinical reasoning. Injury severity is a critical variable that must guide acute management decisions. While PEACE and LOVE provide a valuable rehabilitation-oriented framework, CARE offers a more logical and clinically applicable acute-stage strategy for moderate-to-severe soft-tissue injuries, in which pain and swelling are significant. A severity-based approach that integrates CARE in the acute phase and transitions toward progressive loading and exercise may represent the most balanced and evidence-informed pathway for optimal recovery.

2.2.5.5 Duration and Reapplication Timing of Cryotherapy Across the Different Stages of Healing in Sports Injuries

Acute Stage (First Hours/Days After Injury)

Cryotherapy is most effective when applied immediately after injury, with the primary goals of reducing pain and limiting edema. The literature consistently states that each cryotherapy session should be short, with recommendations ranging from 10 to 20 min for a breathable size and a frozen zone approximately 1 cm thick.

Table 2.5 Contraindications and precautions of cryotherapy in musculoskeletal rehabilitation

Contraindication category	Clinical condition	Rationale for avoidance
Cold hypersensitivity/ cold intolerance	Cold urticaria; cryoglobulinemia; paroxysmal cold hemoglobinuria	Risk of severe cold-induced immunologic or hemolytic reactions
Peripheral vascular disorders	Raynaud's phenomenon; severe peripheral arterial disease; vascular insufficiency	Cold-induced vasoconstriction may aggravate ischemia and impair tissue perfusion
Sensory impairment/ neuropathy	Peripheral neuropathy; chemotherapy-induced neuropathy; reduced thermal sensation	Inability to perceive excessive cooling increases the risk of frostbite or tissue injury
Compromised tissue perfusion	Postsurgical tissue with impaired circulation; ischemic tissue; graft sites	Further reduction in blood flow may delay healing and increase tissue damage
Open wounds or fragile skin	Ulcers; infected wounds; dermatological lesions; fragile or irradiated skin	Cold exposure may impair healing and increase tissue breakdown
Neurological disorders affecting sensorimotor control	Stroke; multiple sclerosis; central nervous system disorders with proprioceptive deficit	Cooling may further impair proprioception, motor control, and balance
Large-area or prolonged cooling before functional activity	Cooling of major joints or muscle groups before gait or balance tasks	Reduced proprioceptive accuracy and neuromuscular performance may increase injury risk
Whole-body cryotherapy risk conditions	Cardiovascular instability; autonomic dysfunction; severe comorbidities	Extreme cold exposure may provoke adverse systemic cardiovascular responses

Extended use (>10–20 min) may compromise neuromuscular integrity and exacerbate injury risk (Table 2.5) [57].

When the aim of cryotherapy is to reduce pain and swelling in areas with a large cross-sectional diameter—such as major joints (knee, shoulder, hip) and large muscle groups (e.g., knee extensors)—continuous application of cryotherapy for *15–20 min* is recommended, depending on the method of application. In contrast, for smaller joints (e.g., elbow, fingers) and muscle groups with a small cross-sectional area, the recommended application time is approximately *10 min*.

The interval between cryotherapy applications depends on the rate of tissue rewarming. Rewarming typically takes 60–90 min in areas with a large cross-sectional diameter and 20–30 min in smaller anatomical regions.

Rupp et al. [77] and Jutte et al. [39] used tissue temperature measurements from thermocouples and showed that maximal cooling occurs during the first 10–20 min, primarily in the superficial tissues. Longer treatment values offer no therapeutic advantage and may be harmful. For this reason, cryotherapy needs to be administered in a repetitive, intermittent fashion (cryotherapy followed by a period of rest, then reapplication) to maintain tissue cooling while preventing skin or neural injury.

Subacute Stage (Days–Weeks After Injury)

By this stage, the early inflammatory response will have begun to subside. Still, some edema, pain, and local tissue hypersensitivity may persist—especially after a period of loading or therapeutic exercise. Here, cryotherapy is used chiefly as an adjunct in pain relief and the control of reactive inflammation that may be sensitized by a slow return to Table 2.5 [51].

2.2.5.6 Duration and Reapplication Timing of Cryotherapy Using Cold Packs During the Acute Stage of Sports Injuries

The duration of cryotherapy application is shorter in the subacute phase than in the acute phase and typically ranges from 10 to 15 min, depending on the anatomical area and tissue depth. Therapeutic exercise or functional activities are often followed by cryotherapy to reduce postexercise pain and increase tissue tolerance to loading. Application times of up to 15 min are recommended for sizable muscle groups and joints, with shorter durations more appropriate for small anatomical areas [38].

Clinical and tissue responses guide the timing of repeat cryotherapy during the subacute phase and are typically 30–60 min after continued discomfort. Care should be taken during successive applications to avoid over-suppressing blood flow and the reparative mechanisms at this stage of healing [71].

In the early subacute phase, cryotherapy should not be regarded as a substitute for therapeutic exercise. Instead, it should be used as a supportive modality to facilitate therapy scheduling and allow for gradual increases in loading. In this way, it helps manage pain and tissue sensitivity, creating more favorable conditions for safe and effective participation in the rehabilitation program. There are certain subacute and chronic sports-related disorders in which cryotherapy can be used in cryokinetics, the controlled application of cold to facilitate a temporary analgesic and/or anesthetic effect, so that therapeutic exercise may be performed with greater intensity or range of movement.

In cryotherapy, treatment is typically applied for a relatively short duration (usually 5–10 min) until pain relief or numbness in the area is achieved. This is then followed directly by dynamic exercise or functional loading to increase range of motion, muscle recruitment, and neuromuscular endurance. Cryotherapy can provide transient analgesia, thereby increasing sustained load tolerance and enabling the performance of modified (otherwise painful) exercises that can be broken down into small progressions with graded intensity and complexity.

Cryotherapy is most commonly used in the subacute phase, when pain impairs rehabilitation and residual soreness or tenderness persists, reducing functional acceptance and return to training. However, the use of cryokinetics is not without caution. Exercise at the time of cryotherapy must be carefully monitored, as the transient analgesic effect may reduce loading more than is desirable and lead to overloading beyond tissue tolerance, resulting in secondary injury. As a result, cryokinetic treatment should be used within physiotherapy under the guidance of a specialist [6].

2.2.6 Sports Recovery and Performance

Cryotherapy is commonly administered in athletic settings to aid recovery after intense training or competition. Athletes often use cold-water immersion (CWI) and whole-body cryotherapy (WBC) to reduce muscle soreness, fatigue perception, and perceived readiness to return to performance. Objective performance outcomes differ between individual studies, and subjective recovery, DOMS, and inflammation have been reported to show some alterations [13]. The literature also supports the idea that cryotherapy could reduce muscle soreness and enhance recovery perception in several athletes, which explains why it is still widely used in applied sports science as a recovery method [5, 65, 91].

Although short-term muscle soreness and perceived recovery may be enhanced by reducing inflammation, chronic attenuation of the inflammatory response may, in some circumstances, affect training adaptations. Hence, clinical and sports practitioners often recommend a personalized approach based on the training phase, competition program, and rehabilitation goals [5, 65, 91].

2.2.7 Postoperative Pain Management

Cryotherapy is increasingly utilized in the postoperative recovery to reduce pain levels as an optional intervention, and a possible role within the same gateway of opioid utilization might be suggested. Postoperative refrigeration may help reduce acute inflammation and provide focal analgesia, thereby making the patient more comfortable during early postoperative mobilization and physiotherapy. There is a consistent reduction in pain and opioid consumption following various surgeries that suggest cryotherapy as an effective element in multimodal analgesia protocols [18, 63]. The integration of this approach into postoperative protocols is often justified by its low cost, relative safety, noninvasive characteristics, and potential for application in rehabilitation facilities [50].

2.2.8 Chronic Inflammatory Conditions

In addition, cryotherapy is employed as adjuvant therapy for chronic inflammatory diseases like rheumatoid arthritis (RA) and multiple sclerosis (MS). Hence, in such situations, the use of cryotherapy, particularly whole-body cryotherapy, has been reported to reduce inflammation, relieve pain, and improve overall quality of life. These systemic effects can also be associated not only with anti-inflammatory cytokine modulation but also with neuroendocrine and autonomic regulation, which could affect fatigue, mood, and perceived disease burden [69]. Results also suggest a possible benefit in symptom-related well-being, and identify cryotherapy as an adjunctive, rather than alternative, therapy for the medical treatment of these patients [67, 68].

2.2.9 Contraindications and Clinical Precautions in Cryotherapy

The analgesic mechanism of cryotherapy is believed to involve a combination of tissue cooling and functional deactivation, resulting in decreased vascularity, reduced local blood flow, inhibition of cellular metabolism, and slowed nerve conduction velocity. Together, these physiological responses are responsible for pain modulation, dampening of inflammation, and short-term symptomatic relief after injury or surgery. Cryotherapy is not risk-free, particularly when delivered without proper screening, dosing, and monitoring, despite its well-established clinical benefits.

An exposure period that is too long, or an exposure level that exceeds the approved safety limit, at temperatures above the approved safety limit, will considerably increase the likelihood of adverse effects. Continuous or repeated cycles of freeze-thaw/freezing, as well as exposure to extreme cold, can cause frostbite, tissue ischemia during rewarming, irreversible skin damage, or delayed nerve injury arising from prolonged vasoconstriction and its associated impairment in neural conduction. These hazards are particularly pertinent in short-term musculoskeletal rehabilitation and postoperative settings where tissue perfusion, sensation, and healing could already be compromised [51].

Cryotherapy contraindications are mostly due to tissue sensitivity or susceptibility of physiological systems to cold stress (Table 2.5). One such risk group is patients with impaired distal sensibility (e.g., peripheral neuropathy), who may not "sense" the degree of cooling or even the progression of tissue damage. The issue in this population becomes one of guarding against the unknown—i.e., the possibility of unseen exposure to excessive cooling or early tissue injury. Evidence from oncology rehabilitation also shows that cold intolerance is a common symptom in chemotherapy-induced peripheral neuropathy patients; the preventive use of cryotherapy in this population should be approached with caution and likely reserved for therapy [30].

In neurorehabilitation practice, exposure to cooling stimuli may evoke a short-term antispastic or muscle-relaxant effect, but the effects that carry over into improved functional activity (e.g., gait performance or motor control) are not evident. In the poststroke period, there is a risk that the ubiquitous use of cryotherapy may mask subtle neurological deficits and/or perturb sensorimotor feedback (in a manner inconsistent with motor relearning strategies). Also, in patients with multiple sclerosis, cryotherapy transiently reduces fatigue and spasticity, but proprioception and joint position sense may be impaired after short-term use, thereby increasing the risk of balance disturbances during functional training [83].

A few patient groups deserve increased attention and may constitute relative or absolute contraindications to cryotherapy. Cold-induced vasoconstriction can worsen ischemia in conditions such as peripheral arterial disease, Raynaud's phenomenon, cold hypersensitivity, or other circulatory disorders. This is especially important in lower-limb rehabilitation settings, such as after total knee arthroplasty, for which cryotherapy would otherwise be recommended for pain relief but is contraindicated due to compromised vascular function [30]. In the same way, cryotherapy should not be performed on damaged skin (open wounds, ulcers, infections, or fragile skin), as exposure to cold can delay healing, increase the risk of infection, and worsen tissue damage. For tendon rehabilitation regimens (including those for conditions such as Achilles tendinopathy), cryotherapy should be used only if the skin is healthy and without inflammatory dermatosis.

Neurological and sensory deficits also require cautious use. Local cooling of large muscle groups and major joints, for example, quadriceps or knees, has been shown to diminish proprioceptive accuracy, and special attention should be paid when treating individuals with sensory loss, disturbed proprioception, or central nervous system pathology. Therefore, cryotherapy should be avoided just before activities that involve balance, coordination, or fine motor control [35]. While complications (i.e., skin irritation, blistering, nail-fold inflammation) have been rare, their presence adds to the need for diligent monitoring in medically complicated cohorts such as cancer rehabilitation.

For risk minimization and safe clinical application, cryotherapy must follow well-defined principles. Treatment times are generally 10–20 min, and temperatures remain within tolerable levels, usually between 0 and 10 °C for ice packs. Longer treatment durations are not more efficacious and increase the risk of neural and cutaneous side effects. Before treatment, a full clinical examination is necessary, including vascular status, skin quality and integrity, sensibility, and pertinent medical history. For athletic and postsurgical recovery, it is advised to begin with conservative dosing and carefully assess skin response and client input.

Equally important is the choice of a proper cryotherapy modality. In daily clinical practice, local applications such as cold gel packs or ice packs are most frequently used due to their ability to target specific treatment sites and the limited risk of systemic adverse reactions. In whole-body cryotherapy, on the other hand, the brief exposure to very low temperatures is controversial and presents absolute contraindications: cardiovascular instability, autonomic dysfunction, and severe comorbidities. When employed, use must be limited to individuals carefully screened and supervised by a physician.

2.2.10 Critical Appraisal and Clinical Perspective on Cryotherapy

Despite its widespread use in musculoskeletal rehabilitation and sports medicine, the current body of evidence raises important questions regarding the clinical effectiveness of cryotherapy beyond short-term symptom relief. While cryotherapy consistently demonstrates an analgesic effect through reductions in nerve conduction velocity and nociceptive transmission, its impact on tissue healing remains uncertain. Contemporary evidence, including systematic reviews and meta-analyses, suggests that any observed improvements in pain and range of motion are generally small and may not be clinically meaningful.

Importantly, the theoretical rationale for cryotherapy in acute injury management—namely, the reduction of inflammation and metabolic activity—should be interpreted with caution. Inflammation is a critical component of the tissue healing process, and excessive suppression of this response may delay regeneration, as suggested by experimental and animal studies. However, high-quality human evidence confirming these effects remains limited.

In the context of sports recovery, cryotherapy may provide short-term reductions in muscle soreness and perceived fatigue, which can be beneficial in congested competition schedules. Nevertheless, repeated or routine use—particularly following resistance training—may attenuate long-term neuromuscular adaptations by interfering with anabolic signaling pathways.

Therefore, cryotherapy should not be considered a primary therapeutic intervention aimed at accelerating tissue healing, but rather an adjunct modality for short-term pain management and symptom control. Clinical decision-making should be individualized, taking into account injury severity, stage of healing, patient characteristics, and rehabilitation goals. A balanced, evidence-informed approach supports the selective and time-limited use of cryotherapy, integrated within a comprehensive rehabilitation program centered on progressive loading and functional recovery.

Despite the widespread use of cryotherapy in clinical practice, the current evidence base remains limited. High-quality, well-powered randomized controlled trials investigating its effects on tissue healing and long-term outcomes are still lacking. As a result, ongoing debates regarding the clinical effectiveness of cryotherapy should be interpreted with caution, and definitive conclusions cannot yet be drawn.

2.2.11 Case Studies

2.2.11.1 Cryotherapy: A Case Study 1 (Acute Sprain to the Ankle)

A 22-year-old amateur basketball player was admitted to the hospital 12 h after being injured with an inversion ankle sprain during a game. The patient presented with lateral ankle pain, increased warmth, and obvious perimalleolar swelling. Clinical examination revealed pain on palpation of the anterior talofibular ligament and inability to bear weight.

Intervention: Local cryotherapy was performed with an ice pack for 15–20 min each time, 3–5 times per day in the first 48–72 h. It was supplemented with external compression, limb elevation, and early protected weight-bearing as tolerated.

Reasons: During the acute inflammatory phase, cryotherapy reduces nociceptive transmission by decreasing nerve conduction velocity, limits secondary hypoxic injury by lowering local metabolic demand, and prevents excessive edema by causing vasoconstriction and decreasing capillary permeability.

Results: At 72 h, the pain and swelling decreased significantly, allowing for gentle ROM exercises, partial weight-bearing, and functional rehabilitation exercises.

2.2.11.2 Cryotherapy: Example Two (Chronic Tendinopathy)

A 45-year-old office worker presented with a 6-month history of chronic lateral elbow tendinopathy pain that was aggravated by grip activities and typing. The patient had been adhering to a prescribed daily eccentric loading regimen for the wrist extensors.

Intervention: A local cryotherapy protocol was provided on symptomatic days and immediately after exercise sessions for 10–15 min, with intensity adjusted to the level of postexercise soreness and irritability.

Reasons: Cryotherapy has no effect on the degenerative tendon matrix in chronic tendinopathy. It works primarily by reducing postrun pain and reactive hyperemia and by increasing short-term pain tolerance, allowing runners to resume running and thereby promoting adherence to therapeutic loading.

Outcome: Over 4 weeks, the patient reported decreased postactivity soreness, increased tolerance to eccentric loading, and improved functional capacity during daily tasks, supporting continuation of rehabilitation.

2.3 Thermotherapy

Thermotherapy is the use of heat as a physical therapy intervention to relieve pain, muscle stiffness, and disease-related limitations, based on several physiological and neurophysiological mechanisms. By raising the temperature of the skin and underlying tissues, thermotherapy promotes local blood flow through vasodilation, increases the metabolic rate at which tissues require nutrients, decreases muscle spindle sensitivity, and makes connective tissues more pliable. Taken together, these effects help reduce pain, decrease muscle guarding, and enhance movement, thereby establishing thermotherapy as a widely applied modality in musculoskeletal and neurological rehabilitation.

In clinical and sports medicine practices, thermotherapy is commonly used in the subacute and chronic phases of injury, once inflammation has subsided (including trigger points). At the same time, goals are now geared toward restoring function through mobility, flexibility, and neuromuscular function. Local heat applications, or Thermotherapies, are widely used by physiotherapists and typically include hot packs/moist heat packs, paraffin wax baths, infrared radiation, and superficial heating modalities (whirlpool therapy and fluidotherapy) for the treatment of localized muscle tightness, joint stiffness, and soft-tissue restriction. Because superficial heat primarily affects cutaneous and subcutaneous tissues, it can be applied to specific anatomical sites to reduce systemic effects.

In addition to its localized effects, thermotherapy is commonly used as a preparatory modality before other forms of treatment, including exercises and hands-on therapy. The use of heat may also play a role in tolerance to stretching, joint mobilization, and strength exercises by reducing pain and increasing tissue compliance, thereby promoting greater effectiveness of rehabilitation programs. In patients with neurological conditions, thermotherapy also appears to help reduce muscle tone and spasticity in some cases; its use should be considered judicious to avoid fatigue or symptom exacerbation.

In summary, local thermotherapy methods are common and attractive approaches due to their convenience, low cost, ease of use, and overall good safety profile when appropriately prescribed. They are mainly used in clinical practice to manage transient pain relief, soft-tissue extensibility, and, therefore, functional movement and exercise ability. However, the effectiveness of thermotherapy as a treatment depends on critical parameters such as temperature, duration, and frequency of application, as well as other factors, including the stage of injury and the patient's condition (circulatory state and thermal sensitivity). Thus, thermotherapy should not be used as a stand-alone or general modality, but rather as an organized, goal-oriented element of a comprehensive rehabilitation program.

2.3.1 Biophysics of Thermotherapy

Thermotherapy is among the most common modalities used in neuromusculoskeletal rehabilitation to treat pain, muscle spasms, stiffness, and other pathologic conditions, such as skeletal muscle adaptation, through local and systemic application. Its biophysical impact is mediated by changes in tissue perfusion, tissue mechanics, and cellular signaling processes, which act on remodeling and repair.

An elevation in tissue temperature of 2–5 °C, which is applied through superficial or deep heating techniques, results in increased blood flow and metabolic activity (vasodilation), with an increase in the extensibility of collagen and a decrease in the viscoelastic resistive forces within soft tissue around muscles [37, 58, 64, 84]. These benefits lead to increased ROM and reduced mechanical stiffness when applied during treatments.

The therapeutic application of heat significantly alters the viscoelastic properties of collagen-rich tissues. By increasing tissue temperature, thermotherapy reduces the viscosity of the ground substance and increases the compliance of connective tissues. This reduces joint stiffness and increases extensibility, creating an optimal "therapeutic window" for subsequent stretching, joint mobilization, and functional exercise [58, 64].

Thermal therapy can also influence neuromuscular function, altering muscle tone and spasm by altering muscle spindle activity and nerve conduction velocity. At the same time, heat increases tolerance to pain and interrupts physiological responses in the pain-spasm-pain cycle: thus enhancing active movement and exercise [8, 37, 58, 64]. Computational simulation of myofascial trigger points at the microstructural level indicates that heating may result in mechanical decoupling between thermal expansion and soft tissue at the fibrous level, with reduced local mechanical stresses within the trigger point locus, including modified transverse compression and passive strain. Cooling, on the other hand, temporarily amplifies these stresses, which may also explain different clinical effects of heating and cooling [53].

2.3.1.1 Muscle Regeneration, Atrophy, and Adaptation

Indeed, long-term heat treatment has been shown to increase the expression of heat shock proteins (HSPs) and to activate their angiogenic, hypertrophic, and mitochondrial signaling pathways in muscle tissue [45, 46]. On the other hand, postinjury heat modalities, such as warm-water immersion in murine models, reduce histological muscle damage and oxidative stress and accelerate the regeneration process [27, 45, 46].

Hot water immersion postexercise, with induced muscle trauma in humans, reduces pain perception and plasma markers of muscle damage while increasing HSP27 and HSP70. Despite such molecular adaptations, cold exposure seems to attenuate them [22]. Long-term exposure to WBH has also been observed to reduce muscle atrophy and decrease in strength during immobilization, which may be due, at least in part, to a reduction of catabolic signaling pathways such as NF-κB and Forkhead (FoxO) following temporary disuse [52].

2.3.1.2 Neuromuscular Performance and Rehabilitation Outcomes

Thermal interventions could prevent muscle mass loss and increase strength gains during rehabilitation programs when long-duration thermal stimuli were applied. A good prescription is FITT—frequency, intensity, time, and type of heating—to raise muscle temperature [45, 46, 75]. There is evidence that isokinetic torque and a pro-angiogenic environment within skeletal muscle can be enhanced after 8 weeks of localized thigh heating in humans [45, 46]. However, the results are inconsistent and can be negative, especially when heating intensity or duration is low or when heating occurs after (preceding) exercise. The discrepancy in these findings supports the need for accurate dosage and the incorporation of thermotherapy into rehabilitation routines [75, 88].

2.3.1.3 Thermal Modalities and Biophysical Characteristics

Surface-heating modalities (e.g., hot packs and warm baths) depend primarily on conductive and convective heat transfer and affect depths of approximately 1–2 cm below the surface. These modalities are often utilized to relieve pain, reduce muscle spasm, and enhance joint mobility [8, 37, 58, 64, 84].

Deep-heating modalities (diathermy and therapeutic ultrasound) increase the depth of heating by delivering electrical or acoustic energy that is converted into heat deep within the muscle. Specifically, they are highly effective in increasing tissue extensibility and preparing tissues for stretching or exercise [58, 64, 84, 88].

Generally, whole-body passive heating techniques, such as saunas and hot-water immersion, increase both muscle and core temperatures. The former may be related to angiogenic adaptations, anti-atrophic effects, and improvements in neuromuscular performance, at least when interventions are applied repeatedly over time (McGorm et al. 2018) [22, 45, 46, 52].

2.3.1.4 Conclusion

During neuromusculoskeletal rehabilitation, the biophysical mechanisms associated with thermotherapy include elevated muscle and connective tissue temperatures and augmented perfusion. Modulating neural conduction and tissue mechanical properties. Thermal interventions, when delivered acutely and at appropriate doses, activate molecular pathways that limit muscle wasting, promote tissue regeneration, and help restore functional potential. The correct prescription and application of thermotherapy in a full rehabilitation plan is important for successful treatment.

2.3.2 Methods and Techniques of Thermotherapy

In outpatient rehabilitation, thermotherapy includes superficial-to-deep, high-tech heating applications intended to increase the temperature of the tissue under treatment in a controlled manner, not for oncologic or ablative purposes (Table 2.6). Response to treatment is in part due to specific mechanical effects, including circulation, neuromuscular function, connective tissue mechanics, and cellular signaling mediators. They are the most commonly used thermal modalities in musculoskeletal rehabilitation. Deep heating modalities such as therapeutic ultrasound (Chap. 3), diathermy (Chap. 4), and HILT (Chap. 5) are discussed in detail in separate chapters and therefore are not analyzed in this cryotherapy–thermotherapy chapter. Tecar is out of the scope of the present book.

2.3.2.1 Hot Packs

Hot packs, which can be made of moist heat, electrical heating, or self-heating materials, are a simple yet effective method in physical therapy for thermotherapy (Fig. 2.4).

These treatments are commonly utilized to relieve low back pain, muscle spasm, stiffness, and chronic musculoskeletal pain. Their therapeutic efficacy has been linked to various factors, such as vasodilatation leading to increased local blood flow, decreased muscle tone, and a rise in pain thresholds, resulting in easier movement and the ability to undergo other treatment modalities [58, 64].

Table 2.6 Thermotherapy modalities and equipment in musculoskeletal physiotherapy

Hot packs/heat wraps	Superficial conductive heat	Myalgia, low back pain, muscle spasm
Warm baths/whirlpool	Superficial + hydrotherapy	Joint stiffness, rheumatic conditions
Paraffin bath	Superficial	Hand and foot osteoarthritis, scars
Diathermy (SW/MW)	Deep electromagnetic heating	Chronic tendinopathies, joint stiffness
Therapeutic ultrasound	Deep thermal and mechanical	Tendons, capsules, scar tissue
TECAR therapy	Deep endogenous RF heating	Low back pain, tendinopathies, OA, sports injuries
High-intensity laser (HILT)	Deep photothermal + photobiomodulation	Knee OA, shoulder pain, epicondylitis

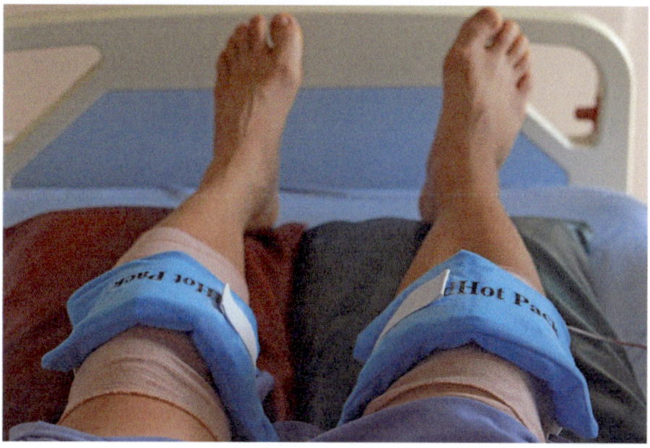

Fig. 2.4 Hot packs. (© Pakkapol Kunanon/Dreamstime.com)

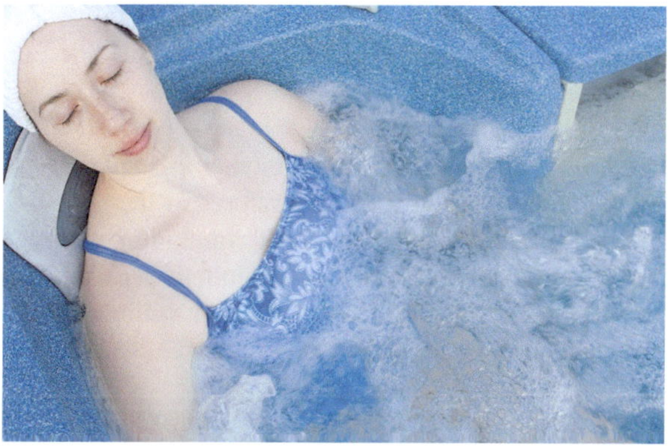

Fig. 2.5 Warm baths/whirlpool. (© Davidcrehner/Dreamstime.com)

Warm Baths/Whirlpool

Hydrotherapy, in the form of pools, tubs, or whirlpool systems, as a means of continuous superficial heat, involves adding thermal energy to that provided by buoyancy and hydrostatic pressure (Fig. 2.5). Submersion at either the local or whole-body level relaxes muscles, reduces joint load, and improves ease of movement. Additionally, these are extremely advantageous within posttraumatic joint stiffness states, juvenile idiopathic arthritis (JIA) conditions, and in chronic pain situations where gentle mobilization has to be given concomitant with thermal analgesia [64].

Paraffin Bath

A paraffin bath is another type of superficial heat that produces a long-lasting elevation in tissue temperature, with published evidence of deep penetration and uniform heating (Fig. 2.6). Application of the hands or feet to warm, melted paraffin wax is a widely accepted therapy for managing hand and foot osteoarthritis, as well as for

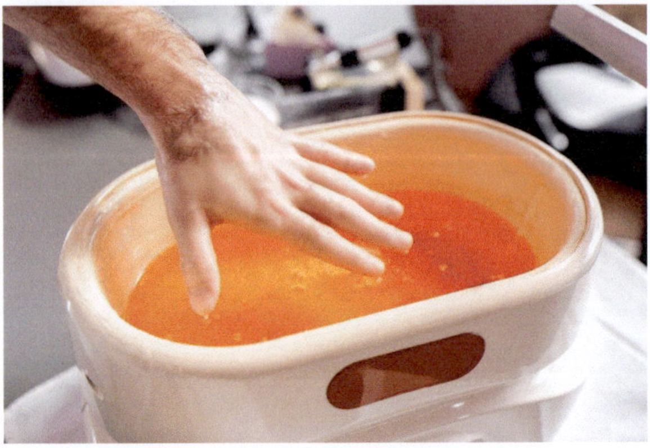

Fig. 2.6 Paraffin bath. (© Didesign021/Dreamstime.com)

painful scar tissue and small-joint stiffness. Sustained heat increases connective tissue extensibility and reduces pain during subsequent mobilization or exercise [58].

2.3.2.2 Infrared Radiation

Infrared radiation is a form of superficial thermotherapy that delivers heat via electromagnetic waves, thereby increasing temperatures in the skin and subcutaneous tissue. It produces vasodilation, enhances local circulation, and may contribute to pain relief and muscle relaxation. However, its depth of penetration is limited compared with other thermotherapeutic modalities, and its clinical use has declined as more targeted and effective interventions have become available. Care should be taken to avoid excessive heating and potential skin burns.

High-Intensity Laser Therapy

High-intensity laser therapy (HILT) (Fig. 2.7) may also produce thermal effects in deeper tissues due to its high power output and penetration capabilities (Normand-Gravier et al. 2024) [88]. However, its mechanisms of action, clinical indications, and therapeutic applications differ substantially from conventional thermotherapy modalities and are discussed in detail in a dedicated chapter (Chap. 5). There is evidence for its use in knee osteoarthritis, shoulder disorders, lateral elbow tendinopathy, plantar fasciitis, muscle strains, and chronic low back pain, with benefits for pain and function. The combination of HILT with exercise therapy or TECAR appears to be even more beneficial for rehabilitation outcomes, as it shortens recovery time and improves symptom resolution.

In clinical practice, any thermotherapy modality should be considered an adjuvant or complementary to other treatments. Their main purpose is to alleviate pain, reduce muscle spasm, improve tissue extensibility, and prepare the neuromusculoskeletal system for active rehabilitation, manual therapy, and patient education. The optimal benefit derives from the appropriate selection of modality, the correct dose, and integration into a structured rehabilitation exercise program.

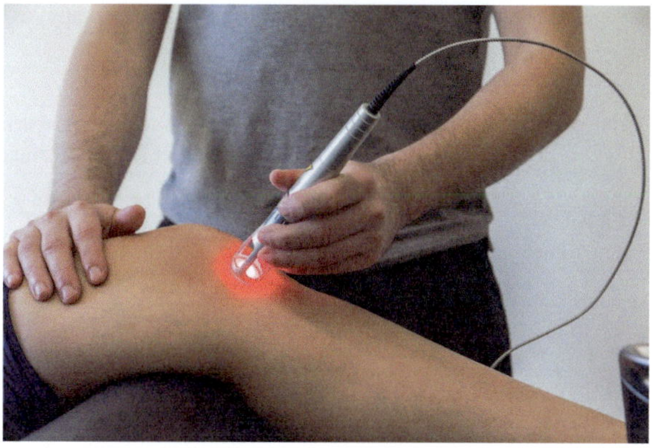

Fig. 2.7 High-intensity laser therapy. (© Vasilis Ververidis/Dreamstime.com)

General Principles of Application and Treatment Duration
Superficial thermotherapy modalities are typically applied for 15–20 min, depending on the treatment goal, the size of the area, and patient tolerance. The method of application should ensure uniform heat distribution while minimizing the risk of thermal injury. Adequate insulation and regular monitoring of skin response are essential to prevent burns, particularly in patients with impaired sensation or circulation. The selection of treatment duration and intensity should be individualized based on the stage of healing, clinical objectives, and patient feedback.

2.3.3 Mechanisms of Action of Thermotherapy in Musculoskeletal Rehabilitation

Thermotherapy exerts its effects through a complex interplay of vascular, neurophysiological, and cellular mechanisms, far beyond mere tissue heating (Table 2.7). Whereas short-term increases in tissue temperature elicit rapid physiological responses that reduce pain and neuromuscular excitability, long-term thermal treatments induce molecular adaptations that promote recovery, metabolic adaptation, and resistance to atrophy. Such mechanisms may help explain the universal appeal of heat-induced treatments in musculoskeletal rehabilitation.

At the acute level, increased temperature in local muscle tissue results in vasodilation and increased local blood flow. This increased perfusion supports the delivery of oxygen and nutrients to musculoskeletal tissues, as well as the removal of metabolic waste products and inflammatory mediators. Additionally, and more importantly from a physiological point of view, these vascular responses would contribute directly to an inhibition of pain and set the stage for tissue recovery in sub-acute and chronic musculoskeletal disorders [24, 58, 64, 76].

The metabolic activity of the cells and mechanics of their surrounding connective tissues are also modified in response to thermal exposure. An increase in tissue

Table 2.7 Acute and chronic mechanisms of action of thermotherapy in musculoskeletal rehabilitation

Mechanism	Physiological effect	Clinical outcome
Vasodilation and increased perfusion	↑ Blood flow, oxygen, and nutrient delivery	Promotion of tissue healing, metabolite clearance
Activation of thermoreceptors (TRPV1)	Modulation of nociceptive signaling	Analgesia, reduced muscle tone
Increased metabolism and tissue elasticity	↓ Stiffness, ↑ connective tissue compliance	Improved ROM, preparation for exercise/manual therapy
Intramuscular Ca^{2+} kinetics	Faster cross-bridge cycling	Improved contractile function and power
Heat shock proteins (HSP27/70)	Protein protection and repair	Muscle regeneration, reduced damage
mTOR and anti-catabolic signaling	↑ Protein synthesis and ↓ degradation	Hypertrophy or attenuation of atrophy

temperature reduces the viscoelastic response of collagenous tissues, leading to more extensible and less passive stiffened tissues. These effects enhance joint movement and lead to it being described as a "preparatory" treatment prior to static stretching, mobilization, or exercise-based rehabilitation [24, 58, 64].

From a neurophysiological perspective, thermotherapy exerts analgesic effects in several ways. The activation of thermosensitive receptors, especially TRPV1 channels, also reduces peripheral and central nociceptive input by interfering with the transmission of painful information and enhancing anti-nociceptive descending pathways. At the same time, stimulation of cutaneous mechanoreceptors by heat also potentiates spinal "gate control," inhibiting pain sensation to an even greater extent. This combined action increases pain thresholds and decreases muscular tone, allowing the free execution of movement/exercise, or functional activities [76, 92].

High muscle temperature also influences neuromuscular function via changes in the contractile properties. Increased calcium sensitivity in muscle fibers speeds cross-bridge cycling and eliminates the sluggish phase of cross-bridge activation. These adaptations might lead to acute improvements in muscle strength and power production and could improve performance during rehabilitation sessions if the positive effects of thermotherapy occur immediately before the exercises [45, 46] (McGorm et al. 2018), or overall [74].

In addition to those acute effects, repeated or prolonged thermal exposures also induce chronic cellular and molecular adaptations that are of great concern during recovery from musculoskeletal damage. One of the most striking responses is the upregulation of heat shock proteins, specifically HSP27 and HSP70. These are molecular chaperones that stabilize the protein structure of the cell, protect it against oxidative and mechanical damage, and aid in muscle fiber regeneration after injury. Animal and human studies indicate that regular exposure to heat increases HSP expression, resulting in an environment that protects against further cellular damage and supports tissue repair [22, 45, 46] (McGorm et al. 2018; Normand-Gravier et al. 2024).

Thermotherapy also modulates anabolic and anti-catabolic pathways. The Akt–mTOR pathway (involving 4E-BP1 and S6 kinase) is activated by passive heating, leading to elevated protein expression. Concomitantly, thermal treatments inhibit catabolic mediators, including FoxO and NF-κB, thereby reducing protein breakdown. These mechanisms are of particular interest in situations of immobilization or unloading, where heat therapy is also reported to attenuate muscle atrophy and strength loss (McGorm et al. 2018; Normand-Gravier et al. 2024).

Further to long-term adaptations, mitochondrial biogenesis and angiogenesis are activated. The enhanced muscle oxidative capacity and fatigue resistance are due to increased muscle VEGF, mitochondrial density, capillary supply, and function resulting from heat exposure. These adaptations would enhance metabolic economy and may be beneficial for stamina and rehabilitative functional recovery [44–46].

Thermotherapy also has a context-dependent effect on inflammatory signaling. Cytokine profiles, such as TNF-α, IL-1β, IL-6, and IL-10, are affected by heat exposure, with the overall effect depending on the treatment intensity/duration and timing. There is evidence that heat, at appropriate doses, induces anti-inflammatory or immunoregulatory effects that are more likely to promote regeneration than to perpetuate a positive feedback loop of tissue damage [47, 76, 92].

In pathological conditions like DOMS or microtrauma, thermotherapy can help to keep high blood-flow levels, promoting oxidative metabolism and inhibiting mechanical hyperalgesia. In humans, sitting in hot water after an experimental muscle-damaging protocol, likewise, reduces pain and systemic indices of muscle damage while elevating cytoprotective protein levels (HSPs/IL-10). Animal research on the effects of early and repeated exposure to such heat has revealed that it accelerates the appearance of regenerating muscle fibers and tissue repair markers [22, 27, 85].

2.3.4 Clinical Indications of Thermotherapy in Musculoskeletal Rehabilitation

Thermotherapy is commonly used in musculoskeletal rehabilitation as an adjunctive intervention to modulate pain, enhance tissue healing, and improve functional performance (Table 2.8). There is evidence for its use in various MSK pain conditions when incorporated into multimodal rehabilitation approaches, including exercise, manual therapy, patient education, and, to a lesser extent, pharmacological treatment [19, 58, 92].

Chronic nonspecific musculoskeletal pain, for instance, neck or low back pain, and generalized muscle aches and stiffness are among the oldest clinical indications for thermotherapy. Thermotherapy modalities (e.g., hot packs and heat wraps) consistently produce analgesia, reduced muscle stiffness, and short-term gains in ROM and function. Clinical trials have shown that continuous low-level heat wraps can decrease pain intensity and disability in acute, subacute, or chronic low back pain

Table 2.8 Clinical indications of thermotherapy in musculoskeletal rehabilitation

Condition	Clinical purpose of thermotherapy	Level/type of evidence
Chronic nonspecific musculoskeletal pain (neck pain, low back pain, muscle stiffness)	Analgesia, muscle relaxation, increased ROM, functional improvement	RCTs show heat wraps reduce pain and disability in acute and subacute low back pain and may outperform cold in DOMS
Knee and peripheral joint osteoarthritis	Symptomatic relief of pain and stiffness, support of exercise therapy	Superficial heat and thermal baths improve pain and function as adjuncts to usual care
Posttraumatic muscle injuries and sprains (subacute/chronic phase)	Muscle relaxation, analgesia, preparation for manual therapy, and exercise	Heat is recommended after the initial inflammatory phase, often following early cryotherapy
DOMS and postexercise recovery	Reduction of muscle pain, facilitation of recovery	Heat wraps and diathermy before or after exercise reduce soreness in selected protocols
Muscle spasm and hypertonicity	Reduction of spasm and tone, improved flexibility	Superficial heat is effective in low-back and neck muscle spasm
Immobilization-related muscle atrophy	Adjunct intervention to attenuate atrophy and support regeneration	Passive heat reduces muscle loss and increases protective molecular responses
Rheumatic and chronic degenerative conditions	Short-term pain and stiffness relief	Recommended as a palliative adjunct, particularly paraffin for hands
Athletic warm-up and injury prevention	Passive tissue warming, reduced stiffness	Heat modalities may complement multimodal warm-up strategies

and provide greater symptom relief than cold application for delayed onset muscle soreness based on randomized controlled trials [8, 19, 58, 64].

Thermotherapy is also frequently integrated into the care of knee and other peripheral joint osteoarthritis as a symptomatic supplement to exercise training. Devices that deliver superficial heat, thermal baths, and spa treatments have also been shown to reduce pain and stiffness and improve the tolerability of therapeutic exercise and functional retraining. Heat does not alter disease pathogenesis; however, its role in comfort and active rehabilitation is well established [10, 19, 92].

Thermotherapy is widely accepted for the care of subacute and/or chronic musculoskeletal traumas, including muscular strains and ligamentous sprains. Once acute inflammation and edema are under control, cryotherapy and heating are used to promote muscle relaxation, analgesia, and to prepare the patient for manual techniques and progressive loading. Guideline recommendations propose avoiding heat in the first inflammatory phase and supporting its use after 48–72 h of tissue response [58, 64, 86, 88].

Heat application has also been explored for exercise recovery and the delayed onset of muscle soreness. There is limited evidence that the use of heat (heat wraps and deep-heating modalities) may reduce perceived muscle soreness and improve recovery when applied postintervention in certain protocols. Although results are mixed and depend on the protocol, some research suggests that heat may be as effective as, or more effective than, cold for managing postexercise pain (McGorm et al. 2018) [22, 88].

Muscle spasm and hypertonicity are other typical indications for heat. By decreasing muscle stiffness and altering neuromuscular excitability, superficial heat modalities are highly effective at reducing spasm in areas such as the cervical and lumbar spine, thereby enhancing comfort and readiness to move and exercise [8, 58]. The literature provides evidence supporting a beneficial effect of warm therapy in reducing muscle atrophy during deconditioning and load reduction. Nonexercise heat exposure has been shown to attenuate muscle atrophy and enhance recovery through molecular response mechanisms, including increased expression of heat shock proteins. Heat cannot be a substitute for mechanical loading, but it can be an interesting complement when access to exercise is limited (McGorm et al. 2018) [22].

In rheumatic and chronic degenerative disease, including RA, thermotherapy is mainly used for symptomatic relief in the short term but not as a disease modifier. Hand paraffin baths are frequently prescribed for pain and stiffness when acute inflammatory flares are absent. In these cohorts, heat should be considered with prudence and as part of the whole for individualized management [10, 64, 73].

Third, thermotherapy can be used in athletes either as part of the exercise warm-up or to prevent injury, as a method of passively warming tissue. Heat modalities may complement active warm-up protocols in cold conditions or in the early stages of rehabilitation programs by increasing tissue extensibility and reducing stiffness (McGorm et al. 2018) [88, 92].

2.3.4.1 General Principles of Clinical Use

Thermotherapy, regardless of indication, should be administered with due regard for timing and clinical setting. Cryotherapy is commonly used in the acute inflammatory stage of an injury, while heat may be most useful once swelling and active inflammation begin to recede. In chronic pain and stiffness, superficial heat modalities have the strongest evidence for immediate symptom relief. Notably, when teaching thermal therapy, it has always been meant to be an adjunctive intervention in the context of a multi-modal and comprehensive rehabilitation approach; hence, never as an isolated and unique means of treatment [19, 58, 86, 92].

2.3.5 Contraindications and Precautions of Thermotherapy in Musculoskeletal Rehabilitation

Thermotherapy is an important complement to musculoskeletal rehabilitation, but must be applied with caution, as contraindications and precautions are well described (Table 2.9). The lead hazards of heat treatment include acute inflammation, sensory or vascular insufficiency, and skin breakdown. Failure to recognize these conditions may lead to worsening symptoms or complications.

Table 2.9 Contraindications and precautions of thermotherapy in musculoskeletal rehabilitation

Contraindication category	Clinical condition	Reason for avoidance
Acute inflammatory phase	Acute joint inflammation, recent injury with edema/hematoma (first 48–72 h)	Heat may exacerbate inflammation and swelling; cryotherapy is preferred initially
Acute structural injury	Fractures, ligament or tendon ruptures, acute muscle tears	Risk of increased bleeding and delayed stabilization
Sensory impairment/ neurological disorders	Peripheral neuropathy, spinal cord injury, reduced thermal sensation	Increased risk of burns due to impaired feedback
Circulatory disorders	Severe peripheral vascular disease, venous insufficiency, heart failure	Potential hemodynamic burden and edema aggravation
Skin lesions or infection	Open wounds, burns, dermatitis, herpes zoster	Compromised skin integrity increases the risk of complications
Active inflammatory arthritis	Acute flare of rheumatoid or inflammatory arthritis	Deep heat may intensify inflammatory activity
Malignancy in the treatment area	Direct heat over the active tumor	Precautions due to a potential increase in tumor perfusion

During the acute inflammatory phase of musculoskeletal injury, heat application is typically not indicated, especially in the first 48–72 h posttrauma. Vasodilation, edema, and the release of inflammatory mediators are dominant features of the early-phase induction, with hyperthermia-induced vasodilation contributing to increased swelling and discomfort. In this case, we usually recommend applying cryotherapy before the inflammatory phase resolves, followed by thermotherapy [56, 64, 66].

Acute injuries with structural (fractures, ligament or tendon ruptures) also probably represent either a relative or transient contraindication of deep versus superficial thermotherapy. Application of heat may also impede recovery or increase tissue damage until integrity can be restored and active bleeding or edema controlled. For that reason, clinical guidelines recommend avoiding heat therapy and using a protective or anti-inflammatory treatment during the early postinjury phase instead [66, 88].

Another major contraindication is neurological diseases with diminished sensation. In patients with peripheral neuropathy, spinal cord injury, or regional sensory deficits, there may be impaired sensation of excessive heat perception and thus a high risk for thermal burns. These risks are particularly significant with excessive use of heat wraps or home applications without supervision and can be exacerbated by caution or contraindication in this population [64, 79, 92].

Peripheral or systemic circulatory disorders should also be carefully considered. Marked peripheral arterial disease, severe chronic venous insufficiency, and decompensated heart failure may restrict the body's ability to compensate for vasodilation brought about by heat. In some of these cases, thermotherapy (whole-body and/or long exposure to heat) can increase edema or put too much strain on the circulatory system, when it should be used after a medical examination or perhaps even contraindicate its use [78, 92].

Before thermotherapy, the skin should be free of open wounds and abrasions to mitigate anticipated risks. Do not employ heat over open wounds, in highly infected or "hot" skin diseases, over burns, or herpes zoster. There is also a potential increase in the risk of tissue injury and infections in compromised skin; therefore, thermotherapy should be avoided until the affected area has recovered [64, 92].

During the acute surge of the disease, thermotherapy should be avoided in patients with inflammatory rheumatic diseases like rheumatoid arthritis. Deep-heating agents, such as those used in ultra-shortwave therapy, may induce inflammation and exacerbate joint symptoms. In the stable or long-term phase, shallow heat may be used with circumspection for symptom management and is at the clinical judge's discretion [64].

In general, malignancy in the treatment site is a relative contraindication to local thermotherapy. While there is no direct evidence, many clinical protocols discourage applying heat over a tumor for theoretical reasons related to increased local blood flow and stimulation of tumor metabolism [87, 92].

However, pregnancy should be taken with caution. Local or systemic heat (e.g., over the lumbar spine or abdomen) should not be used without medical consultation. Developers of continuous heat technology and clinical positions recommend consulting a physician before using their heat therapy during pregnancy [87].

2.3.5.1 General Precautions in Rehabilitation Practice

In addition to contraindications to cryotherapy, some patients require special care during thermotherapy. Geriatric patients with comorbidities, such as diabetes and cardiovascular or rheumatic pathology, should be treated with heat under professional supervision, with attention to cutaneous and systemic reinfection. Shallow heating is well tolerated in the pediatric or adolescent population when used conservatively under adult supervision. Elderly people and the mentally impaired are particularly vulnerable to misuse, supercooling, and extended exposure, causing burn injuries or late recognition of complications.

2.3.5.2 Conclusion

Contraindications to the use of thermotherapy in musculoskeletal rehabilitation include acute inflammation, recent trauma with edema, loss of sensation or circulation, and open or infected skin. In susceptible subjects, heat treatment should be performed with careful control of temperature and duration, under strict clinical surveillance. These precautions ensure that thermotherapy remains a safe and useful adjunct to the overall rehabilitation process.

2.4 Clinical Reasoning in the Selection of Cryotherapy and Thermotherapy in Musculoskeletal Rehabilitation

The selection between cryotherapy and thermotherapy is an important component of clinical reasoning in musculoskeletal rehabilitation. It should be guided by the stage of tissue pathology, the presence and extent of inflammation, the patient's symptoms, and the patient's general therapeutic goals. Acutely, cryotherapy is best utilized in the first 48–72 h, or the acute inflammatory phase, postinjury, when there are clinical signs of pain, heat, and/or swelling. During that phase, cold contributes to diminished nerve conduction velocity, modulates the flow of nociceptive input, and is assumed to help limit excessive edema formation and secondary tissue damage. Thus, cryotherapy primarily serves as a symptom-modulating technique rather than an accelerant of tissue repair, and is most beneficial when used in conjunction with compression, elevation, and early protected mobility.

The widespread use of cryotherapy should be re-evaluated as the inflammatory phase diminishes and the tissue enters the proliferative stage. Cold can still be applied intermittently at this point, for pain control after exercise or manual therapy. Yet, it should not be seen as a substitute for active rehabilitation therapies that focus on regaining movement, strength, and function. Extended or nonspecific application of cold (cryotherapy) beyond the acute state could unnecessarily restrict blood flow (BF), metabolic activity, and tissue extensibility, thereby potentially decreasing functional recovery.

Thermotherapy is usually indicated for subacute and chronic conditions in which acute inflammation is absent, and stiffness, muscle guarding, or limited tissue extensibility are major clinical symptoms. Heat raises tissue temperature, increases blood flow, decreases muscle tone, and improves the viscoelastic properties of collagen, making tissues more pliable in response to stretching, mobilization, and exercise. Therefore, thermotherapy is frequently administered as a preparatory modality before therapeutic exercise, joint mobilization, or soft-tissue procedures for conditions such as osteoarthritis, chronic low back pain, and prolonged muscle tightness.

However, thermotherapy is contraindicated for ongoing inflammation, swelling that is uncontrolled, recent trauma, or suspected hemorrhaging, as a rise in tissue temperature increases edema and pain. For mixed presentations, such as chronic inflammation with intermittent inflammatory flares, we may switch between hot and cold based on day-to-day clinical observations, underscoring the importance of regular reassessment rather than fixed protocols.

The recovery status must be clearly determined.

We need to clarify the following questions:

- Is the area of injury warm when you touch it?
- Is the area tender to palpation?
- Is the degree of swelling stable during the recovery process?
- Is the swelling activity-related?
- Does pain limit joint movement?
- Do you think there may be inflammation?
- Does the patient benefit from cryotherapy?

If the answer is "no" to all, then thermotherapy can be used safely.

For most of the above questions, if your answer is "yes," cryotherapy should be utilized.

However, it is critical to understand that cryotherapy and thermotherapy should not be considered stand-alone treatments. Their role in clinical care is to be included in a multifaceted, task-oriented rehabilitation plan that focuses on active involvement, exercise, patient instruction, and reassessment of the response to the intervention. It is thus evident that the decision regarding cold or heat is dynamic and individualized, based on both biophysical principles and patient-centered clinical reasoning.

2.5 Critical Appraisal and Clinical Perspective on Thermotherapy

Thermotherapy is widely used in musculoskeletal rehabilitation due to its beneficial effects on pain modulation, tissue extensibility, and joint mobility. The available evidence supports its role primarily in the subacute and chronic phases of injury, where increased tissue temperature facilitates blood flow, reduces muscle stiffness, and enhances the viscoelastic properties of connective tissues. These effects contribute to improved range of motion and may optimize conditions for therapeutic exercise and manual interventions.

However, the clinical benefits of thermotherapy should be interpreted within an evidence-based framework. While heat consistently improves short-term flexibility and reduces pain perception, its effects on underlying tissue pathology and long-term functional outcomes remain limited. Thermotherapy does not directly accelerate tissue healing but rather serves as a preparatory and supportive modality that enhances patient comfort and mobility.

Furthermore, inappropriate use—particularly during the acute inflammatory phase—may exacerbate swelling and delay recovery by increasing blood flow and metabolic activity. Therefore, careful consideration of injury stage, patient characteristics, and treatment goals is essential.

In contemporary rehabilitation models, thermotherapy should be applied as an adjunct to active interventions, such as exercise and manual therapy, rather than as a stand-alone treatment. A targeted, time-specific, and individualized approach maximizes its therapeutic value while minimizing potential adverse effects.

2.6 Clinical Case Studies-Thermotherapy

2.6.1 Thermotherapy: Case Study 1 (Knee Osteoarthritis)

A 68-year-old patient with knee osteoarthritis, as shown on X-ray, reports severe morning stiffness and decreased joint range of motion, which gradually improves during the day. On physical examination, there is synovial crepitus and mild periarticular tenderness that limits active knee flexion in the early morning, without evidence of acute synovitis.

Intervention: Superficial thermotherapy application with a moist hot pack to the anterior knee area for 15–20 min, immediately before active range of motion exercises, quadriceps strengthening activities, and functional sit-to-standing.

Rationale: Superficial heat elevates periarticular temperature, which may increase the extensibility of collagen and decrease passive joint stiffness, in addition to promoting local circulation and neuromuscular relaxation. Performing heat before exercise prepares the periarticular structures for loading and allows the athlete to move more comfortably during rehabilitation.

Outcome: Patient gains knee flexion throughout subsequent sessions, experiences less stiffness with therapeutic exercise, and is more comfortable with activities such as walking and getting up from a chair.

2.6.2 Thermotherapy: Case Study 2 (Chronic Low Back Tightness)

A 35-year-old manual worker reports insidious, nonspecific low back muscle tightness over several months, aggravated by prolonged lifting and sustained flexed postures. Examination shows increased paravertebral/lumbar paraspinal tone and decreased trunk flexion, without inflammatory signs or radicular symptoms.

Intervention: Local application of moist heat to the lumbar area for 15 min, plus focusing soft tissue mobilization technique on paraspinals and thoracolumbar fascia, along with delayed stretching of posterior chain musculature.

Thermotherapy not only increases superficial tissue temperature, which decreases muscle spindle sensitivity and protective guarding but also increases the viscoelastic compliance of myofascial tissues. This thermal priming reduces the discomfort of any subsequent patient's deep massage and stretching treatments.

Outcomes: After three treatment sessions, the patient demonstrates improved lumbar flexion and extension, reduced palpable muscle tone, and reduced tightness during occupational activities, suggesting clinical benefit from continued mobility exercises.

2.7 Research Evidence

2.7.1 Key Message 1: Cryotherapy

Existing evidence supports the application of cryotherapy for immediate pain relief and symptom management in acute musculoskeletal trauma, especially early after injury (48–72 h). In this early inflammatory phase, cooling decreases nerve conduction velocity and inhibits nociceptive transmission, leading to analgesia and symptomatic relief. Cryotherapy is also widely believed to help limit excessive edema formation and secondary tissue damage; however, direct effects on structural tissue repair remain insufficiently supported by current evidence.

The available literature indicates very little evidence that cryotherapy accelerates biological healing processes. Its dominant therapeutic effect appears to be symptom modification and edema reduction rather than tissue regeneration. Clinical outcomes are best when cryotherapy is used as part of a multimodal acute injury regimen, namely, compression, elevation, and early protected mobilization; in this way, we provide effective pain control while allowing functional recovery.

2.7.2 Key Message 2: Thermotherapy

There is also moderate-quality evidence for the use of thermotherapy in chronic musculoskeletal disorders, as evidenced by persistent pain, joint stiffness, and muscle tightness, particularly when administered before therapeutic exercise or manual therapy. Application of heat raises local tissue temperatures and blood flow, decreases muscle guarding, and improves the viscoelasticity of collagen tissues. These effects increase tissue extensibility and promote movement, thereby enhancing functional rehabilitation.

As a result, thermotherapy is often used as a pretreatment modality to enhance tissue for stretching, mobilization, and active rehabilitation exercises. By contrast, thermotherapy is generally not indicated in acute inflammatory conditions or immediately postinjury, as elevating tissue temperature may increase edema and pain. In this way, the therapeutic potential of heat is largely determined by the stage of tissue injury and by the presence of current inflammation.

2.7.3 Key Message 3: Overall Interpretation

In conclusion, both cryotherapy and thermotherapy should be considered adjunct treatments within a classical exercise-plus musculoskeletal rehabilitation program rather than as a single form of therapy. They are most clinically useful for pain management, tissue modulation, and the patient's in vivo involvement in developing active rehabilitation and functional recovery.

The current state of the evidence is heterogeneous in methodological quality, and outcomes vary across treatment protocols, application times, and measurement criteria. Accordingly, the clinical decision-making process must not be based solely on modality-specific evidence. Still, it should consider knowledge exchange through a combination of research results and individual patient presentation (stage of tissue healing), symptom behavior, and rehabilitation goals. This view maintains a dynamic, patient-oriented approach, and the choice between cryotherapy and thermotherapy may change over the course of rehabilitation.

2.8 Review Questions

1. Explain the difference between heat and temperature in clinical terms.
2. How do specific heat capacity and thermal conductivity influence the depth of heating or cooling in different tissues?

3. Why is cryotherapy recommended in the acute inflammatory stage of injury?
4. Under what circumstances is thermotherapy contraindicated?
5. Describe how cryotherapy affects nerve conduction velocity and pain perception.
6. Explain why thermotherapy is often used before exercise in chronic conditions.
7. Compare the roles of cryotherapy and thermotherapy in range of motion restoration.
8. Why should cryotherapy and thermotherapy be considered adjuncts rather than stand-alone treatments?

Declarations

Competing Interests The author(s) have no competing interests to declare that are relevant to the content of this manuscript.

References

1. Açık C. The comprehensive evolution of cryotherapy: a review on mechanisms, applications and the future of cold therapy from sports medicine to metabolic health. Asian J Med Health. 2025;23:96–105.
2. Adamczyk JG, Krasowska I, Boguszewski D, Reaburn P. The use of thermal imaging to assess the effectiveness of ice massage and cold-water immersion as methods for supporting post-exercise recovery. J Therm Biol. 2016;60:20–5.
3. Alexander J, Selfe J, Greenhalgh O, Rhodes D. Cryotherapy and compression in sports injury management: a scoping review. Int J Ther Rehabil. 2021;10:0141. https://doi.org/10.12968/ijtr.2020.0141.
4. Allan R, Malone J, Alexander J, Vorajee S, Ihsan M, Gregson W, Kwiecien S, Mawhinney C. Cold for centuries: a brief history of cryotherapies to improve health, injury and post-exercise recovery. Eur J Appl Physiol. 2022;122:1153–62. https://doi.org/10.1007/s00421-022-04915-5.
5. Angelopoulos P, Diakoronas A, Panagiotopoulos D, Tsekoura M, Xaplanteri P, Koumoundourou D, Saki F, Billis E, Tsepis E, Fousekis K. Cold-water immersion and sports massage can improve pain sensation but not functionality in athletes with delayed onset muscle soreness. Healthcare. 2022;10:2449.
6. Bahniuk B. How cryokinetics affect sensory perception, range of motion and postural stability of uninjured ankles and previously injured ankles. Doctoral dissertation, University of Manitoba. 2021.
7. Banfi G, Lombardi G, Colombini A, Melegati G. Whole-body cryotherapy in athletes. Sports Med. 2010;40:509–17. https://doi.org/10.2165/11531940-000000000-00000.
8. Behera D, Shetty A. Effectiveness of heat and cold therapy in muscle spasm: a review. Int J Phys Educ Sports Health. 2023;10:196–200. https://doi.org/10.22271/kheljournal.2023.v10.i3c.2948.
9. Belitsky R, Odam S, Hubley-Kozey C. Evaluation of the effectiveness of wet ice, dry ice, and cryogenic packs in reducing skin temperature. Phys Ther. 1987;67:1080–4. https://doi.org/10.1093/PTJ/67.7.1080.
10. Bernetti A, Mangone M, Alviti F, Paolucci T, Attanasi C, Murgia M, Di Sante L, Agostini F, Vitale M, Paoloni M. Spa therapy and rehabilitation of musculoskeletal pathologies: a proposal for best practice in Italy. Int J Biometeorol. 2019;64:905–14. https://doi.org/10.1007/s00484-019-01731-z.

11. Bleakley CM, Davison GW. What is the biochemical and physiological rationale for using cold-water immersion in sports recovery? A systematic review. Br J Sports Med. 2010;44:179–87. https://doi.org/10.1136/bjsm.2009.065565.
12. Bleakley C, McDonough S, MacAuley D. The use of ice in the treatment of acute soft-tissue injury: a systematic review of randomized controlled trials. Am J Sports Med. 2004;32:251–61.
13. Bleakley CM, Glasgow P, MacAuley DC. PRICE needs updating, should we call the POLICE? Br J Sports Med. 2012;46:220–1.
14. Bracciano AG, Bracciano E. Cryotherapy. In: Physical agent modalities. London: Routledge; 2024. p. 117–48.
15. Bugaj R. The cooling, analgesic, and rewarming effects of ice massage on localized skin. Phys Ther. 1975;55:11–9. https://doi.org/10.1093/PTJ/55.1.11.
16. Burkov I, Kolishkin L, Pushkarev A, Shakurov A, Tsiganov D, Zherdev A. Experimental and computational thermal analysis of partial-body cryotherapy. Int J Heat Mass Transf. 2021;183:122194. https://doi.org/10.1016/j.ijheatmasstransfer.2021.122194.
17. Chesterton LS, Foster NE, Ross L. Skin temperature response to cryotherapy. Arch Phys Med Rehabil. 2002;83:543–9. https://doi.org/10.1053/apmr.2002.30926.
18. Chumkam A, Pongrojpaw D, Chanthasenanont A, Pattaraarchachai J, Bhamarapravatana K, Suwannarurk K. Clinical study cryotherapy reduced postoperative pain in gynecologic surgery: a randomized controlled trial. Pain Res Treat. 2019;2019:2405159.
19. Clijsen R, Stoop R, Hohenauer E, Aerenhouts D, Clarys P, Deflorin C, Taeymans J. Local heat applications as a treatment of physical and functional parameters in acute and chronic musculoskeletal disorders or pain. Arch Phys Med Rehabil. 2021;103:505–22. https://doi.org/10.1016/j.apmr.2021.06.015.
20. Collins NC. Is ice right? Does cryotherapy improve outcome for acute soft tissue injury? Emerg Med J. 2008;25:65–8.
21. Costello J, Selfe J, Hayes G, McInerney C, Donnelly A. The effects of cold air (−110 degrees C) and water (8 degrees C) cryotherapy on knee skin temperature. Med Sci Sports Exerc. 2013. (Conference Abstract).
22. Dablainville V, Mornas A, Normand-Gravier T, Al-Mulla M, Papakostas E, Olory B, Fermín T, Zampeli F, Nader N, Alhammoud M, Bayne F, Sanchez A, Cardinale M, Candau R, Bernardi H, Racinais S. Muscle regeneration is improved by hot water immersion but unchanged by cold following a simulated musculoskeletal injury in humans. J Physiol. 2025;603:7603–25. https://doi.org/10.1113/jp287777.
23. de Oliveira Mianutti G, Milioni VL, Pesenti FB, Macedo CDSG. Effects of different cryotherapy techniques on skin surface temperature, agility and balance-comparison between cold water immersion, game ready®, and ice pack: a randomised clinical trial. Biomed J Sci Tech Res. 2021;39:31011–7.
24. Dmochowski J, Khadka N, Cardoso L, Meneses E, Jin Y, Bikson M. Computational modeling of deep tissue heating by an automatic thermal massage bed: predicting the effects on circulation. Front Med Technol. 2022;4:925554. https://doi.org/10.3389/fmedt.2022.925554.
25. Dubois B, Esculier JF. Soft-tissue injuries simply need PEACE and LOVE. Br J Sports Med. 2020;54:72–3.
26. Elfahem R, Bouchet B, Abbès B, Legrand F, Polidori G, Beaumont F. Investigating heat transfer in whole-body cryotherapy: a 3D thermodynamic modeling approach with participant variability. Fluids. 2024;9:61. https://doi.org/10.3390/fluids9030061.
27. El-Sheikh A, El-Kordy E, Issa S. Influence of heat treatment on muscle recovery after skeletal muscle injury in rats: histological and immunohistochemical studies. J Microsc Ultrastruct. 2021;10:63–71. https://doi.org/10.4103/jmau.jmau_85_20.
28. Fachin K, De Estéfani D, Lima K, Haupenthal D, Haupenthal A. Comparison of cryotherapy performed with ice or gel and superficial skin cooling of older women: a randomized, crossover, clinical trial. J Geriatr Phys Ther. 2024;47:155–61. https://doi.org/10.1519/JPT.0000000000000412.
29. Fousekis K, Tsepis E. Minor soft tissue injuries may need PEACE in the acute phase, but moderate and severe injuries require CARE. J Sports Sci Med. 2021;20:799.

30. Garcia C, Karri J, Zacharias NA, Abd-Elsayed A. Use of cryotherapy for managing chronic pain: an evidence-based narrative. Pain Ther. 2021;10:81–100.
31. Hatfield H, Pugh L. Thermal conductivity of human fat and muscle. Nature. 1951;168:918–9. https://doi.org/10.1038/168918a0.
32. He X, Bischof JC. Quantification of temperature and injury response in thermal therapy and cryosurgery. Crit Rev Biomed Eng. 2003;31:355–422. https://doi.org/10.1615/critrevbiomedeng.v31.i56.10.
33. Higgins TR, Greene DA, Baker MK. Effects of cold water immersion and contrast water therapy for recovery from team sport: a systematic review and meta-analysis. J Strength Cond Res. 2017;31:1443–60.
34. Mirkin G, Hoffman M. The Sports Medicine Book. 1978 Boston, MA: Little, Brown and Company.
35. Imray C, Grieve A, Dhillon S, Caudwell Xtreme Everest Research Group. Cold damage to the extremities: frostbite and non-freezing cold injuries. Postgrad Med J. 2009;85:481–8.
36. Janwantanakul P. The effect of quantity of ice and size of contact area on ice pack/skin interface temperature. Physiotherapy. 2009;95:120–5. https://doi.org/10.1016/j.physio.2009.01.004.
37. Jeon J, Kim S, Kang D, Kim B, Koo J, Moon O, Lee J. Change of isometric contractile force and muscle activity applying heat according to the time on biceps brachii muscle. J Int Acad Phys Ther Res. 2013;4:505–9. https://doi.org/10.5854/jiaptr.2013.05.25.505.
38. Jinnah AH, Luo TD, Mendias C, Freehill M. Cryotherapy duration is critical in short-term recovery of athletes: a systematic review. J ISAKOS. 2019;4:131–6.
39. Jutte LS, Merrick MA, Ingersoll CD, Edwards JE. The relationship between intramuscular temperature, skin temperature, and adipose thickness during cryotherapy and rewarming. Arch Phys Med Rehabil. 2001;82:845–50.
40. Kalli K, Fousekis K. The effects of cryotherapy on athletes' muscle strength, flexibility, and neuromuscular control: a systematic review of the literature. J Bodyw Mov Ther. 2020;24:175–88.
41. Kanlayanaphotporn R, Janwantanakul P. Comparison of skin surface temperature during the application of various cryotherapy modalities. Arch Phys Med Rehabil. 2005;86:1411–5. https://doi.org/10.1016/J.APMR.2004.11.034.
42. Kellett J. Acute soft tissue injuries—a review of the literature. Med Sci Sports Exerc. 1986;18:489–500.
43. Keskin C, Aksoy A, Kalyoncuoğlu E, Keleş A, İlik AA, Kömeç O, Yüzgüleç E, Akgün H, Alak SG, Tokur O. Effect of intracanal cryotherapy on the inflammatory cytokine, proteolytic enzyme levels and post-operative pain in teeth with asymptomatic apical periodontitis: a randomized clinical trial. Int Endod J. 2023;56:932–42.
44. Kim K. Impact of heat therapy on skeletal muscle structure and function. 2019. https://doi.org/10.25394/pgs.11336294.v1.
45. Kim K, Monroe J, Gavin T, Roseguini B. Skeletal muscle adaptations to heat therapy. J Appl Physiol. 2020;128:1635–42. https://doi.org/10.1152/japplphysiol.00061.2020.
46. Kim K, Reid B, Casey C, Bender B, Ro B, Song Q, Trewin A, Petersen A, Kuang S, Gavin T, Roseguini B. Effects of repeated local heat therapy on skeletal muscle structure and function in humans. J Appl Physiol. 2020;128:483–92. https://doi.org/10.1152/japplphysiol.00701.2019.
47. Klemm P, Schulz N, Boettger P, Lange U. Heat therapy in rheumatic and musculoskeletal diseases—an overview of clinical and molecular effects. Int J Hyperth. 2024;41:2322667. https://doi.org/10.1080/02656736.2024.2322667.
48. Kolishkin L, Shakurov A. Heat transfer between a human and a fluid under extreme conditions of partial-body cryotherapy. J Phys Conf Ser. 2020;1683:022021. https://doi.org/10.1088/1742-6596/1683/2/022021.
49. Kowal MA. Review of physiological effects of cryotherapy. J Orthop Sports Phys Ther. 1983;5:66–73. https://doi.org/10.2519/jospt.1983.5.2.66.
50. Kunkle BF, Kothandaraman V, Goodloe JB, Curry EJ, Friedman RJ, Li X, Eichinger JK. Orthopaedic application of cryotherapy: a comprehensive review of the history, basic science, methods, and clinical effectiveness. JBJS Rev. 2021;9:e20.

51. Kwiecien SY, McHugh MP. The cold truth: the role of cryotherapy in the treatment of injury and recovery from exercise. Eur J Appl Physiol. 2021;121:2125–42.
52. Labidi M, Alhammoud M, Mtibaa K, Ihsan M, Elhusseiny R, Deldicque L, Nader N, Nasir N, Papakostas E, Olory B, Cruz F, Farooq M, Sanchez A, d'Hooghe P, Tourny C, Racinais S. The effects of heat therapy during immobilization and rehabilitation on muscle atrophy and strength loss at return to sports in healthy humans. Orthop J Sports Med. 2024;12:23259671241281727. https://doi.org/10.1177/23259671241281727.
53. Lamsfuss J, Bargmann S. Mechanisms of thermal treatments in trigger points of the skeletal muscle: computational microstructural modeling. Eur J Mech A/Solids. 2022;99:104906. https://doi.org/10.1016/j.euromechsol.2022.104906.
54. Lindsay A, Othman MI, Prebble H, Davies S, Gieseg SP. Repetitive cryotherapy attenuates the in vitro and in vivo mononuclear cell activation response. Exp Physiol. 2016;101:851–65.
55. Lombardi G, Ziemann E, Banfi G. Whole-body cryotherapy in athletes: from therapy to stimulation. Front Physiol. 2017;8:258298.
56. Lubrano E, Mazas P, Freiwald J, Krüger K, Grattagliano I, Mur E, Silva R, Maruri G, De Medeiros L. An international multidisciplinary Delphi-based consensus on heat therapy in musculoskeletal pain. Pain Ther. 2022;12:93–110. https://doi.org/10.1007/s40122-022-00419-4.
57. Mac Auley DC. Ice therapy: how good is the evidence? Int J Sports Med. 2001;22:379–84.
58. Malanga G, Yan N, Stark J. Mechanisms and efficacy of heat and cold therapies for musculoskeletal injury. Postgrad Med. 2015;127:57–65. https://doi.org/10.1080/00325481.2015.992719.
59. Merrick MA, Jutte LS, Smith ME. Cold modalities with different thermodynamic properties produce different surface and intramuscular temperatures. J Athl Train. 2003;38:28–33.
60. Metzman L, Gamble J, Rinsky L. Effectiveness of ice packs in reducing skin temperature under casts. Clin Orthop Relat Res. 1996;1996:217–21. https://doi.org/10.1097/00003086-199609000-00029
61. Miranda J, Silva HJ, Correa FG, Figueiredo R, Fonseca G, Oliveira VG, Silva SSBF, Santos SP, Lamas IM, Ataíde F, Santons A. Effects of cryotherapy on function, pain intensity, swelling, and dorsiflexion range of motion in acute ankle sprain: protocol for the FROST randomised controlled trial. PLoS One. 2025;20:e0325456.
62. Morley M. Thermal conductivities of muscles, fats and bones. Int J Food Sci Technol. 2007;1:303–11. https://doi.org/10.1111/j.1365-2621.1966.tb02019.x.
63. Muaddi H, Lillie E, Silva S, Cross JL, Ladha K, Choi S, Mocon A, Karanicolas P. The effect of cryotherapy application on postoperative pain: a systematic review and meta-analysis. Ann Surg. 2023;277:e257–65.
64. Nadler SF, Weingand K, Kruse RJ. The physiologic basis and clinical applications of cryotherapy and thermotherapy for the pain practitioner. Pain Physician. 2004;7:395.
65. Naylor AS. Perceptions and current practice vs evidence-based effects of whole-body cryotherapy on fatigue and recovery in elite rugby players. Doctoral dissertation, University of Bolton. 2022.
66. Nossa F, Franco M, Magni A, Raimondo E, Ventriglia G, Gervasoni F. Heat therapy for musculoskeletal pain conditions: actionable suggestions for pharmacists from a panel of experts. Pharmacy. 2025;13:63. https://doi.org/10.3390/pharmacy13030063.
67. Panchenko OA. Methodology of cryotherapy use in medical practice. Probl Cryobiol Cryomed. 2019;29:137–47.
68. Pawik M, Kowalska J, Rymaszewska J. The effectiveness of whole-body cryotherapy and physical exercises on the psychological well-being of patients with multiple sclerosis: a comparative analysis. Adv Clin Exp Med. 2019;28:1477–83.
69. Peyronnel C, Totoson P, Petitcolin V, Bonnefoy F, Guillot X, Saas P, Verhoeven F, Martin H, Demougeot C. Effects of local cryotherapy on systemic endothelial activation, dysfunction, and vascular inflammation in adjuvant-induced arthritis (AIA) rats. Arthritis Res Ther. 2022;24:97.

70. Racinais S, Dablainville V, Rousse Y, Ihsan M, Grant ME, Schobersberger W, Budgett R, Engebretsen L. Cryotherapy for treating soft tissue injuries in sport medicine: a critical review. Br J Sports Med. 2024;58:1215–23.
71. Raja R, Huddar V. Effectiveness of cryokinetics in comparison with effectiveness of ultrasound therapy in treatment of acute supraspinatus tendonitis. Biomed Pharmacol J. 2021;14:2249–55.
72. Ritter H, Beuermann R, Unkelbach V, Bang H, Feist E. Analgesia by cryotherapy in patients with chronic pain with analysis of pain-modulating and pro-inflammatory parameters—a clinical controlled pilot study. J Clin Med. 2025;14:7567.
73. Robinson V, Brosseau L, Casimiro L, Judd M, Shea B, Wells G, Tugwell P. Thermotherapy for treating rheumatoid arthritis. Cochrane Database Syst Rev. 2002;2:CD002826.
74. Rodrigues P, Trajano G, Stewart I, Minett G. Potential role of passively increased muscle temperature on contractile function. Eur J Appl Physiol. 2022;122:2153–62. https://doi.org/10.1007/s00421-022-04991-7.
75. Rodrigues P, Minett G, Orssatto L. Turning up the heat on skeletal muscle adaptations and neuromuscular function: key considerations for passive heating prescription and best practices. Eur J Appl Physiol. 2025;125:2741–50. https://doi.org/10.1007/s00421-025-05917-9.
76. Rossi R. Heat therapy for different knee diseases: expert opinion. Front Rehab Sci. 2024;5:1390416. https://doi.org/10.3389/fresc.2024.1390416.
77. Rupp KA, Herman DC, Hertel J, Saliba SA. Intramuscular temperature changes during and after 2 different cryotherapy interventions in healthy individuals. J Orthop Sports Phys Ther. 2012;42:731–7.
78. Sastriques-Dunlop S, Elizondo-Benedetto S, Zayed M. Sauna use as a novel management approach for cardiovascular health and peripheral arterial disease. Front Cardiovasc Med. 2025;12:1537194. https://doi.org/10.3389/fcvm.2025.1537194.
79. Scheel-Sailer A, Aliyev N, Jud D, Annaheim S, Harder Y, Krebs J, Wildisen A, Wettstein R. Changes in skin-physiology after local heat application using two different methods in individuals with complete paraplegia: a feasibility and safety trial. Spinal Cord. 2020;58:667–74. https://doi.org/10.1038/s41393-019-0408-8.
80. Scialoia D, Swartzendruber AJ, Scialoia Sainth Joseph D. The RICE protocol is a myth: a review and recommendations. Sport J. 2020;24:1–19.
81. Stefan N, Tomozei R, Tanasa R, Moraru C. Study regarding increased range of motion and muscular force in knee joint sprains. Discobolul. 2022. https://doi.org/10.35189/dpeskj.2022.61.1.12.
82. Szabo D, Neagu N, Teodorescu S, Predescu C, Sopa I, Panait L. TECAR therapy associated with high-intensity laser therapy (Hilt) and manual therapy in the treatment of muscle disorders: a literature review on the theorised effects supporting their use. J Clin Med. 2022;11:6149. https://doi.org/10.3390/jcm11206149.
83. Thibaut A, Chatelle C, Ziegler E, Bruno MA, Laureys S, Gosseries O. Spasticity after stroke: physiology, assessment and treatment. Brain Inj. 2013;27:1093–105.
84. Tomlinson J, Goldberg M. Modalities part 1: thermotherapy. In: Physical rehabilitation for veterinary technicians and nurses. Hoboken, NJ: Wiley Blackwell; 2017. p. 218–30. https://doi.org/10.1002/9781119389668.ch14.
85. Tsuboshima K, Urakawa S, Takamoto K, Taguchi T, Matsuda T, Sakai S, Mizumura K, Ono T, Nishijo H. Distinct effects of thermal treatments after lengthening contraction on mechanical hyperalgesia and exercise-induced physiological changes in the rat muscle. J Appl Physiol. 2020;128:296–306. https://doi.org/10.1152/japplphysiol.00355.2019.
86. Ventriglia G, Gervasoni F, Franco M, Magni A, Panico G, Iolascon G. Musculoskeletal pain management and thermotherapy: an exploratory analysis of Italian physicians' attitude, beliefs, and prescribing habits. J Pain Res. 2023;16:1547–57. https://doi.org/10.2147/jpr.s401550.
87. Ventriglia G, Franco M, Magni A, Gervasoni F. Treatment algorithms for continuous low-level heat wrap therapy for the management of musculoskeletal pain: an Italian position paper. J Pain Res. 2024;17:4075–84. https://doi.org/10.2147/jpr.s452661.

88. Vrindten K, Lonati D, Mazzocca J, Matzkin E. Thermal modalities including hot baths and cold plunges play a unique role in injury prevention and recovery. Arthrosc Sports Med Rehabil. 2024;7:101143. https://doi.org/10.1016/j.asmr.2025.101143.
89. Wallace P, Hartley G, Nowlan J, Ljubanovich J, Sieh N, Taber M, Gagnon D, Cheung S. Endurance capacity impairment in cold air ranging from skin cooling to mild hypothermia. J Appl Physiol. 2023;136:58–69. https://doi.org/10.1152/japplphysiol.00663.2023.
90. Ward K, Thain PK, Bate G, Woodward M. Therapeutic modalities in sports and exercise therapy. In: Routledge handbook of sports and exercise therapy. London: Routledge; 2024. p. 507–98.
91. Wilson LJ, Cockburn E, Paice K, Sinclair S, Faki T, Hills FA, Gondek MB, Wood A, Dimitriou L. Recovery following a marathon: a comparison of cold water immersion, whole body cryotherapy and a placebo control. Eur J Appl Physiol. 2018;118:153–63.
92. Zanoli G, Albarova-Corral I, Ancona M, Grattagliano I, Hotfiel T, Iolascon G, Krüger K, Maruri G. Current indications and future direction in heat therapy for musculoskeletal pain: a narrative review. Muscles. 2024;3:212–23. https://doi.org/10.3390/muscles3030019.
93. Zare P, Ghoraishian M, Khorasani F. A three-dimensional model of transient bioheat transfer in the lower extremity during cryotherapy. Proc Inst Mech Eng H J Eng Med. 2021;235:1413–20. https://doi.org/10.1177/09544119211035855.
94. Zemke JE, et al. Intramuscular temperature responses in the human leg to two forms of cryotherapy: ice massage and ice bag. J Orthop Sports Phys Ther. 1998;27:301–7. https://doi.org/10.2519/jospt.1998.27.4.301.
95. Zhao G, Zhang H, Guo X, Luo D, Gao D. Effect of blood flow and metabolism on multidimensional heat transfer during cryosurgery. Med Eng Phys. 2007;29:205–15. https://doi.org/10.1016/j.medengphy.2006.03.005.

3 Therapeutic Ultrasound and Low-Intensity Pulsed Ultrasound: A Critical Synthesis of Biophysics, Mechanisms, and Clinical Evidence

Konstantinos Papadopoulos

3.1 Introduction

3.1.1 Defining Therapeutic Ultrasound: From Diagnostic Imaging to Therapeutic Intervention

Therapeutic ultrasound (TUS) delivers high-frequency sound energy to living tissue, producing predictable physiological changes (Fig. 3.1). Unlike diagnostic ultrasound—which fires brief pulses and "listens" for echoes to build an image—TUS is designed to act on tissue, not to visualize it. In practice, clinicians use it to deliver a controlled acoustic dose that can promote healing responses, reduce pain, and alter tissue properties to support rehabilitation goals. That distinction in purpose shapes everything from machine design to parameter selection and has kept ultrasound near the center of physiotherapy and rehabilitation practice for more than six decades across a wide range of musculoskeletal presentations [17].

At the heart of every therapeutic unit is a handheld transducer containing piezoelectric crystals. When an alternating electric current is applied, these crystals deform and generate inaudible pressure waves. Because air reflects almost all incident ultrasound, a coupling gel is applied to the skin to eliminate the air interface and enable efficient energy transfer from the transducer face into the tissues (Fig. 3.2). Without that coupling layer, most of the wave would reflect off the skin surface and never reach the intended target [17].

K. Papadopoulos (✉)
School of Health, Medicine and Lifestyle, University of Hertfordshire, Hatfield, UK
e-mail: k.papadopoulos2@herts.ac.uk

D. Stasinopoulos (ed.), *Application of Electrophysical Agents in Physiotherapy*,
https://doi.org/10.1007/978-3-032-32144-2_3

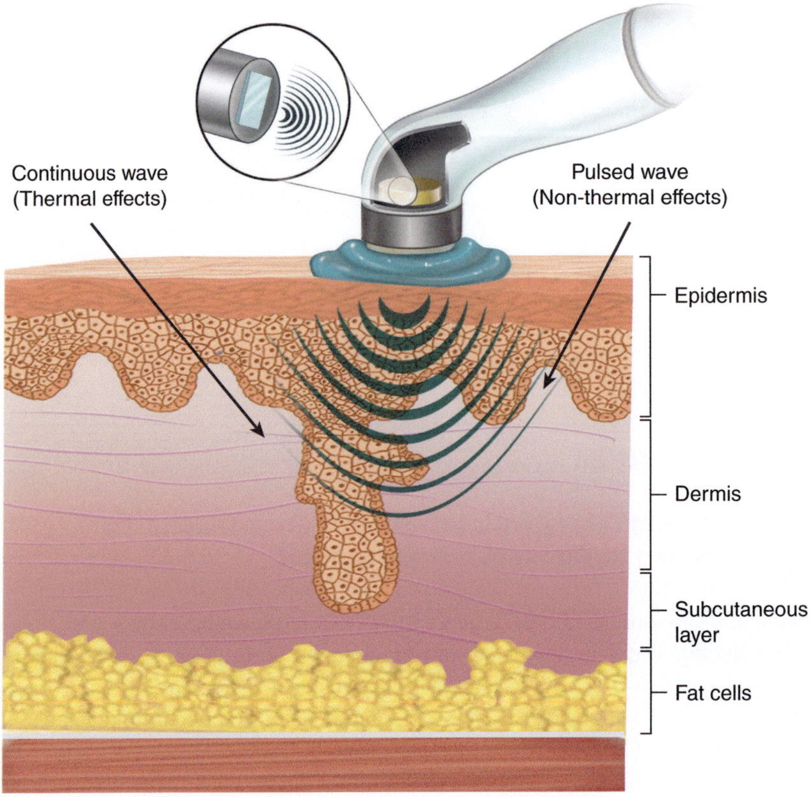

Fig. 3.1 The principle of TUS

3.1.2 Historical Context and Clinical Evolution

The therapeutic use of high-frequency sound waves has roots stretching back more than seven decades, and by the 1950s, ultrasound had already become a familiar part of physiotherapy practice. Early clinicians adopted it for conditions such as tendinitis and bursitis, and over time, it steadily became one of the most widely used electrophysical agents internationally. Despite this long history and its routine presence in clinics, its true clinical value has been repeatedly questioned. The conversation has evolved significantly as the expectations for research evidence have risen, especially with the increasing emphasis on robust methodology and transparent reporting.

What makes ultrasound unusual is the persistent gap between how commonly it is used and how contested its efficacy remains. Generations of clinicians have been trained to include it as a standard tool, yet systematic scrutiny has repeatedly highlighted inconsistencies and methodological limitations in the research base. This

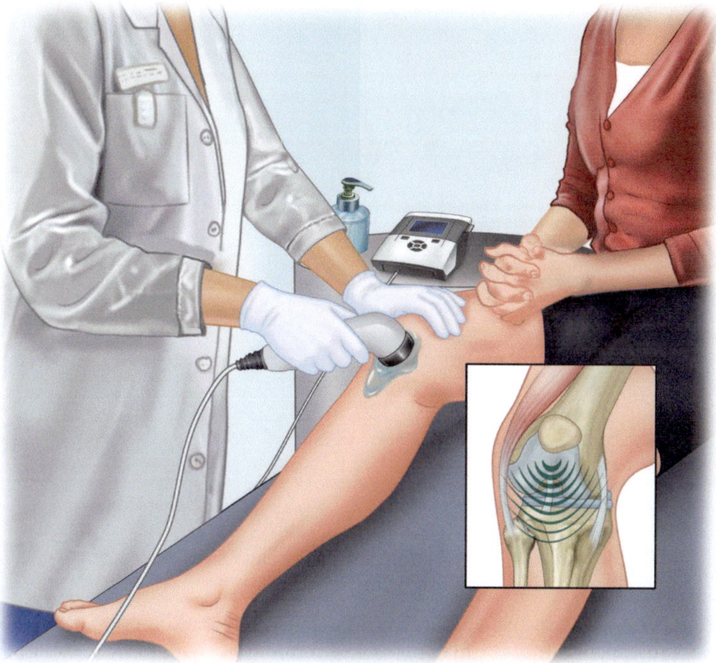

Fig. 3.2 TUS application

tension—between tradition and emerging evidence—continues to shape debate within the field and sets the stage for the later critical examination in Sect. 3.6 [17].

3.1.3 Introduction to Low-Intensity Pulsed Ultrasound (LIPUS) as a Distinct Modality

Within the spectrum of ultrasound-based interventions, low-intensity pulsed ultrasound (LIPUS) stands apart as a clearly specialized technique with its own rationale, design, and clinical indications. Unlike conventional therapeutic ultrasound, which often aims to produce measurable thermal effects in soft tissues, LIPUS operates at a very low spatial-average–temporal-average intensity—typically about 30 mW/cm^2—and is always pulsed [12]. Its purpose is not to heat tissue but to provide a subtle mechanical stimulus that can trigger cellular signaling pathways involved in tissue repair, particularly in bone healing and regeneration [30].

The distinction between TUS and LIPUS goes beyond a simple adjustment of parameters. Each rests on a different therapeutic philosophy. Conventional ultrasound is often applied as a "top-down" modality: clinicians use comparatively high intensities to provoke broad physiological changes such as deep heating, increased

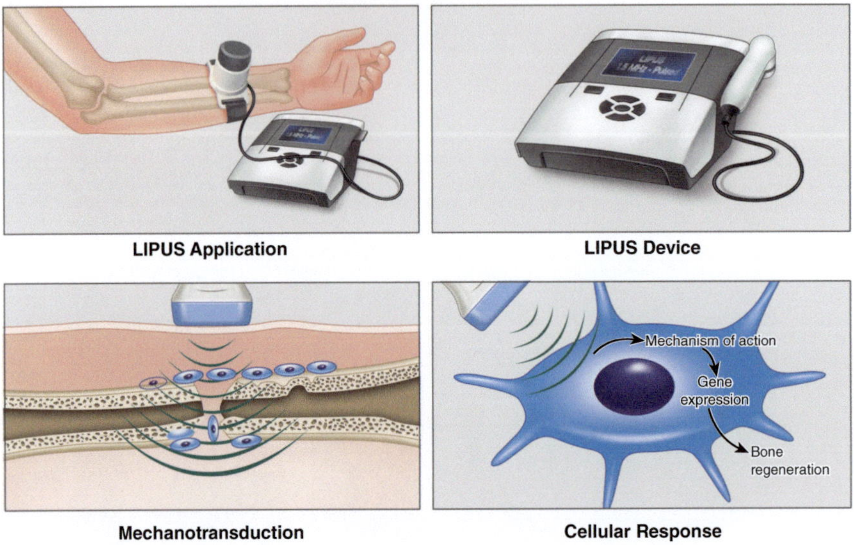

Fig. 3.3 LIPUS: Physiological Effects on Bone Healing and Device Application

circulation, or enhanced tissue extensibility. LIPUS takes the opposite approach. It relies on "bottom-up" mechanotransduction—using extremely low-energy acoustic signals to initiate precise molecular cascades within cells [12] (Fig. 3.3).

This mechanistic divergence has practical consequences. LIPUS parameters are standardized to an unusual degree, and its regulatory approvals—for instance, those granted by the U.S. Food and Drug Administration for specific fracture types—reflect this narrow, targeted therapeutic intent. Treating LIPUS simply as another form of "ultrasound therapy" obscures its unique biophysical properties and its distinct evidence base. The two modalities differ in purpose, underlying science, and clinical justification, and evaluating them together can lead to confusion in both research interpretation and clinical application [30].

3.2 Biophysics

3.2.1 The Piezoelectric Effect: Converting Electrical to Mechanical Energy

Ultrasound waves are longitudinal mechanical waves characterized by alternating phases of compression and rarefaction as they propagate through biological tissues. These pressure oscillations produce molecular vibration and energy transfer, forming the basis for both thermal and nonthermal effects.

Therapeutic ultrasound consists primarily of longitudinal mechanical waves, in which particles vibrate parallel to the direction of wave propagation. This differs from transverse (electromagnetic) waves, in which particle oscillations occur perpendicular to the direction of wave propagation. In biological tissues, ultrasound energy is transmitted mainly as longitudinal pressure waves.

A piezoelectric crystal within the transducer head produces ultrasound energy in therapeutic units.

The generation of all ultrasound, whether for diagnostic or therapeutic purposes, is predicated on the piezoelectric effect. This phenomenon, co-discovered by Pierre and Jacques Curie in the late nineteenth century, describes the ability of certain crystalline materials to generate an electrical charge when subjected to mechanical stress. Therapeutic ultrasound transducers harness the inverse piezoelectric effect, whereby applying an alternating electrical field to these crystals causes them to deform—rapidly expanding and contracting in synchrony with the electrical current. The transducer head contains one or more piezoelectric crystals, typically made of natural quartz or, more commonly, synthetic polycrystalline ceramics such as lead zirconate titanate (PZT). When the high-frequency alternating current from the ultrasound generator is applied, the crystal's oscillations produce a series of mechanical compressions and rarefactions in the adjacent medium. These mechanical vibrations are, in essence, high-frequency sound waves that propagate away from the transducer face. Thus, the piezoelectric crystal acts as a motor, efficiently converting electrical energy into the mechanical energy of the sound wave that forms the basis of the therapy [4].

3.2.2 Characteristics of the Ultrasound Wave: Frequency, Wavelength, and Velocity

The sound wave produced by the transducer can be described by several fundamental properties that govern its behavior in tissue:

- *Frequency (f)*: This is the number of compression-rarefaction cycles that occur per second, measured in hertz (Hz). Therapeutic ultrasound typically employs frequencies of 1 megahertz (MHz) or 3 MHz. This parameter is the single most important determinant of the depth to which ultrasound energy penetrates.
- *Wavelength (λ)*: This is the physical distance the wave travels during one complete cycle. It is inversely proportional to the frequency. In an average soft tissue, the wavelength at 1 MHz is approximately 1.5 mm, while at 3 MHz it is approximately 0.5 mm.
- *Velocity (v)*: This is the speed at which the sound wave propagates through a medium. While it varies slightly between different tissue types, the velocity of ultrasound in most soft tissues is relatively constant, averaging around 1540 m/s, similar to that in saline.

These properties are linked by the fundamental wave equation: $v = f\lambda$. Because velocity is relatively constant in soft tissue, the frequency chosen by the clinician directly determines the wavelength of the sound energy being applied [4].

3.2.3 Interaction with Biological Tissues: Acoustic Impedance, Absorption, Reflection, and Attenuation

When ultrasound energy leaves the transducer and enters the body, it does not behave in a simple or predictable way. It interacts with each tissue it meets, and these interactions ultimately decide how much energy reaches the intended target.

- *Acoustic Impedance (Z)*: Every tissue presents a characteristic resistance to the passage of sound, known as its acoustic impedance. It is a product of the tissue's density and the speed of sound within it. When an ultrasound wave encounters an interface between two tissues with different acoustic impedances (e.g., fat and muscle, or muscle and bone), a portion of the wave's energy is reflected, and a portion is transmitted across the boundary. The greater the impedance mismatch, the greater the percentage of energy that is reflected. This principle is most starkly illustrated at the interface between the transducer head (steel) and air, where the impedance mismatch is so large that approximately 99.9% of the energy is reflected. This is why a coupling medium (gel) is essential; it displaces the air and provides a medium with an impedance closer to that of skin, allowing for efficient transmission of energy into the body [4]. It is also important to note that the nature of the wave itself can change depending on the medium. Due to the fluid nature of soft tissues, ultrasound typically travels in longitudinal waves, causing compression and rarefaction. However, when these waves encounter a rigid boundary, such as bone, they can also generate transverse, or "shear," waves, which involve particle displacement perpendicular to the direction of wave propagation [11]. Reflection of ultrasound at tissue interfaces may lead to the formation of standing waves, which arise from interference between incident and reflected waves. Standing waves can produce localized areas of increased energy concentration, which has historically supported the recommendation to move the transducer continuously during treatment to avoid potential tissue irritation.
- *Absorption and Attenuation*: Attenuation refers to the progressive reduction in the intensity of the ultrasound beam as it passes through tissue. This loss of energy is due to a combination of absorption, reflection, and scattering. Absorption is the most clinically relevant component of attenuation, as it involves the conversion of the mechanical energy of the sound wave into heat. This absorption process is not linear; it follows an exponential pattern, meaning that superficial tissues absorb more energy than deeper ones. The rate of absorption is highly dependent on both the tissue type and the ultrasound frequency. Tissues with high protein and collagen content, such as muscle, tendon, ligament, joint capsule, and bone, are efficient absorbers of ultrasound energy. Tissues with high water content, such as fat and blood, are poor absorbers and thus allow the energy to pass through with less attenuation.

A key practical point is that higher-frequency ultrasound gets absorbed much faster than lower-frequency energy. A 3 MHz beam is absorbed approximately three times

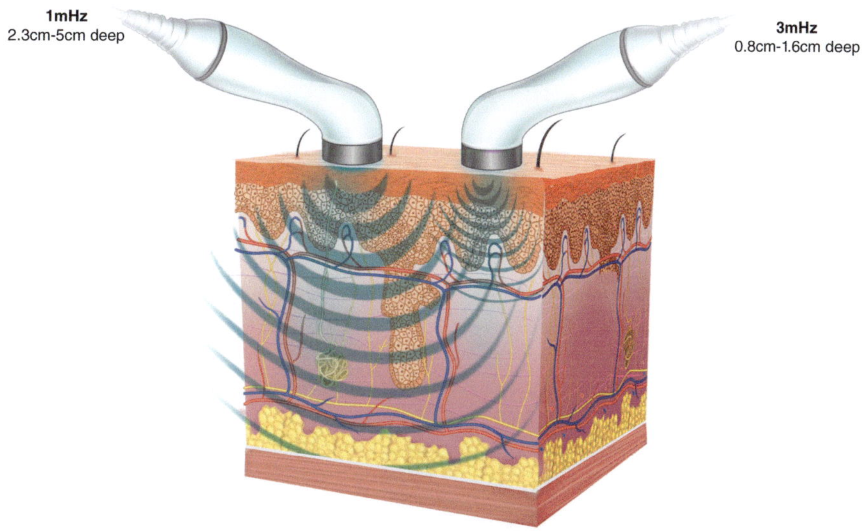

Fig. 3.4 Relationship between ultrasound frequency and tissue penetration depth

faster than a 1 MHz beam. This physical reality dictates the clinical use of frequency: 3 MHz is used for superficial targets (1–2 cm deep) because its energy is absorbed quickly, while 1 MHz is used for deeper targets (up to 5 cm deep) because its energy is absorbed more slowly, allowing it to penetrate further into the body (Fig. 3.4). This creates an inherent trade-off between penetration depth and heating efficiency. To heat a deep structure like the piriformis muscle, a clinician must select 1 MHz. However, because this frequency is absorbed less avidly, a higher intensity or longer treatment time will be required to achieve a therapeutic temperature rise at that depth compared with heating a superficial structure such as the patellar tendon at 3 MHz. The choice of frequency is therefore not arbitrary but rather a direct clinical application of the laws of acoustics, which in turn influences all other dosimetric decisions [1, 4].

3.2.4 The Near Field and Far Field: Understanding the Ultrasound Beam

The ultrasound beam emitted from the transducer is not a perfectly uniform cylinder of energy. It has a complex spatial structure divided into two distinct zones (Fig. 3.5):

- *The Near Field (Fresnel Zone)*: This is the region closest to the transducer face. Here, the beam is relatively collimated (parallel-sided) but exhibits significant spatial intensity variations. Interference patterns from the vibrating crystal surface produce multiple peaks and troughs of varying intensities. Therapeutic applications are conducted within this near field.

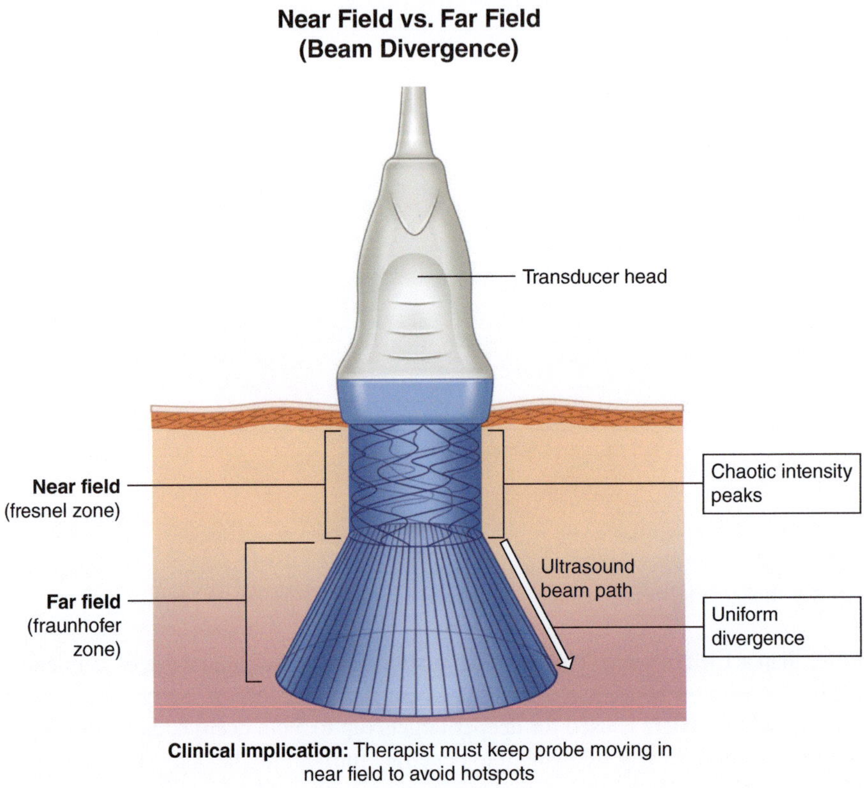

Fig. 3.5 Diagram of ultrasound beam profile illustrating near field (chaotic intensity) versus far field (uniform divergence)

- *The Far Field (Fraunhofer Zone)*: Beyond the near field, the beam begins to diverge, and the intensity becomes more uniform but progressively weaker.

The existence of high-intensity peaks within the near field is a critical safety and efficacy consideration. The degree of this nonuniformity is quantified by the beam nonuniformity ratio (BNR), a key dosimetric parameter discussed in the following section [4].

3.3 Dosage and Parameters

3.3.1 The Challenge of Dosimetry: Toward a Standardized Framework

If you ask ten clinicians how they dose ultrasound, you will probably hear ten different answers. That lack of consistency points to a deeper problem: the field has never settled on a reliable, standardized dosimetry system. In therapeutic modalities like ionizing radiation, dosimetry is well-defined, with units such as the absorbed dose (Gray) and the equivalent dose (Sievert) providing a quantifiable measure that relates the applied energy to a predictable biological effect. No such universally accepted dose parameter exists for ultrasound. The descriptive parameters commonly used in research and clinical practice—such as spatial peak temporal average intensity (I_{SPTA}) or spatial average temporal average intensity (I_{SATA})—characterize the acoustic field to which the target tissue is exposed but do not quantify the energy actually absorbed by the target tissue. This makes it exceptionally difficult to compare results across studies, plan treatments to achieve a specific biological endpoint, or establish clear dose-response relationships [17].

3.3.2 Key Treatment Parameters for Conventional Ultrasound

Despite the overarching challenge of dosimetry, clinical application is guided by the manipulation of several key parameters. According to recent systematic reviews, the effectiveness of ultrasound depends on proper application and appropriate parameter selection [23].

- *Frequency (1 vs. 3 MHz)*: As established in the biophysics section, the choice of frequency is dictated by the depth of the target tissue. A frequency of 1 MHz is selected for deeper injuries (3–5 cm), while 3 MHz is used for more superficial lesions (1–2 cm) [4]. This clinical rule is based on the physical principle that the 1 MHz frequency exhibits greater penetration and is absorbed less readily by superficial tissues. In contrast, the 3 MHz frequency is absorbed more rapidly, concentrating its energy at shallower depths [8].
- *Intensity (W/cm^2)*: Intensity represents the rate at which energy is being delivered per unit area of the transducer, typically expressed in watts per square centimeter (W/cm^2). The clinically relevant measure is the spatial average intensity (SAI), defined as the total power (in watts) divided by the transducer's effective radiating area (ERA) in cm^2. Therapeutic intensities generally range from 0.1 to 2.0 W/cm^2. Common clinical guidelines recommend tailoring the intensity to the stage of injury. For acute conditions where nonthermal effects are desired, a low intensity of 0.1–0.3 W/cm^2 is recommended. In the subacute stage, this may be increased to 0.2–0.5 W/cm^2, and for chronic conditions where a mild thermal effect may be beneficial, intensities of 0.3–0.8 W/cm^2 are often used [28]. Physiotherapy ultrasound devices typically have a maximum intensity of approximately 3 W/cm^2, in accordance with IEC and FDA specifications. Notably, the WHO does not establish a specific intensity limit for therapeutic ultrasound [1].

Common transducer head sizes used clinically range from approximately 1–10 cm^2, most commonly between 1 and 5 cm^2 effective radiating area (ERA). Smaller heads are suited to focal or irregular anatomical regions, whereas larger

Table 3.1 Conventional ultrasound parameter guidelines by injury stage (based on common clinical heuristics)

Injury stage	Recommended pulse ratio	Recommended intensity range (W/cm^2)
Acute	1:4 (20% duty cycle)	0.1–0.3
Subacute	1:2 or 1:1 (33–50% duty cycle)	0.2–0.5
Chronic	1:1 or continuous (50–100% duty cycle)	0.3–0.8

heads are selected for broader treatment areas. In clinical practice, the treatment area should generally not exceed two to three times the ERA of the ultrasound head.

Intensity may be expressed as spatial average intensity (SAI) or spatial peak intensity (SPI). Because the ultrasound beam is not perfectly uniform, local peaks can exceed the average intensity, making it important to consider beam nonuniformity during treatment.

The total acoustic energy delivered depends on intensity, treatment area, and duration. Although energy density (J/cm^2) is less commonly reported in ultrasound research than in photobiomodulation literature, it remains clinically useful for understanding cumulative dose.

- *Mode and Duty Cycle (Continuous vs. Pulsed)*: The mode of ultrasound delivery determines the temporal characteristics of energy application and is the primary control for achieving thermal versus nonthermal effects.
  - *Continuous Mode*: The ultrasound wave is delivered without interruption, corresponding to a 100% duty cycle. This mode maximizes energy delivery and is typically used when the primary therapeutic goal is tissue heating, making it most suitable for chronic conditions.
  - *Pulsed Mode*: The ultrasound delivery is periodically interrupted, creating 'on' and 'off' periods. The duty cycle is the ratio of the 'on' time to the total time, expressed as a percentage (e.g., 20% or 50%). Pulsing the beam allows the heat generated during the 'on' phase to dissipate via blood flow during the 'off' phase, thus minimizing the net thermal effect. This mode is selected when the intended therapeutic mechanisms are primarily nonthermal [27]. Clinical heuristics often link the pulse ratio to the chronicity of the injury. For instance, in acute injuries, a 1:4 pulse ratio (equivalent to a 20% duty cycle) is commonly used to minimize thermal effects. In contrast, in chronic injuries, a 1:1 ratio (50% duty cycle) may be selected to introduce a mild thermal component alongside mechanical effects [28].

Lower duty cycles reduce thermal accumulation and are traditionally used when nonthermal mechanical effects are desired, particularly during early stages of tissue healing.

To illustrate the relationship between duty cycle and clinical application, Table 3.1 summarizes recommended settings across the acute-to-chronic spectrum.

- *Treatment Duration and Area*: The duration of treatment is typically between 5 and 10 min. A common clinical heuristic is to treat an area approximately two to three times the transducer's ERA. A more specific formula-based approach is also used to standardize application time based on the treatment area and pulse ratio. The equation is:

$$\text{Treatment time}(\text{min}) = 1 \times \begin{pmatrix} \text{Number of times the treatment} \\ \text{head fits onto the target tissue} \end{pmatrix} \times (\text{Pulse factor})$$

  To calculate the *pulse factor*, add the two numbers in the pulse ratio together. For example:
  - A 1:4 ratio gives a pulse factor of 1 + 4 = 5.
  - A 1:1 ratio gives a pulse factor of 1 + 1 = 2.

  This means that a larger treatment area or a more heavily pulsed application (e.g., 1:4) will require a proportionally longer treatment time to deliver an equivalent amount of energy [28].

  When continuous therapeutic ultrasound is applied at an intensity of approximately 2 W/cm^2 and a frequency of 1 MHz, a treatment duration of around 10 min is commonly used to achieve a meaningful thermal effect. A temperature increase of approximately 4 °C is generally considered necessary for optimal therapeutic heating. Experimental data suggest that under these parameters, tissue temperature may increase by approximately 0.4 °C/min, which supports the use of longer application times to reach the desired thermal threshold.

  If the applied intensity is reduced due to patient discomfort or intolerance to thermal effects, treatment duration should be adjusted accordingly to achieve a comparable thermal outcome. Indicatively, the rate of temperature increase depends on both intensity and frequency. For example, at an intensity of 0.5 W/cm^2, the temperature rise is approximately 0.04 °C/min at 1 MHz and 0.3 °C at 3 MHz. At 1.0 W/cm^2, the increase is approximately 0.2 and 0.6 °C respectively; at 1.5 W/cm^2, 0.3 and 0.9 °C; and at 2.0 W/cm^2, approximately 0.4 °C at 1 MHz and 1.4 °C at 3 MHz.
- *Frequency of Treatments*: The recommended frequency of ultrasound sessions also varies with the stage of injury. There is no consensus on session frequency. Emphasize delivering an 'adequate dose per session' and reassess after three to four treatments; subsequent frequency should follow clinical response rather than fixed daily schedules. The total number of sessions is not fixed but is determined by the patient's response to the intervention [27].

  For a more quantitative understanding of ultrasound dosing, several fundamental relationships can be used to describe the interaction between intensity, time, and delivered energy. Although these calculations are not routinely applied in everyday clinical practice, they provide a useful framework for interpreting treatment parameters and understanding dose–response relationships.

  For continuous therapeutic ultrasound, energy density (ED) is defined as the product of spatial peak intensity (SPI) and treatment time (T), expressed as ED = SPI × T. Total energy (ET) is calculated as ET = SPI × ERA × T, where

ERA represents the effective radiating area of the transducer. The dose per treatment (DT) can then be estimated by dividing the total energy (TE) by the treatment surface area (S), i.e., DT = TE/S.

In pulsed ultrasound, the same relationships apply; however, spatial average intensity (SAI) is used instead of spatial peak intensity. SAI is calculated as SAI = SPI × DC, where DC is the duty cycle, the proportion of time the ultrasound actively delivers energy.

3.3.3 Transducer Characteristics: Effective Radiating Area (ERA) and Beam Nonuniformity Ratio (BNR)

A critical parameter in ultrasound dosimetry is the beam nonuniformity ratio (BNR), which is the ratio of the spatial peak intensity to the spatial average intensity of the ultrasound beam.

The physical characteristics of the transducer head itself are critical dosimetric parameters that are often overlooked.

- *Effective Radiating Area (ERA)*: The ERA is the portion of the transducer's surface that actually produces the sound wave. It is always smaller than the metal faceplate's actual surface area. Since the clinical intensity (W/cm^2) is calculated by dividing the total power output by the ERA, an accurate ERA value is essential for correct dosing.
- *Beam Nonuniformity Ratio (BNR)*: As described previously, the ultrasound beam is not uniform, containing peaks of high intensity. The BNR is the ratio of the spatial peak intensity to the spatial average intensity within the beam. An ideal BNR would be 1:1, but this is physically unattainable. A lower BNR (e.g., 2:1–5:1) is highly desirable because it indicates a more uniform beam. A high BNR (e.g., >6:1) signifies the presence of intense "hot spots," which increase the risk of periosteal pain or tissue damage and require the clinician to move the transducer head more rapidly to average out the energy delivery [4].

The variability—and, in many cases, poor calibration—of clinical ultrasound machines introduces a substantial, often overlooked source of error in both research and everyday practice. Several evaluations of commercially available devices have shown striking discrepancies between the intensity displayed on the unit and the actual acoustic output. In some cases, the true output has been found to deviate anywhere from −43% to +61% from the stated value, largely due to mismatches between the manufacturer's reported effective radiating area (ERA) and the ERA measured independently. The practical implication is difficult to ignore: two clinicians using what appears to be the same protocol—for example, 1.5 W/cm^2 for 8 min—may, in reality, be delivering very different energy doses to the tissue.

This technical instability creates a familiar problem for researchers. If the input is unreliable, the results will inevitably reflect that inconsistency. Systematic reviews may unknowingly synthesize data from studies that used acoustically incomparable interventions, even when they appear identical on paper. This offers a simple, non-biological explanation for why so many findings in the therapeutic ultrasound literature have been inconsistent or inconclusive. As Robertson and Baker [4] argue, when the delivered dose fluctuates substantially, obtaining reproducible effects becomes virtually impossible.

There is also a deeper irony here. Clinical guidelines often present ultrasound dosing as a precise, tightly controlled process, offering specific recommendations such as 0.1–0.3 W/cm^2 for acute conditions. In reality, the accuracy of many machines does not support that level of confidence. A clinician may believe they are delivering a carefully calibrated dose simply because they have followed the "recipe," yet the true output may differ dramatically from what the display indicates. When equipment cannot guarantee reliable delivery, the entire premise of a dose-dependent therapeutic effect becomes unstable. This disconnect between theoretical precision and practical uncertainty makes it extraordinarily difficult to rigorously validate ultrasound protocols.

3.3.4 Specific Dosology for Low-Intensity Pulsed Ultrasound (LIPUS)

In stark contrast to the variable parameters of conventional ultrasound, the dosology for LIPUS is highly standardized and consistent across clinical trials and commercial devices. The FDA-approved and most widely studied parameters are fixed and are not typically altered by the clinician [6]:

- *Frequency*: 1.5 MHz.
- *Intensity* (I_{SATA}): 30 mW/cm^2 (equivalent to 0.03 W/cm^2).
- *Pulse Characteristics*: A 200 μs burst of 1.5 MHz sine waves, repeated at a rate of 1 kHz. This corresponds to a 20% duty cycle (200 μs 'on' time in every 1000 μs period).
- *Treatment Duration*: 20 min, applied once daily.

The vast differences in the core parameters of these two modalities are summarized in Table 3.2. The intensity used in LIPUS, for example, is typically 50–100 times lower than that used in conventional thermal ultrasound, immediately clarifying that they operate on fundamentally different principles and should not be conceptually conflated.

Table 3.2 Comparison of typical dosimetric parameters: conventional ultrasound versus LIPUS

Parameter	Conventional therapeutic US	Low-intensity pulsed US (LIPUS)
Frequency	1 or 3 MHz	1.5 MHz
Intensity (I_{SATA})	0.1–2.0 W/cm^2 (100–2000 mW/cm^2)	30 mW/cm^2
Duty cycle	20–100% (pulsed or continuous)	20% (pulsed only)
Duration	5–10 min/session	20 min/day

3.3.5 Application Technique and Coupling Media

Beyond the machine settings, the transducer's physical application is critical for effective treatment. A coupling medium is essential to eliminate air between the transducer and the skin, which would otherwise reflect nearly all of the acoustic energy. Preferred coupling media for TUS are water-based gels or water immersion; avoid thick creams/oils that impair transmission. For LIPUS (e.g., EXOGEN), mineral oil may be used if gel is unavailable. Ideally, the coupling medium should be fluid enough to fill all available spaces, relatively viscous so that it remains in place, have an acoustic impedance appropriate to the media it connects, and allow transmission of ultrasound with minimal absorption, attenuation, or disturbance.

Water immersion may be used as an alternative coupling medium for irregular anatomical surfaces, as ultrasound transmission through water reduces air-interface reflections and allows more uniform energy delivery.

Furthermore, the transducer's angle relative to the skin surface is a critical factor. In addition to reflection caused by differences in acoustic impedance, refraction (bending of the wave) will occur if the ultrasound beam does not strike the boundary at a 90° angle (Fig. 3.6). To maximize energy transmission into the target tissue and minimize unpredictable scattering and refraction, the transducer should be kept perpendicular to the skin surface throughout the treatment [28].

The transducer should be moved slowly and continuously (approximately 3–4 cm/s) using overlapping circular or longitudinal motions to produce a light, massage-like movement. This minimizes the formation of standing waves and prevents localized energy concentration.

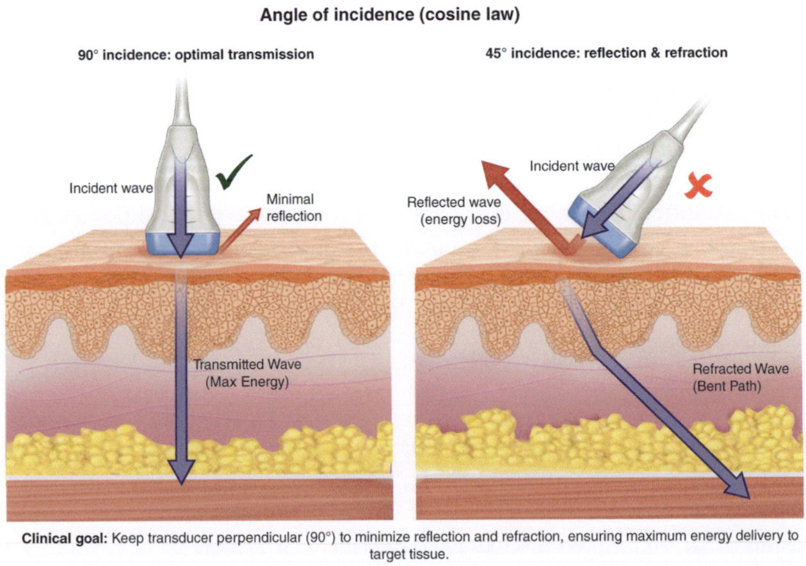

Fig. 3.6 Therapeutic ultrasound angle of incidence diagram

3.4 Mechanism of Action: Physiological and Therapeutic Effects

3.4.1 Thermal Effects of Conventional Ultrasound

The best-understood and least controversial mechanism of action of continuous therapeutic ultrasound is its ability to produce deep-tissue heating.

- *Mechanism of Deep Heating*: As tissues absorb the mechanical energy of the ultrasound wave, it causes the tissue's molecules to vibrate, and this increased kinetic energy manifests as a rise in temperature. The magnitude of this temperature increase is dependent on the treatment parameters (intensity, duration, and continuous mode) and the acoustic properties of the tissue itself. Tissues with high collagen content, such as tendons, ligaments, joint capsules, and scar tissue, are preferential absorbers of ultrasound energy and therefore heat more effectively than tissues like muscle or fat. This property enables selective heating of deep periarticular structures to a therapeutic temperature range (40–45 °C) without excessively heating the overlying skin and subcutaneous fat [4]. Experimental studies [8] suggest that continuous ultrasound at appropriate intensities may increase intramuscular temperature by approximately 1, 2–3, or >4 °C, depending on frequency, intensity, and treatment duration, with greater temperature rise generally observed within the first 5–10 min.
- *Physiological Responses to Heat*: The local increase in tissue temperature elicits several well-established physiological responses that are believed to be therapeutic:
  - *Increased Blood Flow (Hyperemia)*: Heating causes local vasodilation, which increases blood perfusion to the treated area. This enhanced circulation delivers more oxygen and nutrients, removes metabolic waste products, and can help resolve chronic inflammatory processes [4].
  - *Pain Reduction*: The application of heat can reduce pain through several mechanisms, including altering nerve conduction velocity, increasing the pain threshold of nociceptors, and modulating pain transmission via the spinal gating mechanism [4].
  - *Reduction of Muscle Spasm*: Heat can reduce the firing rate of muscle spindle afferents, leading to a decrease in motor neuron activity and a subsequent reduction in muscle spasm.
  - *Increased Collagen Extensibility*: This is perhaps the most significant and clinically utilized thermal effect. Heating collagenous tissues like tendons, joint capsules, and scar tissue to the therapeutic range of 40–45 °C decreases their viscosity and increases their extensibility. When combined with stretching, this effect can lead to greater and more permanent increases in range of motion and tissue flexibility [4].

3.4.2 Nonthermal (Mechanical) Effects of Conventional Ultrasound

In addition to thermal effects, therapeutic ultrasound is proposed to exert biological effects through mechanical mechanisms, which are thought to predominate when ultrasound is applied in pulsed mode or at very low intensity. The two primary proposed mechanisms are cavitation and acoustic streaming.

- *Cavitation*: Cavitation is the formation, growth, and behavior of microscopic gas bubbles (or "voids") within tissue fluids, which are subjected to the alternating compression and rarefaction phases of the sound wave.
  - *Stable Cavitation*: At lower therapeutic intensities, bubbles are thought to form and oscillate in size around an equilibrium radius without collapsing (Fig. 3.7). This stable pulsation of the bubbles is believed to be beneficial, as it induces microstreaming of the fluid around the bubbles' surfaces [4].
  - *Unstable (Transient) Cavitation*: At higher intensities, the bubbles can expand to an unstable size during the rarefaction phase and then collapse violently during the compression phase. This implosion releases a tremendous amount of localized energy in the form of shock waves and high temperatures, which are destructive to adjacent cells. Unstable cavitation is not thought to occur at standard therapeutic intensities. Still, it is the intended mechanism in high-intensity applications such as extracorporeal shockwave lithotripsy (ESWL) for breaking up kidney stones [13].
- *Acoustic Streaming and Microstreaming*: Acoustic streaming is the unidirectional movement of fluids along cell membranes and tissue interfaces, driven by the pressure gradient of the ultrasound field. Microstreaming refers more

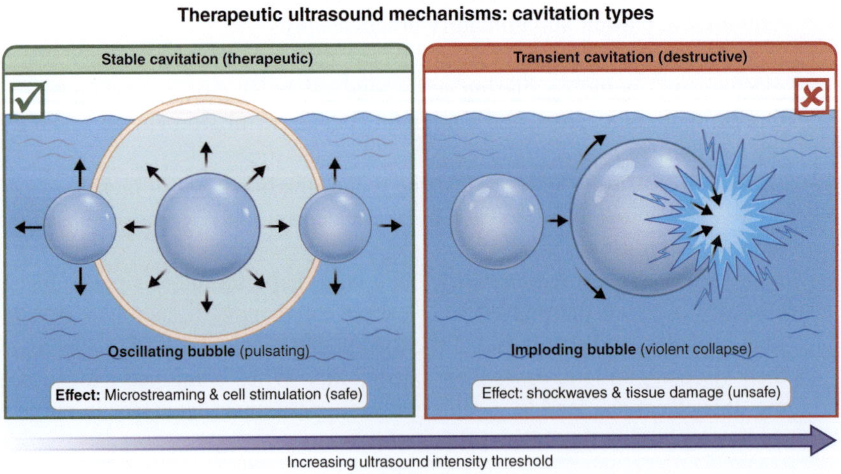

Fig. 3.7 Comparison of stable (therapeutic) and transient (destructive) cavitation mechanisms in ultrasound therapy

specifically to the small-scale eddying of fluid that occurs in the immediate vicinity of an oscillating object, such as a stable cavitation bubble. Together, these fluid movements are purported to exert mechanical shear stresses on cell membranes, leading to a range of biological effects, including increased cell membrane permeability, altered ion transport (particularly calcium ions), and stimulation of cellular activities like protein synthesis and the degranulation of mast cells [13].

- *The In Vitro Versus In Vivo Debate*: The clinical relevance of these nonthermal mechanisms is a subject of intense scientific debate. In a highly influential 2001 review, Baker, Robertson, and Duck argued that many of the proposed nonthermal effects, particularly cavitation and the powerful microstreaming it causes, have been demonstrated primarily in in vitro laboratory settings (i.e., on cells in a culture dish). They contended that there is little to no direct evidence that these phenomena actually occur in intact, living tissue (in vivo) at the intensities used in standard therapy. The complex homeostatic mechanisms, tissue pressures, and fluid dynamics within a living organism are thought to significantly increase the threshold for cavitation, making it a highly improbable event [4]. The World Federation for Ultrasound in Medicine and Biology (WFUMB) has explicitly cautioned against directly extrapolating in vitro findings to clinical practice, noting that the likelihood of cavitation is much greater under laboratory conditions [29]. This critique fundamentally challenges the scientific rationale for using pulsed ultrasound to achieve nonthermal effects.

3.4.3 The Molecular Mechanism of LIPUS: Mechanotransduction in Tissue Repair

The mechanism of action for LIPUS is entirely distinct from the thermal and cavitational effects described for conventional ultrasound. LIPUS operates via a nonthermal, nondestructive process called mechanotransduction, whereby cells convert a very low-energy mechanical signal into a cascade of specific biochemical events that promote tissue repair. This model aligns well with what modern cell biology tells us and is much more specific than the mechanisms proposed for conventional ultrasound. The proposed mechanisms for TUS and LIPUS are not only different but are based on almost mutually exclusive principles. The nonthermal effects of TUS are theorized to rely on physical disruption—bubble oscillations and forced fluid motion—to perturb the cellular environment. In contrast, the mechanism of LIPUS relies on a highly specific, nondisruptive biological signal delivered at an energy level well below the threshold where significant cavitation is expected in vivo.

- *Activation of Integrins and Stretch-Activated Ion Channels*: The process begins at the cell surface. The mechanical pressure waves from the LIPUS signal are sensed by mechanoreceptors embedded in the cell membrane, primarily cell-surface proteins called integrins and stretch-activated ion channels. This mechanical stimulation causes a conformational change in these receptors, initiating intracellular signaling. A key early event is the clustering of integrins to form focal adhesion plaques, which act as signaling hubs [12].

- *Key Signaling Pathways in Bone Healing*: The activation of these surface receptors triggers a series of well-defined downstream intracellular signaling pathways that are known to be critical for osteogenesis (bone formation):
  - *Integrin/PI3K/Akt Pathway*: This is a central pathway that is activated following integrin stimulation, leading to a cascade of protein phosphorylation events inside the cell [12].
  - *Rho/ROCK/Src/ERK Pathway*: This pathway is involved in regulating the cytoskeleton and gene expression and is activated by LIPUS to promote cell proliferation [30].
  - *Wnt/β-catenin Pathway*: A crucial pathway for skeletal development and bone mass regulation, which LIPUS can activate to promote the differentiation of bone marrow stem cells into osteoblasts [30].
- *Upregulation of Osteogenic and Angiogenic Factors*: Ultimately, the activation of these signaling cascades converges on the cell's nucleus, altering gene expression and leading to the increased production and release of key molecules that orchestrate the bone healing process:
  - *Upregulation of COX-2 and PGE2*: LIPUS stimulation leads to increased expression of the enzyme cyclooxygenase-2 (COX-2) and subsequent production of prostaglandin E2 (PGE2), molecules that are critical mediators in the early inflammatory and reparative stages of bone healing [12].
  - *Increased Osteogenic Transcription Factors*: The expression of master-switch transcription factors for bone formation, such as Runt-related transcription factor 2 (RUNX2) and Osterix, is upregulated, driving mesenchymal stem cells to differentiate into bone-forming osteoblasts [12].
  - *Increased Growth Factor Production*: LIPUS has been shown to increase the local production of essential growth factors, including bone morphogenetic proteins (BMPs), which are powerful stimulants of osteogenesis, and vascular endothelial growth factor (VEGF), which promotes angiogenesis (the formation of new blood vessels) necessary to supply the healing fracture site [12].

In summary, LIPUS acts as a biophysical stimulus that effectively "switches on" the cell's own genetic machinery for bone repair.

3.5 Indications, Contraindications, Precautions, and Side Effects

3.5.1 Therapeutic Ultrasound

- *Primary Indications*: Based on its established thermal and proposed nonthermal physiological effects, conventional therapeutic ultrasound is commonly indicated for a range of musculoskeletal conditions. These include conditions that benefit from deep heat, such as pain relief, muscle spasms, and joint contractures. Specific examples include soft-tissue shortening (to increase the extensibility of joint contractures, adhesions, and scar tissue before stretching), subacute and chronic inflammation (e.g., bursitis, capsulitis, epicondylitis, ligament sprains, tendinitis, and muscle strains), and promoting the healing of scar tissue [3, 10]. It is also used to promote healing in chronic wounds such as venous leg ulcers and pressure injuries.
- *Absolute and Relative Contraindications*: The application of therapeutic ultrasound is contraindicated in certain situations due to the potential for serious adverse reactions. These absolute contraindications include application over:
  - *Malignant Tumors: Due to the risk of increasing metabolic activity and blood flow, which could potentially promote tumor* growth or metastasis.
  - Pregnancy: Over the abdomen, pelvic region, or low back, due to unknown effects on the developing fetus.
  - *Pacemakers/ICDs*: Avoid insonation over the device or thorax; elsewhere consider case-by-case use with precautions and liaison with cardiology.
  - *The Eye and Gonads*: The high fluid content and sensitivity of these organs make them susceptible to damage.
  - *Thrombophlebitis/Deep Vein Thrombosis (DVT)*: Due to the risk of dislodging a thrombus, leading to an embolus.
  - *Active Infection or Tuberculosis*: Due to the risk of spreading the infection.
  - *Hemorrhagic Conditions: In areas of active bleeding or in patients with hemophilia*, due to the risk of exacerbating bleeding.
  - *Vascular Problems*: In areas with significantly compromised circulation.
    - *Active Growth Plates (Epiphyses)*: In skeletally immature individuals [1].
- *Precautions for Safe Application*: In certain situations, ultrasound may be applied, but with extra caution. These precautions include application over:
  - *The Spinal Cord*: Particularly after a laminectomy, where the protective bone has been removed.
  - *Anesthetized Areas or Altered Sensation*: In patients who cannot provide feedback about excessive heat or pain.
  - *Areas with Impaired Circulation*: The reduced blood flow may not be able to dissipate heat effectively, increasing the risk of burns.
  - *Subcutaneous Bony Prominences*: Bone is highly reflective of ultrasound, which can lead to the creation of standing waves and rapid overheating of the periosteum if the transducer is held stationary.

  - *Metal Implants*: While older concerns existed, modern practice generally considers it safe to apply ultrasound over metal implants, as the metal dissipates heat effectively and the risk of selective heating is low, provided the transducer is kept moving [1].
- *Potential Side Effects and Adverse Events*: When applied correctly by a trained therapist, therapeutic ultrasound has a low risk of complications. However, improper technique can lead to adverse events. The most common side effect is a superficial skin burn, which can occur if the transducer is held stationary during a continuous application, if the intensity is too high, or if there is insufficient coupling gel. Patients may also experience a sharp, deep ache if the beam is held stationary over bone, which is due to overheating of the periosteum [13].

Phonophoresis refers to the use of ultrasound to enhance transdermal drug delivery. Although proposed mechanisms include increased tissue permeability and acoustic streaming, clinical evidence remains inconsistent, and routine use is not universally recommended.

3.5.2 Low-Intensity Pulsed Ultrasound (LIPUS)

- *FDA-Approved and Off-Label Indications*: The primary indications for LIPUS are narrower and more specific than for conventional ultrasound, focusing almost exclusively on bone. FDA-approved indications include the following:
  - Accelerating Healing of Fresh Fractures: Specifically for fresh, closed, posteriorly displaced distal radius fractures and fresh, closed or Grade I open tibial diaphysis fractures.
  - Treatment of Established Nonunions: For fractures that have failed to show signs of healing, excluding the skull and vertebrae [6].
  - Other common off-label uses include the treatment of delayed unions, stress fractures, and as an adjunct in distraction osteogenesis procedures.

  Beyond these orthopedic applications, recent research has begun to explore the neuromodulatory potential of LIPUS. A pivotal trial rationale published in 2025 outlines the use of transcranial LIPUS for early Alzheimer's disease, proposing that it may upregulate endothelial nitric oxide synthase (eNOS) to slow cognitive decline [21]. While experimental, this marks a significant expansion of LIPUS indications.
- *Contraindications and precautions from manufacturer guidelines*: The safety information provided by manufacturers of leading LIPUS devices, such as Exogen and Melmak, uses specific and important terminology. Both manufacturers state that there are "no known contraindications" for their devices. However, this statement is immediately followed by a list of populations and conditions in which "safety and effectiveness have not been established." This list, which functions as a set of strong precautions or relative contraindications, typically includes the following:

Table 3.3 Summary of key contraindications and precautions for therapeutic ultrasound and LIPUS

Condition/area	Therapeutic ultrasound	LIPUS
Malignancy	Absolute contraindication	Precaution (not for pathological fractures)
Pregnancy	Absolute contraindication	Precaution (safety not established)
Pacemaker	Absolute contraindication	Precaution (safety not established)
Open epiphyses	Absolute contraindication	Precaution (safety not established)
DVT/ thrombophlebitis	Absolute contraindication	Precaution (vascular insufficiency)
Eyes/gonads	Absolute contraindication	Not applicable

- Individuals lacking skeletal maturity (i.e., children and adolescents with open epiphyseal plates).
- Pregnant or nursing women.
- Patients with cardiac pacemakers or other active electronic implants.
- Application over fractures caused by bone cancer (pathological fractures).
- Patients with poor blood circulation (vascular insufficiency) or clotting problems [15].

This distinction between "no known contraindications" and "safety not established" is a crucial medico-legal point. A formal contraindication implies that evidence of harm exists. The manufacturer's phrasing indicates an absence of evidence of safety in these specific groups, not necessarily evidence of its absence. This places the legal and ethical responsibility for a risk-benefit analysis squarely on the prescribing clinician. Prescribing LIPUS to a pregnant patient, for example, is not technically against a stated contraindication but constitutes an off-label use in a population with unevaluated risk.

Additional precautions include the following:

- LIPUS is not intended to treat the skull or vertebrae.
- In accordance with manufacturer guidance, the transducer must be positioned adjacent to—rather than directly over—metallic fixation hardware. This ensures that the beam provides adequate penetration to the fracture site (Table 3.3).

3.6 Research Evidence: A Critical Appraisal

The clinical use of therapeutic ultrasound has been underpinned by a body of research that is both extensive and contentious. A critical examination of this evidence reveals a field marked by methodological challenges, conflicting results, and a significant evolution in scientific consensus over time.

3.6.1 The Foundational Critique: Robertson and Baker's 2001 Systematic Reviews

In 2001, two companion systematic reviews, published in the journal *Physical Therapy* by Valma Robertson and Kerry Baker, fundamentally challenged the prevailing assumptions about therapeutic ultrasound's efficacy and scientific basis. These papers remain landmark critiques in the field.

- "*A Review of Therapeutic Ultrasound: Effectiveness Studies*": This review systematically examined the clinical evidence for therapeutic ultrasound in treating pain and musculoskeletal injuries. The authors identified 35 English-language randomized controlled trials (RCTs) published between 1975 and 1999. Each trial was critically appraised for methodological quality using rigorous criteria based on the work of Sackett et al., which included requirements for adequate placebo controls, proper blinding of patients and therapists, and sufficient statistical power. Of the initial 35 trials, only 10 were judged to have acceptable methodology. The results from these 10 high-quality studies were stark:
  - Two trials suggested that active therapeutic ultrasound was more effective than placebo ultrasound for treating carpal tunnel syndrome and calcific tendinitis of the shoulder.
  - Eight trials found that active ultrasound was no more effective than placebo for a range of other conditions, including epicondylitis, osteoarthritis of the knee, shoulder pain, and pressure sores.

  The authors' conclusion was unequivocal and practice-changing: "There was little evidence that active therapeutic ultrasound is more effective than placebo ultrasound for treating people with pain or a range of musculoskeletal injuries or for promoting soft tissue healing" [17]. They also noted that the dosages used across the studies varied considerably, often for no discernible reason, highlighting the lack of a clear dose-response relationship.
- "*A Review of Therapeutic Ultrasound: Biophysical Effects*": The companion review questioned the very scientific foundation upon which the modality's use was based. It argued that the most frequently cited biophysical effects—particularly the nonthermal mechanisms of cavitation and acoustic streaming—were derived almost exclusively from in vitro studies on isolated cells. The review presented a compelling case that there was insufficient evidence to prove these effects actually occurred in the complex environment of living tissue (in vivo) at therapeutic intensities. The conclusion was as damning as that of its companion paper: "there is currently insufficient biophysical evidence to provide a scientific foundation for the clinical use of therapeutic ultrasound" [4].

Together, these two reviews established a high bar for future research and cast a long shadow of doubt over a widely used therapy.

3.6.2 The Evolving Evidence for Conventional Ultrasound (Post-2001)

In the years since the Robertson and Baker reviews, researchers have continued to investigate the efficacy of conventional ultrasound, with mixed results that have done little to resolve the central controversy.

- *Evidence in Musculoskeletal Soft-Tissue Injuries*: The evidence for one of its most common applications, tendinopathy, remains conflicted. For plantar fasciitis, a 2025 systematic review and meta-analysis by Li et al. included 13 trials and concluded that ultrasound, whether applied alone or in combination with conventional exercises, did not reduce pain intensity compared to control groups. It did, however, find that ultrasound combined with exercise may improve foot function. In contrast, another 2024 systematic review on the same topic by Shrestha et al. [22], which included only five RCTs, reached a more positive conclusion, stating that the review supports the use of ultrasound therapy to reduce pain and improve functional disability. The existence of two contemporary systematic reviews on the same topic reaching different conclusions underscores the ongoing ambiguity in the evidence base.
- *Evidence in Other Conditions*: For osteoarthritis of the knee and hip, a Cochrane systematic review concluded that ultrasound therapy appears to have no benefit over placebo or other active therapies like shortwave diathermy for pain or function [18]. However, the authors of the Cochrane review tempered this conclusion by noting the generally low methodological quality of the included trials. This persistent problem has plagued research in this field for decades. More recent syntheses suggest a small-to-moderate pain benefit in knee OA [2, 10]. A 2024 protocol published in BMJ Open outlines an ongoing trial to assess whether adding LIPUS to conventional physiotherapy improves outcomes in knee osteoarthritis. Results are currently pending [7].

3.6.2.1 The Challenge of Establishing Effective Parameters: The Case of Lateral Elbow Tendinopathy

The detailed dosimetric guidelines presented in Sect. 3.3 reflect a widespread clinical belief that the effectiveness of ultrasound is highly dependent on the correct choice of parameters. This belief, however, presupposes that a set of "effective parameters" has been scientifically established. A systematic review by Stasinopoulos, Cheimonidou, and Chatzidamianos [23] directly investigated this presupposition for one of the most common applications of ultrasound: lateral elbow tendinopathy (LET). The review's specific aim was not to determine if ultrasound was effective per se, but to identify the *appropriate parameters* for its use in managing LET based on high-quality evidence.

The review's methodology was designed to identify randomized controlled trials (RCTs) that not only demonstrated a positive effect of ultrasound but also provided detailed descriptions of the parameters used. After searching six major databases, the authors found that no RCT met their inclusion criteria. Their conclusion was stark: "it is impossible to find out the appropriate ultrasound parameters in the management of LET based on previously conducted RCTs" [23]. Any recommendations for parameters had to be extrapolated from animal studies or from studies on conditions with similar clinical or histopathological characteristics.

This finding reveals a profound disconnect between clinical practice and the evidence base. It demonstrates that for at least one major indication, the detailed clinical heuristics for selecting frequency, intensity, and duty cycle are not derived from high-quality human clinical trials. They are based on tradition, theoretical reasoning, or extrapolation. This represents a form of inversion of the scientific method, where the "answer" (the specific parameters to use) has been widely adopted and taught before the fundamental question ("what parameters, if any, are effective?") has been answered. This powerfully reinforces the critique that the widespread use of this modality rests on a foundation lacking robust scientific support, extending uncertainty from *whether* it works to *how* it should even be applied.

3.6.3 The Controversial Evidence for LIPUS in Bone Healing

The story of the LIPUS evidence base is a compelling narrative of how scientific consensus can shift dramatically as research quality improves. It serves as a powerful case study in the principles of evidence-based medicine.

- *Early Evidence and Meta-Analyses Suggesting Efficacy*: Initial clinical trials and subsequent meta-analyses of this early work painted a promising picture. The biological rationale was strong; studies demonstrated that low-intensity ultrasound could stimulate osteoblasts, upregulate key genes like COX-2, and increase the production of growth factors crucial for bone repair [9]. Clinical studies reported that LIPUS could accelerate the radiographic healing time of fresh fractures by 24–38% and could successfully heal a high percentage (e.g., 86%) of established nonunions [14]. These positive findings provided the basis for FDA approval and led to the widespread clinical adoption of LIPUS as a noninvasive method to enhance bone healing. However, even during this period, more critical systematic reviews, such as one by Busse et al. [6], highlighted a "substantial level of inconsistency" and "conflicting results" across the available trials, suggesting the evidence was not as robust as it first appeared.
- *The Impact of High-Quality, Low-Bias RCTs: The TRUST Trial*: A pivotal moment in the LIPUS evidence story was the publication of the Tibial Fracture Trial (TRUST) in 2016. This was a large, multicenter, rigorously designed RCT that randomized 501 patients with surgically fixed tibial fractures to receive either a functional LIPUS device or an identical sham (placebo) device. The trial was designed to provide a definitive answer on the efficacy of LIPUS for a common and clinically significant fracture. Its results were unequivocally negative: after 1 year, there was no difference between the LIPUS and sham groups in terms of functional recovery or in the time to radiographic healing [20].

- *Recent Systematic Reviews* (e.g., Schandelmaier et al. [20]): *A Shift in Conclusion*: The most comprehensive and impactful analysis of the LIPUS evidence to date was a systematic review and meta-analysis by Schandelmaier et al. published in *The BMJ* in 2017, which incorporated the data from the TRUST trial. This review analyzed 26 RCTs involving nearly 1600 patients. Its key finding was that when the analysis was restricted to trials with a low risk of bias, LIPUS showed no benefit for patient-important outcomes, including time to return to work, pain levels, or the need for subsequent operations. Furthermore, it likely did not affect radiographic bone healing [20].
- *Synthesizing the Conflict: Risk of Bias as a Key Explanatory Factor*: The crucial contribution of the Schandelmaier et al. [20] review was its exploration of the profound heterogeneity in the literature. Using meta-regression, the authors found a highly significant statistical interaction ($p < 0.001$) between a trial's risk of bias and its reported outcome. Trials at a high risk of bias (e.g., those with inadequate blinding or allocation concealment) consistently suggested a benefit from LIPUS. In contrast, high-quality trials at a low risk of bias consistently did not. This finding strongly implies that the positive effects reported in the earlier LIPUS literature were likely not a true biological effect of the therapy but rather artifacts of methodological flaws, placebo effects, and bias.

The trajectory of LIPUS research thus serves as a powerful cautionary tale. An apparently strong biological rationale and promising results from early, smaller, and often industry-funded studies led to regulatory approval and widespread, expensive clinical use. However, this initial signal of efficacy ultimately proved to be noise when subjected to the highest levels of scientific scrutiny in large, independently funded, methodologically rigorous RCTs. This shift in the evidence base has real consequences for clinicians, policymakers, and the patients who rely on these treatments.

3.6.3.1 Shifting Focus: LIPUS in Postsurgical Soft-Tissue Recovery

In light of the strong evidence against LIPUS for fresh fractures, research in 2024–2025 has pivoted toward soft-tissue applications, where the mechanism of action involves anti-inflammatory modulation rather than calcification.

While the TRUST trial demonstrated inefficacy in bone union, a 2025 randomized study published in International Orthopedics investigated the efficacy of focused LIPUS following total knee arthroplasty (TKA). The trial reported that patients receiving LIPUS had significantly reduced lower-extremity swelling and walking pain during the first 14 days postsurgery compared with controls [26]. This suggests that the future of LIPUS may lie in acute postsurgical rehabilitation, targeting the COX-2/PGE2 inflammatory pathways to manage edema, rather than accelerating bone healing in healthy patients. These findings are preliminary and require replication in adequately powered, low-risk-of-bias randomized controlled trials before definitive clinical recommendations can be made (Table 3.4).

Table 3.4 Evolution of evidence: a summary of key systematic reviews on LIPUS for bone healing

Review (author, year)	Key findings on efficacy	Conclusion on evidence quality/consistency
Busse et al. [6]	Three of seven RCTs showed significantly reduced healing time; four showed no difference.	"Substantial level of inconsistency"; evidence provides "conflicting results."
Tajali et al. [24]	Stimulates radiographic bone healing in fresh fractures. Weak evidence for delayed unions/nonunions.	Paucity of sufficient studies with similar outcome measures for pooling.
Schandelmaier et al. [20]	No benefit on patient-important outcomes (return to work, pain, re-operation) or radiographic healing in low-risk-of-bias trials.	Moderate to high-quality evidence of no effect. Positive findings are associated with high risk of bias.
Radha and Varghese [16]	Inconsistent results for clinical parameters. Positive influence on radiographic/histological parameters is promising for future research.	"Cannot give a definitive conclusion" on clinical effectiveness due to heterogeneity.

3.7 Summary and Conclusion

3.7.1 Synthesizing the Biophysics, Mechanisms, and Evidence

This chapter has navigated the complex and often contradictory landscape of therapeutic ultrasound and its specialized derivative, LIPUS. For conventional therapeutic ultrasound, a plausible biophysical basis for its thermal effects—deep tissue heating leading to increased blood flow and collagen extensibility—remains its most biologically plausible and clinically defensible rationale [4]. However, the proposed nonthermal mechanisms, such as cavitation and acoustic streaming, are based on in vitro phenomena whose occurrence and relevance in living tissue remain highly questionable [4]. This weak mechanistic underpinning is mirrored in the clinical evidence, which, more than two decades after the landmark critiques of Robertson and Baker [4], remains ambiguous and unconvincing for many of its most common applications. Furthermore, this analysis has revealed a deeper issue: even the detailed prescriptive dosimetric guidelines used in daily clinical practice lack a foundation in high-quality clinical evidence, as demonstrated by the systematic review on lateral elbow tendinopathy [23].

For LIPUS, the narrative is different but leads to a similarly sobering conclusion. A strong and elegant molecular mechanism—mechanotransduction—has been well elucidated, providing a compelling biological rationale for its use in bone healing [12]. However, translating these robust in vitro cellular effects into tangible in vivo clinical benefits has not been supported by the highest-quality evidence. The most rigorous, large-scale, and low-bias clinical trials have failed to demonstrate that LIPUS improves patient-important outcomes or accelerates radiographic healing compared to placebo [20]. The history of LIPUS research serves as a stark reminder that a plausible biological mechanism is a necessary, but not sufficient, condition for clinical effectiveness.

3.7.2 The Current Standing of Therapeutic Ultrasound in Clinical Practice

Given the current state of the evidence, the role of these modalities in modern, evidence-based practice requires careful consideration.

- *Conventional herapeutic Ultrasound*: The continued widespread use of this modality for a myriad of musculoskeletal conditions appears to be driven more by historical practice and anecdotal experience than by high-quality scientific evidence. Currently, its most defensible application remains the use of continuous, 100% duty-cycle ultrasound to deliver deep heat to collagenous tissues—such as joint capsules, large tendons, and scar tissue—as an adjunct to manual therapy or stretching, to increase tissue extensibility. However, the use of pulsed ultrasound to achieve purported nonthermal 'healing' effects rests on a tenuous scientific foundation. A consistent body of high-quality clinical evidence does not support it.
- *Low-Intensity Pulsed Ultrasound (LIPUS)*: The routine use of LIPUS for accelerating the healing of fresh fractures is not supported by the best available evidence [5]. While its role in treating established nonunions remains a subject of debate, the lack of effect seen in high-quality trials on fresh fractures makes a significant benefit in nonunions unlikely. Ultimately, clinicians and healthcare systems must weigh the high cost of these devices against the high-quality evidence suggesting a lack of efficacy.

3.7.3 Unresolved Questions and Future Research Directions

Despite several decades of investigation, many fundamental uncertainties remain. For conventional therapeutic ultrasound, the most urgent need is still the same: well-designed, adequately powered randomized controlled trials focused on clearly defined clinical conditions. Any new research must also confront the longstanding dosimetry issue. Without standardized, independently calibrated equipment, it is impossible to know whether the treatment being studied is truly comparable across sites or even within a single trial. If this issue remains unresolved, the field is likely to continue producing results that are contradictory, difficult to interpret, or simply uninformative.

The situation with LIPUS raises an even more intriguing challenge. On the laboratory bench, the biological effects of LIPUS on isolated cells are robust and reproducible. Yet these effects have not translated convincingly into clinical benefit for human patients. One possible avenue for future work is identifying narrowly defined patient subgroups—perhaps individuals with specific genetic, metabolic, or healing impairments—who might still respond to LIPUS despite the disappointing results in the general population. At present, however, the evidence offers little momentum for this line of inquiry.

Understanding why a clear mechanotransductive signal at the cellular level fails to produce meaningful outcomes in vivo may ultimately shed light on the complexity of bone healing itself, which depends on a wide interplay of biological, mechanical, and systemic factors. At the same time, the field is beginning to expand into new territory. Protocols developed in 2024/2025 for the use of LIPUS in neuromodulation—specifically in early Alzheimer's disease [21]—represent a notable shift. These emerging applications will require rigorous testing to avoid repeating the familiar cycle: early biological excitement, rapid clinical adoption, and subsequent disappointment once high-quality trials appear. Ensuring that the next generation of ultrasound interventions does not follow the same trajectory as the bone-healing story will be essential for the field's credibility and future progress.

3.8 Case Studies

3.8.1 Case Study 1: Conventional Therapeutic Ultrasound for Chronic Achilles Tendinopathy

- *Patient Presentation*: A 40-year-old male presents with a 3.5-year history of bilateral mid-substance Achilles tendon pain, rated 6/10 on a Visual Analog Scale (VAS). The pain is worse in the morning upon waking and after periods of running. He has previously undergone physiotherapy, which included therapeutic ultrasound, massage, and stretching, but reports that these interventions provided only temporary relief. Physical examination reveals palpable thickening and tenderness approximately 4 cm proximal to the calcaneal insertion of the left Achilles tendon. There is pain on resisted plantar flexion and with passive dorsiflexion.
- *Intervention*: This hypothetical case illustrates the intended clinical reasoning for applying therapeutic ultrasound, despite the uncertain evidence. The goal is to treat a chronic, superficial tendinopathy. The chosen parameters are:
  - *Frequency*: 3 MHz (for a superficial target).
  - *Mode*: Pulsed, 1:1 ratio (50% duty cycle), consistent with guidelines for a chronic condition where a mild thermal/mechanical stimulus is desired.
  - *Intensity*: 0.8 W/cm^2, at the upper end of the recommended range for chronic conditions.
  - *Duration*: 8 min
  - *Application*: The transducer head is moved in slow, overlapping circles over the most tender and thickened area of the tendon. This treatment is applied three times per week for 4 weeks, in conjunction with a structured eccentric heel-drop exercise program, which is the evidence-based cornerstone of treatment.
- *Discussion*: The selection of 3 MHz is appropriate for the superficial location of the Achilles tendon. The pulsed mode and intensity are chosen based on the traditional (though poorly supported) rationale of stimulating cellular repair in a chronic condition. However, it is critical to acknowledge that the evidence for the

effectiveness of ultrasound in Achilles tendinopathy is weak to nonexistent. The case study by Tumia and Maffulli [25] highlights a patient for whom previous ultrasound treatment was unsuccessful. Therefore, while this protocol represents a common clinical application of ultrasound, any improvement seen in the patient is most likely attributable to the proven efficacy of the eccentric loading program. The additive benefit of the ultrasound itself remains highly uncertain.

3.8.2 Case Study 2: Low-Intensity Pulsed Ultrasound (LIPUS) for a Tibial Delayed Union

- *Patient Presentation*: A 40-year-old female sustained a closed diaphyseal fracture of the tibia, which was treated with an intramedullary nail. She is a smoker, a significant risk factor for impaired bone healing. At her 16-week postoperative follow-up, she continues to experience pain with partial weight-bearing. Radiographs show a persistent, visible fracture line with minimal bridging callus formation. The clinical and radiographic picture is consistent with a delayed union. The patient is anxious to avoid further surgery.
- *Intervention*: The patient is prescribed a LIPUS device (e.g., Exogen) for home use. The treatment protocol is fixed according to the manufacturer's specifications:
  - *Parameters*: 1.5 MHz frequency, I_{SATA} = 30 mW/cm^2 (equivalent to 0.03 W/cm^2), 20% duty cycle.
  - *Duration*: 20 min, once daily.
  - *Application*: The patient is instructed on how to locate the fracture site by palpation and using the markings on her skin. She applies the coupling gel and places the transducer directly over the fracture site, securing it with a strap. The device automatically runs the 20-min treatment cycle. Treatment is continued daily, with radiographic follow-up every 4–6 weeks.
- *Discussion*: This case represents the primary clinical indication for which LIPUS is marketed and prescribed. The rationale is to provide a noninvasive biophysical stimulus to "restart" a stalled healing process via mechanotransduction. Case series and early clinical trials have reported high union rates (over 80%) in such cases, suggesting a high likelihood of a positive outcome for this patient [19]. However, an evidence-based discussion must present the counterargument derived from higher-quality research. The systematic review by Schandelmaier et al. [20], heavily influenced by the large TRUST trial, concluded that LIPUS provides no significant benefit over placebo for fracture healing. This suggests that if this patient's fracture heals while using the LIPUS device, it is highly likely that healing would have occurred anyway as part of the fracture's natural (albeit slow) history. The outcome cannot be reliably attributed to the device. While the patient may perceive a benefit, and the clinician may observe radiographic union, the best available evidence indicates that LIPUS is not an effective intervention. This presents a significant clinical and ethical dilemma regarding the prescription of an expensive therapy with strong evidence of inefficacy.

3.9 Review Questions

1. Explain the piezoelectric effect and how the inverse piezoelectric effect is used to generate an ultrasound wave in a transducer.
2. A patient presents with pain in their piriformis muscle, a deep hip rotator. What frequency (1 or 3 MHz) would you choose for a thermal ultrasound treatment, and what is the biophysical rationale for your choice?
3. Define beam nonuniformity ratio (BNR). Why is a low BNR clinically important for patient safety and treatment efficacy, particularly when using continuous ultrasound?
4. Compare and contrast the proposed mechanisms of action for the thermal effects of continuous ultrasound and the molecular effects of LIPUS.
5. Critically discuss the statement: "The nonthermal effects of therapeutic ultrasound, such as cavitation and acoustic streaming, are well-established mechanisms for promoting tissue healing." Your answer should incorporate the in vitro–in vivo debate.
6. A 25-year-old patient with a fresh scaphoid fracture who has a cardiac pacemaker asks if he can use a LIPUS device to speed up his healing. Based on manufacturer guidelines and the principles of evidence-based practice, how would you advise him?
7. Summarize the main findings and overall impact of the two 2001 systematic reviews by Robertson and Baker on the field of therapeutic ultrasound.
8. Explain the evolution of the evidence for LIPUS in bone healing, from early positive studies to the conclusions of the TRUST trial and the Schandelmaier et al. [20] systematic review. What role did "risk of bias" play in explaining this evolution?
9. What is mechanotransduction, and what are the key cellular and molecular events (including key pathways and proteins) that are thought to be initiated by LIPUS in bone cells?
10. A therapist is treating a patient with an acute ankle sprain. According to common clinical guidelines, what pulse ratio and intensity range would they select for pulsed ultrasound? Critically discuss the quality of evidence supporting these specific parameters, referencing the findings of the systematic review by Stasinopoulos et al. [23].
11. Given the current body of evidence, what is the most scientifically defensible clinical application for conventional therapeutic ultrasound, and what is the current evidence-based recommendation regarding the routine use of LIPUS for fresh fractures?

Declarations

Competing Interests The author(s) have no competing interests to declare that are relevant to the content of this manuscript.

References

1. AIUM. Statement on biological effects of therapeutic ultrasound. 2023. Available at: https://www.aium.org/resources/official-statements/view/statement-on-biological-effects-of-therapeutic-ultrasound. Accessed 23 Oct 2025.
2. Aiyer R, Noori SA, Schlueter R, Chang KV, Osborne JR, Gungor S, Orhurhu V, Abd-Elsayed A, Urits I. Therapeutic ultrasound for chronic pain management in joints: a systematic review. Pain Med. 2019;21:1437–48.
3. Alhakami AM, Babkair RA, Sahely A, Nuhmani S. Effectiveness of therapeutic ultrasound on plantar fasciitis: a systematic review of RCTs. PeerJ. 2024;12:e17147.
4. Baker KG, Robertson VJ, Duck FA. A review of therapeutic ultrasound: biophysical effects. Phys Ther. 2001;81:1351–8.
5. BMJ Rapid Recommendations Panel. Low intensity pulsed ultrasound (LIPUS) for bone healing: a clinical practice guideline. BMJ. 2017;356:j576.
6. Busse JW, Morton E, Lacchetti C, Guyatt GH, Bhandari M. Low intensity pulsed ultrasonography for fractures: systematic review of randomised controlled trials. BMJ. 2009;338:b390.
7. Chen T, He Y, Xia S, Zhou F, Yuan X, Liu X. Evaluation of the effect of low-intensity pulsed ultrasound in pain and dysfunction for knee osteoarthritis: a double-blind, randomised controlled trial protocol. BMJ Open. 2024;14:e082108. https://doi.org/10.1136/bmjopen-2023-082108.
8. Draper DO, Castel JC, Castel D. Rate of temperature increase in human muscle during 1 MHz and 3 MHz continuous ultrasound. J Orthop Sports Phys Ther. 1995;22:142–50.
9. Erdogan O, Esen E. Biological aspects and clinical importance of ultrasound therapy in bone healing. J Ultrasound Med. 2009;28:765–76.
10. Guan H, Zhang C, Lin J, Chen W, Liu C, Chen G. Ultrasound therapy for pain reduction in musculoskeletal disorders: a systematic review and meta-analysis. Ther Adv Chronic Dis. 2024;15:20406223241267217.
11. Haar GT, Dyson M, Oakley S. Ultrasound in physiotherapy in the United Kingdom: results of a questionnaire. Physiother Pract. 1988;4:69–72.
12. Li X, Zhong Y, Zhang L, Xie M. Recent advances in the molecular mechanisms of low-intensity pulsed ultrasound against inflammation. J Mol Med. 2023;101:361–74.
13. Miller DL, Smith NB, Bailey MR, Czarnota GJ, Hynynen K, Makin IRS. Overview of therapeutic ultrasound applications and safety considerations. J Ultrasound Med. 2012;31:623–34.
14. Mundi R, Petis S, Kaloty R, Shetty V, Bhandari M. Low-intensity pulsed ultrasound for fracture healing: a systematic review of the evidence. Indian J Orthop. 2009;43:132–40.
15. NICE. Medical Technologies Guidance MTG12: EXOGEN ultrasound bone healing system for long bone fractures with non-union or delayed healing—review decision and cost update. 2019. Available at: https://www.nice.org.uk/guidance/mtg12. Accessed 23 Oct 2025.
16. Radha V, Varghese SS. Effectiveness of low intensity pulsed ultrasound (LIPUS) on bone healing and regeneration: a systematic review. Rev Gaúch Odontol. 2022;70:e20220051.
17. Robertson VJ, Baker KG. A review of therapeutic ultrasound: effectiveness studies. Phys Ther. 2001;81:1339–50.
18. Rutjes AW, Nüesch E, Sterchi R, Jüni P. Therapeutic ultrasound for osteoarthritis of the knee or hip. Cochrane Database Syst Rev. 2010;1:CD003132. https://doi.org/10.1002/14651858.CD003132.pub2.

19. Rutten S, van den Bekerom MPJ, Sierevelt IN, van Dijk CN. Low-intensity pulsed ultrasound for posttraumatic nonunions of the tibia: a review of patients treated in The Netherlands. J Trauma Acute Care Surg. 2017;82:764–9.
20. Schandelmaier S, et al. Low intensity pulsed ultrasound for bone healing: systematic review of randomized controlled trials. BMJ. 2017;356:j656.
21. Shimokawa H, Akishita M, Ihara M, Teramukai S, Ishiki A, Nagai Y, Fukushima M. Pivotal trial of low-intensity pulsed ultrasound therapy for early Alzheimer's disease: rationale and design. J Alzheimers Dis Rep. 2025;9:1–12. https://doi.org/10.1177/25424823241312108.
22. Shrestha S, Shrestha R, Lama D, Thapa M. Effectiveness of therapeutic ultrasound on reducing pain intensity and functional disability in patients with plantar fasciitis: a systematic review of randomised controlled trials. PeerJ. 2024;12:e17147.
23. Stasinopoulos D, Cheimonidou AZ, Chatzidamianos T. Are there effective ultrasound parameters in the management of lateral elbow tendinopathy? A systematic review of the literature. Int J Phys Med Rehabil. 2013;1:1000117. https://doi.org/10.4172/2329-9096.1000117.
24. Tajali SB, et al. Effects of low-intensity pulsed ultrasound therapy on fracture healing: a systematic review and meta-analysis. Am J Sports Med. 2011;39:2465–73.
25. Tumia N, Maffulli N. Conservative management of a bilateral chronic Achilles tendinopathy. J Sports Sci Med. 2011;10:783–7.
26. Wang Q, et al. Efficacy of focused low intensity pulsed ultrasound in reducing lower-extremity swelling and pain after total knee arthroplasty: a randomised study. Int Orthop. 2025;49:312–20.
27. Watson T, editor. Electrotherapy: evidence based practice. 12th ed. London: Elsevier; 2008.
28. Watson T. Electrotherapy on the Web. 2020. Available at: http://www.electrotherapy.org. Accessed 26 Aug 2020.
29. WFUMB. WFUMB Clinical Safety Statement for Diagnostic Ultrasound – an overview. 2012. Available at: https://wfumb.org/2012/09/29/wfumb-clinical-safety-statement-for-diagnostic-ultrasound-an-overview/. Accessed 23 Oct 2025.
30. Zhou J, Liu Z, Wang Z, Qi W, Wang Y, Chen Y. Effectiveness of low-intensity pulsed ultrasound on osteoarthritis: molecular mechanism and tissue engineering. Front Med. 2024;11:1292473.

4 Diathermy

George Sebastian Iacob

4.1 Introduction

Diathermy is a widely used therapeutic modality that generates heat in tissues using electromagnetic or mechanical energy and is commonly used to treat musculoskeletal and soft-tissue dysfunctions [1, 2]. One of the most widely accepted definitions of diathermy is provided by the US Food and Drug Administration (FDA), which describes diathermy as a therapeutic method that produces deep heating in tissues beneath the skin, muscles, and joints to achieve therapeutic objectives. The general clinical classification includes three main forms: shortwave diathermy (SWD), microwave diathermy (MWD), and ultrasound (US) therapy [3]. Although therapeutic ultrasound is often classified as a distinct electrophysical modality, it is included in this chapter because it can produce diathermic effects via mechanical energy transfer. This approach reflects a functional classification based on tissue heating and therapeutic outcomes, while a detailed analysis of ultrasound is presented in a dedicated chapter.

One of the earliest suggestions for the therapeutic use of high-frequency currents dates back to 1891 and is attributed to Nikola Tesla. He observed that irradiating tissues with high-frequency alternating currents at wavelengths exceeding those of conventional radio waves could have medical applications [4]. The late 1800s saw the first experiments with high-frequency currents, with Jacques-Arsène d'Arsonval exploring the physiological effects of alternating currents in tissues, laying the conceptual foundation for diathermy [5]. In 1909, the German physician K.F. Nagelschmidt formally introduced the term "diathermy," which translates as "heating through." Diathermy began to be implemented in clinical practice during the 1920s and 1930s, primarily using continuous shortwave modalities. Over the course of the twentieth century, the technique evolved through refined dosage

G. S. Iacob (✉)
Department of Physiotherapy, Physiozentrum Däniken, Olten, Switzerland

D. Stasinopoulos (ed.), *Application of Electrophysical Agents in Physiotherapy*,
https://doi.org/10.1007/978-3-032-32144-2_4

protocols, reduced excessive heating, and safer, more precise clinical application. These elements were marked by the development of the pulsed form of SWD, along with technological advancements and improved safety mechanisms [2, 6].

Clinically, diathermy encompasses shortwave, microwave, and ultrasound modalities, which differ in penetration depth, energy transfer mechanisms, and safety considerations [1–3].

In physiotherapy, diathermy refers to the clinical application of high-frequency electromagnetic or mechanical energy to induce therapeutic effects in deep tissues [7]. It applies to a wide range of musculoskeletal conditions, including myofascial pain syndromes [8] and chronic pain [9]. In contemporary practice, diathermy is rarely applied as a standalone treatment; instead, it is integrated into multimodal rehabilitation programs that may include manual therapy, therapeutic exercises, patient education, and functional training. Effective application of diathermy requires structured clinical reasoning. Clinicians should determine whether the primary therapeutic goal is thermal (e.g., increasing tissue extensibility, promoting muscle relaxation) or nonthermal (e.g., modulating pain, supporting cellular repair) and select the appropriate modality and treatment parameters accordingly. It is important to note that diathermy should be integrated into a comprehensive rehabilitation strategy rather than applied in isolation. This chapter focuses primarily on the application of diathermy in musculoskeletal rehabilitation within physiotherapy practice.

Depending on the applied dosage, diathermy can induce controlled biological responses. The literature primarily highlights its use in relieving muscle pain and managing spinal [10] and locomotor [11] conditions, making it a valuable tool in physical medicine, rehabilitation, and physiotherapy. In addition to traditional shortwave and pulsed diathermy, emerging technologies such as TECAR therapy and longwave diathermy (LWD) are gaining interest. TECAR delivers radiofrequency energy to support tissue healing, circulation, and pain modulation, while LWD uses lower frequencies to provide deeper, more comfortable heating for large muscles or joints.

The following sections of this chapter aim to explore in detail the concept of diathermy, its biophysical principles, and precise dosimetry within the context of medical rehabilitation. This integrated perspective supports the rational selection of diathermy modalities and parameters within evidence-based physiotherapy practice.

4.2 Biophysics

Diathermy uses nonionizing electromagnetic energy at radiofrequency and microwave frequencies. The goal of the procedure involves the controlled heating of tissues located in specific superficial or deep layers [1, 2].

The functionality of shortwave diathermy (SWD) is based on the commonly used frequency of 27.12 MHz with a wavelength of approximately 11 meters in free space [1]. Clinically, SWD is primarily used to achieve deep heating of muscles and periarticular structures. The energy transfer mechanisms differ for each type of diathermy applied, depending on the applicator system (inductive or capacitive coupling) [9].

4.2.1 Fundamental Wave Phenomena Relevant to Diathermy

Understanding the interaction between electromagnetic energy and biological tissues requires familiarity with the fundamental wave phenomena and physical laws that govern energy propagation, absorption, and tissue response [12, 13].

Electromagnetic energy propagates through space and biological tissues in the form of oscillating electric and magnetic fields [12]. The relationship between frequency (f) and wavelength (λ) is inverse and is described by the equation $\lambda = c/f$, where c represents the speed of light in the medium [12, 14]. In clinical diathermy, lower-frequency electromagnetic waves (e.g., shortwave diathermy at 27.12 MHz) have longer wavelengths and generally greater tissue penetration. In contrast, higher-frequency waves (e.g., microwave diathermy at 2450 MHz) have shorter wavelengths and are absorbed more superficially [15, 16]. This frequency–wavelength relationship underpins modality selection based on the desired depth of tissue heating.

As electromagnetic waves enter biological tissues, a portion of the energy is absorbed and converted into heat through molecular vibration and ionic movement [17, 18]. This absorption is heavily influenced by the dielectric properties of tissues, including permittivity and conductivity [17]. Tissues with high water content and dielectric constant, such as muscle and blood-rich structures, absorb electromagnetic energy more effectively [15, 17]. Conversely, tissues with low dielectric properties, such as adipose tissue, may exhibit significant heating in capacitive fields due to relative resistive heating [3, 14].

Scattering occurs when electromagnetic waves interact with heterogeneous tissue interfaces, such as transitions between muscle, fat, bone, and connective tissue. This alters the direction of wave propagation and contributes to nonuniform energy distribution within the treatment area [13].

Reflection refers to the redirection of electromagnetic waves at boundaries with marked impedance differences, such as interfaces between soft tissue and bone or metallic objects [14, 15]. Reflected energy does not contribute to therapeutic heating and may increase the risk of localized hot spots. Electromagnetic fields may concentrate at sharp anatomical curvatures or near metallic edges, a phenomenon known as the "Point Effect" or "Edge Effect," which increases the risk of thermal injury [15]. Careful applicator positioning and avoiding metallic objects within the treatment field are essential for safe practice.

Refraction is the change in direction of electromagnetic wave propagation when waves pass between tissues with different dielectric properties [14]. This bending of wave trajectories influences field distribution and heating patterns, particularly in regions with complex anatomy. Reflection, refraction, and scattering together explain why diathermy heating may be nonuniform, reinforcing the importance of clinical monitoring and individualized parameter selection [12, 14].

4.2.2 Fundamental Physical Laws Relevant to Diathermy

Several foundational physical laws provide a conceptual framework for understanding energy delivery and biological response in diathermy and other electrophysical agents [12, 19]:

- *Law of Cosines*: Maximum energy absorption occurs when electromagnetic energy is applied perpendicular to the tissue surface. As the angle of incidence deviates from the perpendicular, effective energy delivery decreases in proportion to the cosine of the angle, highlighting the importance of proper applicator orientation [12, 14].
- *Inverse Square Law*: Energy intensity decreases proportionally to the square of the distance from the source [12]. Small changes in applicator distance can produce substantial reductions in delivered energy, underscoring the importance of consistent positioning.
- *Grotthuss–Draper Law*: Only energy that is absorbed by tissue can produce a biological effect. Energy that is reflected, transmitted, or scattered without absorption does not contribute to therapeutic outcomes, underscoring the importance of selecting appropriate frequencies, applicator types, and treatment parameters [3, 20].
- *Arndt–Schulz Law*: This dose–response principle describes how low-intensity stimuli may stimulate physiological activity, moderate intensities support adaptation, and excessively high intensities may inhibit function or cause tissue damage [19]. In diathermy, this law supports the rationale for Pulsed Shortwave Diathermy (PSWD), where low mean power induces nonthermal cellular effects and promotes healing in the acute stage without risking the deleterious effects of excessive thermal loading [3].

Together, these principles form the biophysical basis for selecting diathermy modality, applicator design, and treatment parameters to optimize therapeutic effects while minimizing risks [12, 15].

4.2.3 Shortwave Diathermy: Inductive Method

The inductive method of SWD is based on the alternating magnetic field generated by an applicator coil or drum, which creates eddy currents in the conductive tissues [3]. A key characteristic is the preferential heating of tissues with high ionic content and consequently high conductivity (blood, muscles) [21].

4.2.4 Shortwave Diathermy: Capacitive Method

The capacitive method of SWD requires placing the desired segment between two capacitor plates to create an electric field through the tissue, which will act as a dielectric [10]. High-impedance tissues such as subcutaneous fat tend to absorb more energy, resulting in greater superficial heating under standard configurations [21].

4.2.5 Emerging Radiofrequency Applications

Modern physiotherapy increasingly uses longwave radiofrequency, such as TECAR therapy (Transfer of Energy Capacitive and Resistive), which typically operates between 300 kHz and 1.2 MHz. While this modality shares the biophysical goal of deep tissue heating with traditional diathermy, it employs a contact-electrode system and is often integrated with manual therapy. A detailed analysis of TECAR therapy and its specific clinical applications is beyond the scope of this chapter.

4.2.6 Microwave Diathermy (MWD)

Microwave diathermy employs electromagnetic radiation at microwave medical frequencies, such as 915 MHz, which typically produces moderate deep heating (approximately 3–5 cm), and 2450 MHz, which is associated with more superficial heating (approximately 1–3 cm) [22]. Tissue penetration can be achieved in several planes, but is characterized by strong absorption in high-water tissues and the risk of hot spots (due to sensitivity to reflection, refraction, and field concentration) [15].

Tissue interaction is characterized by strong absorption in water-rich tissues and increased sensitivity to reflection, refraction, and field concentration, which may result in localized hot spots [15]. As a result, microwave diathermy generally produces more superficial and less uniform heating compared with shortwave diathermy [23]. The applicator is positioned at a fixed distance, perpendicular to the skin surface, without direct contact. The use of towels or additional insulating layers is generally avoided, as they can alter the electromagnetic field's distribution and increase the risk of uneven heating. Careful alignment and continuous patient feed back are essential to ensure safe and effective application.

4.2.7 Portable Diathermy

In recent years, portable diathermy devices have been introduced, offering increased flexibility in clinical and, in some cases, home-based settings. These systems are typically smaller and may operate at lower power outputs than conventional diathermy equipment. While they offer advantages in accessibility and ease of use, their clinical effectiveness may vary with device specifications and treatment parameters. Therefore, clinicians should exercise caution when selecting portable systems and ensure that their use is guided by appropriate clinical reasoning and available evidence, rather than convenience alone.

Ultrasound (US), based on mechanical acoustic waves, typically comprises two modes, with common frequencies of 1 MHz for deep tissues and 3 MHz for superficial tissues [8]. In addition to thermal effects, low-intensity pulsed ultrasound induces nonthermal mechanisms, such as stable cavitation and acoustic streaming, that exert cellular-level effects. The production of heat explains the mode of operation upon absorption of mechanical energy, which leads to molecular vibration and localized frictional heating. The biophysical reasoning presents application possibilities depending on the type of tissue, its structure, and the clinical objective [18]. Although ultrasound is often discussed as a separate modality, it is included here for its ability to induce diathermic thermal and nonthermal effects in deep tissues through acoustic (mechanical) energy absorption rather than electromagnetic fields.

Tissue properties influence heat distribution, which explains why different diathermy modalities have specific clinical indications (Fig. 4.1). Because inductive SWD produces eddy currents in conductive tissues, it effectively heats structures such as muscle and vascularized soft tissues. Deep visceral organs have similar conductive properties but are not intended for clinical heating due to safety considerations [24]. In capacitive SWD, superficial tissues with higher impedance—such as fat and skin—absorb more energy and warm more readily. Bone behaves differently because its density and impedance produce reflections rather than uniform heating [25]. Dielectric properties vary with tissue type [18]. Water-rich tissues optimize dielectric permittivity and facilitate the propagation of radiofrequency fields, whereas fatty tissues limit penetration and sometimes result in only superficial heating [15]. The acoustic properties specific to ultrasound (US) also include different absorption capacities. Tendons and ligaments favor absorption due to their high protein content; muscles have moderate absorption due to their high water content; and bone exhibits high absorption due to its density, which may increase the risk of periosteal pain [23]. Tissue anisotropy, including fiber alignment and directional conductivity in muscles, can modulate local energy absorption and influence the resulting heating pattern [26].

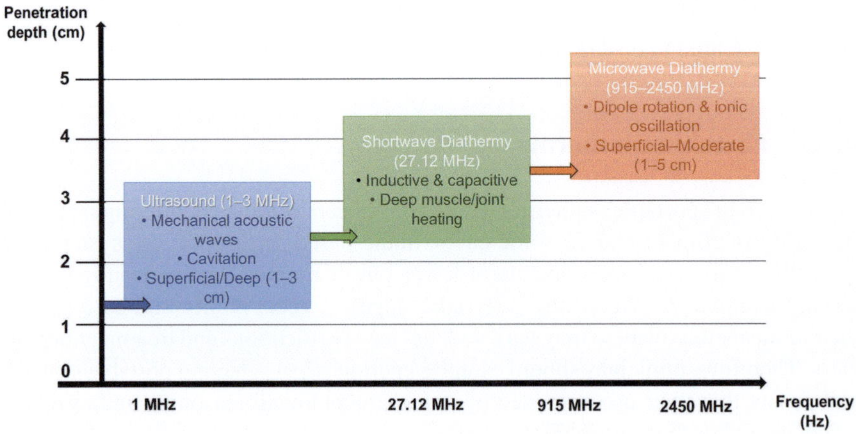

Fig. 4.1 Schematic representation of the spectrum and approximate depth of penetration of common diathermy modalities

Multiple technical and patient-related factors influence the heating pattern and penetration depth. Among the technical parameters, the mode of application of the therapy—continuous output producing stronger thermal effects and pulsed output producing mild or subthermal effects—plays a primary role [3]. Additional determinants include the operating frequency and the applicator design (drum, cable, plates), as well as technical aspects related to the device and the technique itself.

Superficial thermal agents penetrate only up to ~1 cm and usually heat the skin and superficial fascia. In contrast, diathermy has the main advantage of heating to a depth of 3–5 cm, depending on the chosen modality [18]. Other favorable arguments include uniform heating regardless of thermal tolerance or skin type, as well as the presence of both thermal and nonthermal effects [3, 27]. A comprehensive analysis of therapeutic ultrasound, including detailed biophysical mechanisms and clinical applications, is provided in a separate chapter.

4.3 Dosimetry and Treatment Parameters

Dosimetry involves the systematic selection of energy parameters to achieve specific therapeutic results. In physiotherapy, dosimetry refers to the systematic selection and adjustment of treatment parameters to achieve specific therapeutic outcomes while maintaining safety. Clinicians apply a structured clinical reasoning framework, considering the patient's condition, treatment goal, tissue type, pathology stage, and tolerance when selecting parameters. Typical therapeutic objectives include selecting parameters appropriate for pain management, thermal loading, or sub-thermal stimulation, depending on tissue type and stage of pathology [3]. In clinical practice, adherence to safe methodology is essential, including monitoring patient responses, pretesting, identifying potential contraindications or cautionary conditions, and understanding the device's technical specifications, calibration requirements, and recommended dosage ranges [2, 28]. In addition to subjective patient feedback, objective indicators such as treatment duration, device output settings, and clinical outcome measures should be considered when selecting dosage.

The selection of power, frequency, wavelength, duty cycle, and duration is essential for achieving therapeutic objectives. Frequency and wavelength follow well-established principles: lower frequencies generally allow deeper tissue penetration (e.g., SWD at 27.12 MHz is most commonly used, with other frequencies including 13.56 and 40.68 MHz) [15]. Higher frequencies are typically indicated for superficial tissues, as energy absorption occurs predominantly in these layers (e.g., MWD at 2450 MHz for superficial heating, US at 3 MHz for superficial tissues). Additional factors influencing tissue absorption include water content, dielectric permittivity, and electrical conductivity, which determine how effectively energy is converted into heat in different tissues [18].

Continuous SWD is typically selected when a thermal response is desired, whereas PSWD is used when minimal temperature elevation is required [29, 30]. The physiological basis of these responses is discussed in the Sect. 4.4.

The operating cycle significantly affects the heating pattern, particularly when comparing continuous and pulsed modes. Session duration is typically set between 10 and 30 min, depending on tissue location, the chosen modality, and the specific therapeutic objective. The patient's subjective response often guides dosage, as prolonged exposure may cause discomfort or thermal irritation [3].

The methodology of diathermy application requires careful attention to the treatment area and applicator positioning to ensure uniform energy distribution and optimal heating. Placement differs according to the type of diathermy:

- *Inductive SWD*: spiral or drum applicator positioned near the target muscle; avoid air gaps to prevent uneven heating [30].
- *Capacitive SWD*: target tissue placed between capacitor plates; good contact is essential.
- *MWD*: applicator directed perpendicular to the skin, maintaining a constant distance.
- *Ultrasound (US)*: coupling gel applied, with slow and controlled movement over the tissue [1, 29].

Adaptation is essential, as anatomical factors such as curvature, fat-muscle-bone ratio, and body surface area influence the choice of plate or spiral dimensions [29]. Another principle concerns the positioning of the patient, typically in a neutral position, often supine or sitting, which allows a stable, comfortable posture and optimal access to the target tissue [2].

Therapeutic effects of diathermy depend on the selected dose level and target area. Each modality allows adjustment of power, frequency, and duration, with ongoing monitoring of physiological responses and patient feedback [31]. Dose levels are commonly classified as mild, moderate, or vigorous, guiding the clinician in parameter selection and patient monitoring [32].

Tissue composition influences parameter selection, particularly the choice of applicator type, power output, and treatment duration [9]. Patient-related factors such as tolerance, skin integrity, and local sensitivity should always guide dose adjustment [31, 32]. Monitoring can be enhanced using thermometers, infrared imaging, or other objective assessment tools.

There are also differences depending on the distance between the applicator and the treated area, the positioning, angulation, and the quality of the medium coupling (US) [33]. The distribution of fat, muscle, and bone, tissue hydration (which affects dielectric properties), local temperature, anatomical geometry, and blood perfusion collectively determine how electromagnetic energy is absorbed in each patient [27]. Generally, these factors also influence the specific absorption rate (SAR), which quantifies the rate at which electromagnetic energy is converted into heat per unit mass of tissue [24, 33].

Table 4.1 presents representative parameter settings commonly used in clinical practice for different conditions and diathermy modalities, illustrating how specific frequencies, modes, and intensity levels are applied to achieve the desired therapeutic effects.

Table 4.1 Representative diathermy parameter settings for selected musculoskeletal conditions

Diathermy type	Condition and target tissue	Frequency/ mode	Power/ intensity	Duration (min)	Thermal goal	Evidence
SWD	Deep muscle spasm	27.12 MHz, continuous	Mild-mod	15–20	Mod	RCT
SWD	Chronic low back pain	27.12 MHz, pulsed 50%	Mod	20	L mod	SR
MWD	Superficial joint pain	2450 MHz, continuous	Mod	10–15	Mod	RCT
US	Tendon inflammation	3 MHz, pulsed 20–50%	Low-mod	5–10	Mild	RCT
US	Deep joint stiffness	1 MHz, continuous	Moderate	10–15	Mod	SR

Footnote/Notes:
SWD applicator: inductive or capacitive, depending on tissue depth
Chronic low back pain: can be combined with exercise; monitor patient feedback
MWD: maintain distance from skin; superficial heating
US tendon inflammation: use coupling gel, slow circular movement
US deep stiffness: avoid bone prominences
Evidence classification reflects the type and consistency of supporting studies and does not represent guideline-level clinical recommendations
Legend:
Thermal: Mild/Low-Moderate (L-Mod)/Moderate (Mod)/Vigorous (Vig)
Evidence: *RCT* randomized controlled trial, *SR* systematic review

Technical considerations are critical in the safe delivery of diathermy. This includes verifying the functionality and integrity of the applicators (drums, plates, cables) and connectors, as well as ensuring that the device calibration is current and meets manufacturer specifications [32, 34].

The following considerations can guide clinicians in selecting appropriate treatment parameters based on patient presentation and therapeutic goals (Box 4.1):

Box 4.1 Clinical Decision-Making Considerations in Diathermy Application

- Therapeutic goal (thermal vs nonthermal)
- Stage of pathology
- Target tissue depth
- Patient risk profile
- Integration with exercise or manual therapy
- Patient tolerance

4.4 Mechanism of Action (Physiological and Therapeutic Effects)

The therapeutic effects of diathermy are mediated by the interaction of high-frequency electromagnetic energy with biological tissues, eliciting both thermal and nonthermal physiological responses. These responses are determined by the mode of energy delivery (continuous or pulsed), the dosage parameters, and the biological properties of the target tissues. Understanding these mechanisms is essential for safe and effective clinical application and for optimizing preexercise preparation and implementation of the most adequate rehabilitation strategies (Fig. 4.2) [3, 35].

Thermal effects are primarily associated with continuous shortwave and microwave diathermy, which deliver sufficient energy to raise tissue temperature. Elevated tissue temperature induces local vasodilation through direct smooth muscle relaxation and the release of vasoactive metabolites. The resulting increase in blood flow improves oxygen and nutrient delivery, facilitates the removal of metabolic by-products, and contributes to the modulation of inflammatory mediators in chronic conditions [21]. Clinically, this warming effect is particularly useful as a preexercise or premobilization intervention, as it enhances tissue extensibility, reduces stiffness, and prepares muscles and joints for stretching or active therapy.

Heating also accelerates cellular metabolic processes, increases enzymatic activity, and promotes tissue repair. Enhanced metabolism supports fibroblastic activity, collagen remodeling, and soft-tissue recovery.

One of the most relevant effects of diathermy is its ability to increase the viscoelastic properties of collagen-rich tissues, including joint capsules, tendons, and

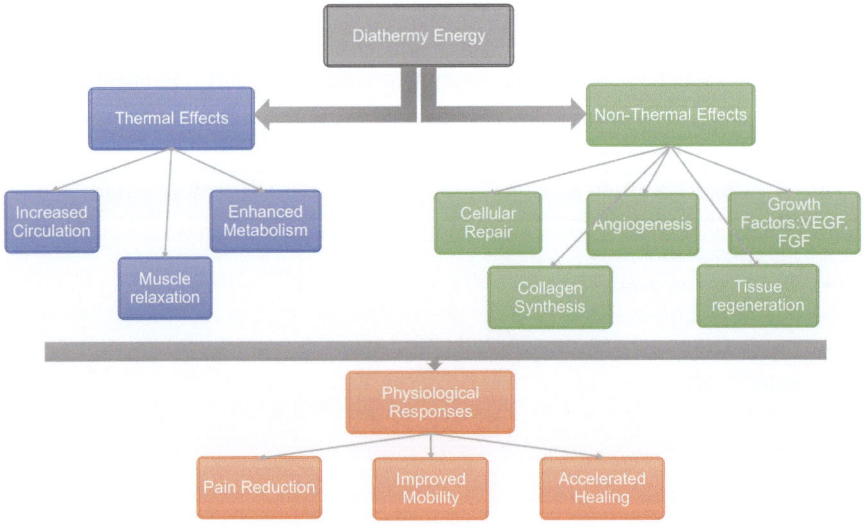

Fig. 4.2 Overview of the thermal and nonthermal mechanisms of action of diathermy and their associated physiological and therapeutic effects

ligaments. When applied before stretching or mobilization, diathermy reduces tissue stiffness, increases range of motion, and enhances the effectiveness of manual therapy and exercise interventions [35]. These effects are temperature-dependent and underscore the importance of appropriate dosage selection.

Nonthermal effects are mainly attributed to pulsed shortwave diathermy (PSWD), in which average power levels are insufficient to cause significant tissue heating. Pulsed electromagnetic fields influence cell membrane permeability and ion exchange, facilitating the transmembrane transport of calcium and other signaling molecules. These mechanisms support cellular repair processes, tissue regeneration, and the release of growth factors such as VEGF, promoting angiogenesis and enhanced microvascularization [36, 37]. While supported by experimental and cellular studies, nonthermal effects are most clinically relevant when pulsed diathermy is used as an adjunct to active rehabilitation rather than as a standalone intervention.

The effects of diathermy follow a dose–response relationship, whereby treatment parameters determine the magnitude of tissue heating and cellular response. Higher thermal doses result in greater temperature elevation and associated physiological effects, whereas low-intensity or pulsed applications primarily elicit nonthermal cellular responses. Tissue characteristics and patient-specific factors further modulate these effects, necessitating individualized dose selection [3, 35].

In clinical practice, the effective use of diathermy depends on combining its thermal and nonthermal effects with careful clinical judgment. Dosing parameters and mode of application should be guided not only by the desired therapeutic outcome (e.g., pain relief, muscle relaxation, or tissue healing) but also by patient-specific safety considerations [3]. These considerations emphasize the importance of understanding the indications, contraindications, and precautions, which are essential for safe and responsible clinical application and are addressed in the following section.

4.5 Indications, Contraindications, Precautions, and Side Effects

4.5.1 Indications

Diathermy is widely used in physiotherapy to support tissue healing, pain management, and functional recovery. Safe application requires careful consideration of clinical indications, contraindications, precautions, and potential adverse effects. Evidence-based clinical indications include:

Chronic inflammatory and degenerative musculoskeletal conditions, such as tendinopathies, bursitis, and osteoarthritis, where pulsed or thermal diathermy may be used to support pain management and tissue recovery, including modulation of inflammatory processes without excessive thermal loading [3, 35–37].

Muscle spasm and chronic musculoskeletal pain, including myofascial pain syndromes, where diathermy may be used to support pain management and muscle relaxation as part of a comprehensive rehabilitation program [3, 37, 38].

Scar tissue remodeling and selected wound-healing applications, including hypertrophic scars, adhesions, and postsurgical recovery. Pulsed shortwave diathermy may be considered in situations where thermal loading is contraindicated [36, 39].

Clinical note: The choice of diathermy parameters (frequency, intensity, duration) should be adapted to the stage of the pathology, tissue type, and patient comfort, ensuring an optimal balance between thermal and nonthermal effects (Fig. 4.1).

Certain conditions are *absolute contraindications*, meaning that diathermy should not be used under any circumstances due to the risk of serious complications (Fig. 4.3):

- Pacemakers or implantable electronic devices: Risk of potentially fatal arrhythmias [35].
- Pregnancy: Diathermy over the abdomen or pelvis is not recommended due to potential risks to the developing fetus [3].
- Malignancy in the treatment area: Heating may promote tumor growth or alter local vascularity.
- Metallic implants in the treatment area: The concentration of electromagnetic energy may cause burns or tissue damage [36].

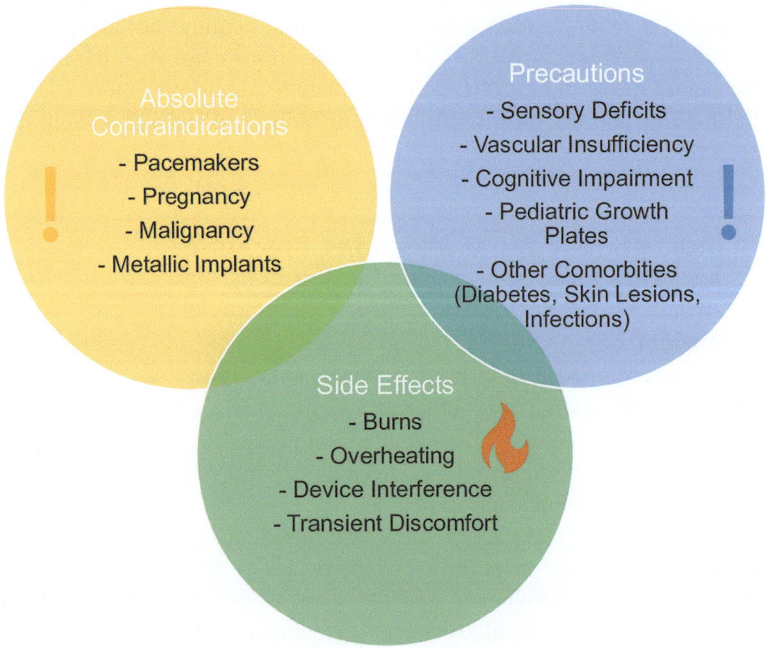

Fig. 4.3 Summary of major contraindications, precautions, and potential adverse effects associated with diathermy application

Beyond these absolute restrictions, the following *relative contraindications and precautions* require careful consideration and adjustment of diathermy treatment to ensure patient safety [40]:

- Impaired thermal sensation: Patients may not perceive overheating.
- Vascular insufficiency: Increased risk of tissue damage.
- Cognitive impairment: Patients may not report discomfort reliably.
- Pediatric growth plates: Avoid excessive heating over epiphyseal regions.
- Other comorbidities: Diabetes, skin lesions, or infections may require adapted protocols.

Clinical tip: Always perform a thorough medical history and examine the treatment area for implants, skin lesions, or vascular compromise.

Side effects of diathermy are generally uncommon, but can occur, especially when parameters exceed safety thresholds (Fig. 4.3):

- Burns typically occur over bony prominences or metal implants [36].
- Tissue overheating: Deep tissue heating can occur without visible surface changes. Objective temperature monitoring is recommended [38].
- Electromagnetic fields may interfere with devices such as pacemakers, insulin pumps, and neurostimulators. Avoid treating these devices [35].
- Transient discomfort: Patients may experience warmth, tingling, or mild erythema, which usually resolves after treatment [37].

4.5.2 Risk Management and Professional Responsibility

The safe use of diathermy requires adherence to risk management principles, professional standards, and institutional regulations, as well as appropriate patient selection and parameter selection.

Diathermy equipment must be regularly maintained and calibrated to ensure accurate energy delivery [40]. Clinicians should minimize occupational exposure to electromagnetic fields by avoiding unnecessary proximity to active applicators and following workplace safety guidelines.

4.5.3 Occupational and Environmental Safety

Safety protocols must address both the patient and the clinician. To minimize occupational exposure to electromagnetic fields (EMFs), therapists are advised to maintain a minimum safety distance of 1–2 m from the unit and its cables during operation. For patient safety, ensuring the treatment area is completely free of moisture or perspiration is critical to prevent "hot spots" and potential burns. Furthermore, rigorous screening for "invisible" contraindications, such as implanted electronic devices (e.g., pacemakers) or internal metal fixations, is mandatory to prevent localized tissue necrosis from rapid overheating [19, 41].

Treatment sessions must be clearly documented, including modality, parameters, applicator placement, patient feedback, and contraindication screening. Diathermy should be applied only within the clinician's scope of practice and in compliance with national regulations, electrical safety standards, and institutional policies [40, 42]. Common clinical errors that may compromise safety and treatment effectiveness are summarized in Box 4.2:

Safe clinical application requires *standardized protocols* and adherence to best practices (Fig. 4.4) [42]:

1. *Patient verification*: Confirm medical history, implants, pregnancy status, and comorbidities.
2. *Treatment area inspection*: Examine skin for lesions, metal, or vascular compromise.
3. *Parameter selection*: Adjust frequency, intensity, duration, and mode based on pathology and patient tolerance.
4. *Patient education*: Explain sensations to expect, and instruct to report discomfort immediately.
5. *Monitoring and documentation*: Record treatment parameters, patient feedback, and skin checks.

Box 4.2 Common Clinical Errors in Diathermy Application

- Using diathermy without integration into an active rehabilitation program
- Inadequate assessment of contraindications and precautions
- Excessive thermal dosing or poor applicator positioning resulting in uneven heating
- Failure to monitor patient feedback during treatment

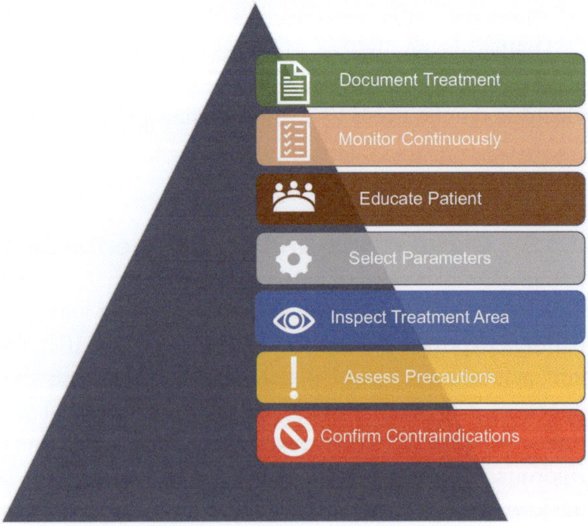

Fig. 4.4 Standardized clinical workflow for the safe application of diathermy in physiotherapy practice

4.6 Research Evidence

This section presents a critical assessment of the existing clinical evidence regarding the use of diathermy in practice. While the literature appears extensive, it is methodologically heterogeneous, underscoring the need to clearly distinguish between well-supported indications and applications with limited or emerging evidence [3, 21, 27]. Therapeutic uses of diathermy have been reported across various contexts, encompassing diverse recovery plans, patient populations, and phases of rehabilitation (Table 4.2). Overall, the levels of evidence include: randomized controlled trials (RCTs) assessing clinical efficacy [9–11]; systematic reviews and meta-analyses providing comprehensive syntheses of the research [3, 37]; comparative studies (e.g., diathermy versus ultrasound or other active therapies, or against placebo) [7, 8]; and observational studies, particularly for the evaluation of novel applications [6, 35, 43].

4.6.1 Evidence for Pain Reduction

Most RCTs have consistently demonstrated therapeutically and statistically significant effects of diathermy when combined with therapeutic exercise or incorporated into a multimodal treatment program, particularly for chronic musculoskeletal conditions affecting the upper and lower limbs [9–11]. Meta-analyses report predominantly moderate yet clinically relevant effects, while also highlighting substantial variability across implemented protocols [3, 21]. Strong evidence is consistently reported for chronic musculoskeletal conditions, including osteoarthritis, chronic low back pain, and various forms of myofascial syndrome [3, 9, 27].

4.6.2 Evidence for Optimization Range of Motion (ROM)

There is sufficient qualitative and quantitative evidence supporting improvements in tissue extensibility and ROM, particularly in the short term [7, 8]. Effective recovery protocols typically involve applying diathermy, followed by stretching or joint mobilization. Notable limitations include the relatively small number of studies assessing long-term outcomes and the variability in ROM measurement methods, which may be either subjective or objective [35, 37].

4.6.3 Evidence for Functional Recovery

Functional recovery encompasses complex outcomes, including factors such as pain reduction and increased mobility that can directly or indirectly influence overall function. Studies indicate consistent improvements, particularly in protocols combining diathermy with physical exercise [9, 11]. Functional recovery is

Table 4.2 Summary of clinical research evidence on the therapeutic use of diathermy

Author (year)	Study design	Population/condition	Diathermy modality	Main outcomes	Strength of evidence
Pollet et al. (2023) [3]	Systematic review and meta-analysis	Musculoskeletal disorders	Electromagnetic diathermy (SWD, RF)	Significant pain reduction; small-to-moderate functional improvement	Moderate to strong
Beninca et al. (2021) [21]	Systematic review	Experimental and clinical studies	Capacitive and inductive SWD	Consistent deep tissue heating; effects dependent on application method	Strong (physiological), moderate (clinical)
Barteau (2024) [27]	Systematic narrative review	Hip and knee osteoarthritis	Multiple modalities, including diathermy	Diathermy supports pain management as an adjunct modality	Moderate
Paolucci et al. (2020) [37]	Systematic review	Musculoskeletal pain conditions	Electromagnetic field therapies/PSWD	Variable pain reduction and anti-inflammatory effects	Limited to moderate
Albornoz-Cabello et al. (2023) [9]	Randomized controlled trial	Patellofemoral pain syndrome	RF diathermy + exercise	Greater pain reduction and functional gains compared with exercise alone	Strong (combined therapy)
Albornoz-Cabello et al. (2024) [11]	Randomized controlled trial	Patellofemoral pain syndrome	Noninvasive RF diathermy + supervised exercise	Sustained pain and functional improvements at follow-up	Strong
Lara-Palomo et al. (2025) [10]	Randomized clinical trial	Chronic low back pain	Monopolar RF diathermy + exercise	Reduced pain and disability; improved functional outcomes	Moderate to strong
Jia et al. (2022) [7]	Randomized comparative trial	Knee osteoarthritis	Pulsed shortwave diathermy vs. pulsed ultrasound	Comparable pain relief and functional improvement between groups	Moderate
Jimenez-Sanchez et al. (2024) [8]	Randomized crossover trial	Myofascial trigger points (upper trapezius)	RF diathermy vs. ultrasound	Both modalities effective; faster pain reduction with diathermy	Moderate
Masiero et al. (2020) [35]	Observational pilot study	Musculoskeletal disorders	Shortwave diathermy	Clinical improvement reported; lack of control group	Limited
Yang et al. (2024) [43]	Clinical study	Pediatric burn wounds	Pulsed shortwave diathermy	Accelerated wound healing and tissue repair	Emerging
Mratskova et al. (2023) [6]	Narrative review	Rehabilitation practice	Shortwave diathermy	Potential therapeutic benefits highlighted; need for robust trials	Limited

Footnote: Evidence classification reflects the type and consistency of supporting studies and does not represent guideline-level clinical recommendations typically assessed using a variety of measures, often relying on subjective scores and standardized scales (e.g., WOMAC, DASH). The overall classification and quantification of results from the main categories of studies with high scientific relevance suggest varying levels of support, depending on the conditions addressed and the modalities of application. Conversely, limited or inconsistent support is observed for therapeutic applications in acute conditions, certain neurological indications, and, more generally, for the use of diathermy as a standalone treatment [6, 35].

4.6.4 Methodological Limitations and Future Research Directions

Several factors currently limit the generalizability of findings on the therapeutic use of diathermy. These include variability in treatment protocols (such as duration, frequency, and intensity), limited reporting of standardized outcome measures, challenges in conducting double-masked studies, and the generally short follow-up periods in most trials [6, 37]. These methodological constraints highlight the need for more rigorous research and the establishment of standardized protocols to ensure reproducibility and clinical relevance.

Building on these findings, future research should focus on areas that show promise but remain underexplored. These include the study of nonthermal effects and the enhancement of regenerative and recovery capacities with pulsed shortwave diathermy, which has been documented primarily in combination with other therapies [3, 21]. Other promising directions may include the treatment of chronic wounds, for which available sample sizes remain limited [43], and strategies to reduce postexertional pain alongside the restoration of soft tissues, where preliminary evidence suggests potential benefits of diathermy. However, the magnitude of its effect within interdisciplinary approaches remains to be determined [8, 35].

To facilitate clinical decision-making and reinforce key concepts, Table 4.3 summarizes the main characteristics of each physical modality, including the type of energy used, primary target tissues, and typical depth of penetration:

Table 4.3 A quick-reference table for students to distinguish between the modalities covered in this chapter

Modality	Physical agent	Primary target tissues	Depth of penetration
Inductive SWD	Magnetic field	High conductivity (muscles, blood)	3–5 cm
Capacitive SWD	Electric field	High impedance (adipose tissue/fat)	Superficial to deep
Microwave diathermy	Electromagnetic waves	Tissues with high water content	1–3 cm
Therapeutic ultrasound	Acoustic energy	Collagen-rich (joint capsules, fascia)	2–5 cm

4.7 Summary/Conclusion

The main practical observations and conclusions are presented below, with an emphasis on clinical relevance and future directions for development and research, which are essential for advancing the field.

4.7.1 Biophysical Principles and Mechanisms of Action

Diathermy exerts its effects through both thermal and nonthermal mechanisms, enhancing blood circulation, stimulating tissue metabolism, and reducing pain. Depending on the clinical context and the individual patient, different types of diathermy—such as pulsed or continuous—may be applied, each offering specific advantages. Correct implementation, including the systematic selection of parameters such as frequency, duration, and intensity, is essential to maximize therapeutic benefits while minimizing risks.

4.7.2 Clinical Evidence and Practical Implications

Research generally supports the valuable contribution of diathermy to a combined rehabilitation program, particularly for chronic musculoskeletal conditions, arthrosis, and painful myofascial syndromes. Clinically and statistically significant evidence indicates that combining diathermy with physical exercise, stretching, or other rehabilitation techniques produces consistent benefits. In contrast, evidence for the use of diathermy as a standalone therapy is limited, especially in acute conditions or neurological applications. These findings highlight the importance of systematic patient selection and the integration of diathermy into comprehensive treatment plans.

4.7.3 Safety and Best Practices

When applied correctly, diathermy is a safe, noninvasive therapy, with adverse effects being rare. Careful monitoring of treatment intensity, adherence to technical and clinical application guidelines, and full awareness of contraindications are essential to prevent adverse complications.

4.7.4 Practical Recommendations for Clinicians

- Implement diathermy as part of a combined treatment (e.g., manual therapies, active physiotherapy, electrotherapy) rather than as a single modality, to enhance synergistic effects.
- Educate patients about the goals of therapy, how it works, and expected outcomes to improve adherence.

- Adjust the mode, parameters, and frequency according to the patient's individual characteristics to ensure personalized treatment.
- Continuously monitor and assess outcomes using validated tools (pain scales, range of motion, functional assessments) to track progress and optimize therapy.
- Focus on chronic musculoskeletal conditions, where evidence suggests the greatest clinical benefit.

Diathermy is a valuable tool in physiotherapy, with consistent clinical evidence supporting pain reduction, improved mobility and flexibility, and enhanced functional recovery across diverse patient groups. Clinically, diathermy is most effectively applied as a short preexercise or premobilization intervention to optimize tissue readiness. Clinicians should integrate diathermy into individualized, multimodal rehabilitation programs, considering both methodological principles outlined in the literature and emerging directions for research and technological development.

Future research should prioritize improved parameter standardization, individualized dosimetry, and real-time monitoring to enhance safety and effectiveness.

4.8 Clinical Case Studies

The following table summarizes the main characteristics, treatment parameters, and outcomes of two illustrative cases demonstrating the clinical application of diathermy in musculoskeletal rehabilitation (Table 4.4).

4.8.1 Case 1: Shortwave Diathermy for Post-traumatic Shoulder Stiffness

Background/Screening

A 45-year-old patient presented with limited mobility and persistent pain in the right shoulder, 3 months following a conservatively treated proximal humerus fracture. The patient underwent a brief assessment, which confirmed limited active and passive shoulder mobility, persistent pain, and difficulty with daily activities. Prior physiotherapy, including myofascial techniques and mobilization, had not fully restored function.

Clinical Reasoning

Shortwave diathermy was selected, given the chronic stage of healing and the depth of capsular restriction, to improve tissue extensibility and modulate pain.

Table 4.4 Treatment summary per case

Case	Condition	Diathermy modality	Frequency/duration	Combined therapy	Outcome
1	Posttraumatic shoulder stiffness	SWD continuous	3×/week, 20 min, 6 weeks	Myofascial techniques Passive and active-assisted mobilization exercises	Pain ↓6 → 2 VAS, flexion ↑90° → 150°, abduction ↑80° → 140°, DASH + 35%
2	Knee osteoarthritis	Pulsed SWD	2×/week, 15 min/side, 8 weeks	Quadriceps and gluteal strengthening, stretching, and low-impact aerobic exercises	Pain ↓7 → 3 VAS, knee flexion ↑100° → 120°, WOMAC function + 40%

Intervention

Continuous shortwave diathermy (27.12 MHz) was applied three times per week for 6 weeks, with each session lasting 20 min. Treatment intensity and frequency parameters were adjusted to patient tolerance to avoid discomfort, hyperemia, or burns. Each session was immediately followed by passive and active-assisted mobilization exercises, in accordance with clinical protocols reported in the recent literature [3, 37].

Outcome

After 6 weeks of treatment:

- Pain decreased from 6/10 to 2/10 on the Visual Analog Scale (VAS).
- Active shoulder flexion improved from 90° to 150°.
- Active abduction increased from 80° to 140°.
- DASH score indicated a 35% improvement in functional ability.

The patient was able to resume professional and recreational activities without discomfort.

Discussion

This case demonstrates the benefits of integrating shortwave diathermy into a multimodal rehabilitation program. The thermal effects of shortwave diathermy enhanced tissue extensibility and increased local circulation, facilitating joint mobility across all planes when combined with mobilization exercises. Nonthermal effects, such as pain modulation, contributed substantially to patient comfort and adherence to therapy, which are critical for functional recovery and quality of life [21]. Limitations include the need for careful parameter monitoring and individualized adjustments based on patient tolerance.

4.8.2 Case 2: Pulsed Diathermy for Pain Associated with Knee Osteoarthritis

Background/Screening

A 62-year-old female patient with bilateral knee osteoarthritis (Kellgren-Lawrence grade II–III) presented with pain, particularly at night or after exertion, stiffness, and difficulty ascending and descending stairs. Assessment confirmed persistent functional limitations despite prior treatments, including NSAIDs and mobility and strengthening exercise programs.

Clinical Reasoning

Pulsed shortwave diathermy (PSWD) was selected to leverage nonthermal analgesic effects and moderate thermal perfusion, supporting pain reduction, tissue recovery, and improved joint mobility in a chronic condition.

Intervention

Pulsed shortwave diathermy (PSWD) was applied twice weekly for 8 weeks, with each session lasting 15 min per knee. The treatment was combined with:

- Quadriceps and gluteal muscle strengthening exercises.
- Lower limb stretching (passive, dynamic, and PNF techniques).
- Low-impact aerobic activity (e.g., stationary cycling).

Treatment parameters were adjusted to patient tolerance to avoid discomfort or adverse effects. This multimodal approach is supported by clinical protocols and evidence reported in the literature [7, 9].

Outcome

After 8 weeks:

- Pain decreased from 7/10 to 3/10 on the VAS.
- Knee flexion improved from 100° to 120°.
- WOMAC function score improved by 40%.
- No adverse effects were reported.

Discussion

PSWD exerts therapeutic effects through a combination of nonthermal mechanisms, such as analgesia and modulation of inflammatory mediators, and moderate thermal effects that enhance local tissue perfusion. When integrated with strengthening exercises and patient education, PSWD contributes to improved clinical outcomes and ensures safe application [35]. This case demonstrates the clinical value of pulsed diathermy as part of a multimodal rehabilitation program for knee osteoarthritis, with potential benefits extending to medium- and long-term management.

4.9 Review Questions

1. Differentiate between the two modes of *shortwave diathermy (inductive vs. capacitive)*, in terms of *mechanism* and *tissue effects*.
2. List three *physiological effects* of *thermal diathermy*.
3. Identify potential *nonthermal effects* of *pulsed diathermy* and discuss their *clinical relevance*.
4. Describe key *contraindications* to *diathermy*, including *metallic implants* and *implanted electronic devices*, and explain why they are important.
5. Why is *skin dryness* considered a critical *safety parameter* during *high-frequency electromagnetic treatments*?
6. What principles should be incorporated to ensure the *safe implementation* of *diathermy therapy*?
7. Explain why *diathermy* is more effective as part of a *multimodal program* rather than as a standalone therapy.

8. Describe the clinical rationale for using *Pulsed Shortwave Diathermy (PSWD)* in the management of *acute injuries*.
9. How does the *depth of penetration* of *therapeutic ultrasound* compare to that of *Inductive SWD*?

Declarations

Competing Interests The author(s) have no competing interests to declare that are relevant to the content of this manuscript.

References

1. Kitchen S, Partridge C. Electrotherapy: evidence-based practice. 13th ed. London: Elsevier; 2013.
2. Robertson V, Ward A, Low J, Reed A. Electrotherapy explained: principles and practice. 5th ed. London: Elsevier; 2019.
3. Pollet J, Ranica G, Pedersini P, Lazzarini SG, Pancera S, Buraschi R. The efficacy of electromagnetic diathermy for the treatment of musculoskeletal disorders: a systematic review with meta-analysis. J Clin Med. 2023;12:3956. https://doi.org/10.3390/jcm12123956.
4. Vucevic D, Dordevic D, Radosavljevic T. Nikola tesla and medicine: 160th anniversary of the birth of the genius who gave light to the world—part II. Med Pregl. 2016;69:391–401. https://doi.org/10.2298/MPNS1612391V.
5. Heidland A, Fazeli G, Klassen A, Sebekova K, Hennemann H, Bahner U, et al. Neuromuscular electrostimulation techniques: historical aspects and current possibilities in treatment of pain and muscle wasting. Clin Nephrol. 2013;79:S12–23.
6. Mratskova G, Cvetanov T, Dimitrov S. Short-wave diathermy – possible therapeutic benefits of high-frequency electromagnetic field therapy in physical practice. Knowl Int J. 2023;61:727–33.
7. Jia L, Li D, Wei X, et al. Efficacy and safety of focused low-intensity pulsed ultrasound versus pulsed shortwave diathermy on knee osteoarthritis: a randomized comparative trial. Sci Rep. 2022;12:12792. https://doi.org/10.1038/s41598-022-17291-z.
8. Jimenez-Sanchez C, Cordova-Alegre P, Carpallo-Porcar B, Burgos-Bragado JM, Sanjuan-Sánchez D, Brandín-de la Cruz N. Effects of transcutaneous radiofrequency diathermy versus ultrasound on latent myofascial trigger points in the upper trapezius: a randomized crossover trial. J Back Musculoskelet Rehabil. 2024;37:1049–58. https://doi.org/10.3233/BMR-230296.
9. Albornoz-Cabello M, Ibáñez-Vera AJ, Barrios-Quinta CJ, Espejo-Antúnez L, Lara-Palomo IC, Cardero-Durán MA. Effects of radiofrequency diathermy plus therapeutic exercises on pain and functionality of patients with patellofemoral pain syndrome: a randomized controlled trial. J Clin Med. 2023;12:2348. https://doi.org/10.3390/jcm12062348.
10. Lara-Palomo IC, Capel-Alcaraz AM, García-López H, Castro-Sánchez AM, Querol-Zaldívar MLA, Fernández-Sánchez M. Effectiveness of monopolar diathermy by radiofrequency combined with exercise in patients with chronic low back pain: a randomized clinical trial. J Back Musculoskelet Rehabil. 2025;38:420–33. https://doi.org/10.3233/BMR-240118.
11. Albornoz-Cabello M, Ibáñez-Vera AJ, Barrios-Quinta CJ, Espejo-Antúnez L, Lara-Palomo IC, Cardero-Durán MA. Non-invasive radiofrequency diathermy neuromodulation added to supervised therapeutic exercise in patellofemoral pain syndrome: a single-blind randomized controlled trial with six months of follow-up. Biomedicine. 2024;12:850. https://doi.org/10.3390/biomedicines12040850.
12. Griffiths DJ. Introduction to electrodynamics. 4th ed. Boston: Pearson Education; 2013.
13. Wait JR. Electromagnetic waves in stratified media. 2nd ed. Piscataway: IEEE Press; 2012.

14. Balanis CA. Advanced engineering electromagnetics. Hoboken: Wiley; 2012.
15. Rossmann C, Haemmerich D. Review of temperature dependence of thermal properties, dielectric properties, and perfusion of biological tissues at hyperthermic and ablation temperatures. Crit Rev Biomed Eng. 2014;42:467–92. https://doi.org/10.1615/CritRevBiomedEng.2015012486.
16. Bowman JR, Batchelor JC. Electromagnetic radiation and scattering. Oxford: Oxford University Press; 1986.
17. Gabriel S, Lau RW, Gabriel C. The dielectric properties of biological tissues: II. Measurements in the frequency range 10 Hz to 20 GHz. Phys Med Biol. 1996;41:2251–69. https://doi.org/10.1088/0031-9155/41/11/002.
18. Gabriel S, Lau RW, Gabriel C. The dielectric properties of biological tissues: III. Parametric models for the dielectric spectrum of tissues. Phys Med Biol. 1996;41:2271–93. https://doi.org/10.1088/0031-9155/41/11/003.
19. Guyton AC, Hall JE. Textbook of medical physiology. 13th ed. Philadelphia: WB Saunders; 2016. p. 741–7.
20. Hecht E. Optics. 5th ed. Boston: Pearson; 2017.
21. Beninca IL, de Estéfani D, Pereira de Souza S, Weisshahn NK, Haupenthal A. Tissue heating in different short wave diathermy methods: a systematic review and narrative synthesis. J Bodyw Mov Ther. 2021;28:298–310. https://doi.org/10.1016/j.jbmt.2021.07.031.
22. Origlia C, Rodriguez Duarte DO, Tobon Vasquez JA, Bolomey JC, Vipiana F. Review of microwave near field sensing and imaging devices in medical applications. Sensors (Basel). 2024;24:4515. https://doi.org/10.3390/s24144515.
23. Martusevich A, Nazarov V, Bocharin I, Surovegina A, Guryanov M, Suldin P. Microwave estimation of dielectric properties of biological tissue under thermal modification. Archiv Euromedica. 2022;12:e1. https://doi.org/10.35630/2199-885X/2022/12/3.4.
24. Firuzalizadeh M, Gaffoglio R, Giordanengo G, Righero M, Vecchi G. Specific absorption rate optimization in microwave cancer hyperthermia via local power synthesis algorithm. Cancers (Basel). 2025;17:2813. https://doi.org/10.3390/cancers17172813.
25. Jeas M, et al. A heuristic model to evaluate the dielectric properties of human tissues at microwave band based on water and solid content. J Eng Appl Sci. 2023;70:43. https://doi.org/10.1186/s44147-023-00187-8.
26. Gu K, Yan S, Wu X. Effect of anisotropy in myocardial electrical conductivity on lesion characteristics during radiofrequency cardiac ablation: a numerical study. Int J Hyperth. 2022;39:120–33. https://doi.org/10.1080/02656736.2021.2022220.
27. Barteau JP. Systematic narrative review of modalities in physiotherapy for managing pain in hip and knee osteoarthritis. Medicine (Baltimore). 2024;103:e38225. https://doi.org/10.1097/MD.0000000000038225.
28. Li Y, Li W, Liu X, Liu X, Zhu B, Guo S, et al. Effects of low-intensity pulsed ultrasound in tendon injuries. J Ultrasound Med. 2023;42:1923–39. https://doi.org/10.1002/jum.16230.
29. Chang KH, Huang CW. Thermal modeling of ultrasound diathermy in tissues with a circular inclusion near a curved interface. Appl Sci. 2022;12:5166. https://doi.org/10.3390/app12105166.
30. Espinoza ANC, Moreira PM, Yamada FT, Meira CP, Paladini LH, de Macedo ACB. Immediate effects of two modes of shortwave diathermy in chronic low back pain: randomized controlled clinical trial. Pain Manag. 2025;15:931. https://doi.org/10.1080/17581869.2025.2570117.
31. Demchak TJ, Stone MB. Effectiveness of clinical ultrasound parameters on changing intramuscular temperature. J Sport Rehabil. 2008;17:220–9. https://doi.org/10.1123/jsr.17.3.220.
32. Lee JH, Do JG, Park HJ, Lee YT, Kim SJ. A comparison of the effect of a 4.4-MHz radiofrequency deep heating therapy and ultrasound on low back pain: a randomized, double-blind, multicenter trial. J Clin Med. 2022;11:5011. https://doi.org/10.3390/jcm11175011.
33. Bevacqua MT, Gaffoglio R, Bellizzi GG, Righero M, Giordanengo G, Crocco L, et al. Field and temperature shaping for microwave hyperthermia: recent treatment planning tools to enhance SAR-based procedures. Cancers (Basel). 2023;15:1560. https://doi.org/10.3390/cancers15051560.

34. Guirro RR, Guirro EC, Alves de Sousa NT. Lack of maintenance of shortwave diathermy equipment has a negative impact on power output. J Phys Ther Sci. 2014;26:557–62. https://doi.org/10.1589/jpts.26.557.
35. Masiero S, Pignataro A, Piran G, Duso M, Mimche P, Ermani M, et al. Short-wave diathermy in the clinical management of musculoskeletal disorders: a pilot observational study. Int J Biometeorol. 2020;64:981–8. https://doi.org/10.1007/s00484-019-01806-x.
36. Al Mandeel MM, Watson T. The thermal and nonthermal effects of high and low doses of pulsed short-wave therapy (PSWT). Physiother Res Int. 2010;15:199–211. https://doi.org/10.1002/pri.460.
37. Paolucci T, Pezzi L, Centra AM, Giannandrea N, Bellomo RG, Saggini R, et al. Electromagnetic field therapy: a rehabilitative perspective in the management of musculoskeletal pain—a systematic review. J Pain Res. 2020;13:1385–400. https://doi.org/10.2147/JPR.S231778.
38. Sousa AMM, Meyer KA, Santpere G, Gulden FO, Sestan N. Evolution of the human nervous system function, structure, and development. Cell. 2017;170:226–47. https://doi.org/10.1016/j.cell.2017.06.036.
39. Fu T, Lineaweaver WC, Zhang F, Zhang J. Role of shortwave and microwave diathermy in peripheral neuropathy. J Int Med Res. 2019;47:3569–79. https://doi.org/10.1177/0300060519854905.
40. Shah SG, Farrow A. Investigation of practices and procedures in the use of therapeutic diathermy: a study from the physiotherapists' health and safety perspective. Physiother Res Int. 2007;12:228–41. https://doi.org/10.1002/pri.382.
41. Stam R, Yamaguchi-Sekino S. Occupational exposure to electromagnetic fields from medical sources. Ind Health. 2018;56:96–105. https://doi.org/10.2486/indhealth.2017-0112.
42. Almalty AR, Abdelnour HM, Hawamdeh M, Alkhob SA. Physiotherapists' understanding of shortwave diathermy contraindications: a questionnaire survey. Risk Manag Healthc Policy. 2023;16:1171–85. https://doi.org/10.2147/RMHP.S413806.
43. Yang R, Li X, Tian X, et al. Efficacy of pulsed shortwave diathermy on wound healing in children with burns. J Army Med Univ. 2024;46:1569–76. https://doi.org/10.16016/j.2097-0927.202312033.

Photobiomodulation

5

Javier Aceituno-Gómez

5.1 Introduction

At the beginning of the twentieth century, Albert Einstein theorized the existence of photons and the possibility of *stimulated emission* [1]. Between this theoretical foundation and the first ruby laser emission achieved by Theodore Maiman in 1960 [2], several intermediate milestones were reached, including the development of the optical maser (using microwaves) by Townes and Schawlow, in parallel with Basov and Prokhorov, and the coining of the term *laser*—an acronym for *light amplification by stimulated emission of radiation*—by Gordon Gould in 1957 [3]. From the second half of the twentieth century to the present, five Nobel Prizes in Physics have been directly related to the research and use of laser emission (1964, 1981, 1997, 2005, and 2018). The potential biological effects of laser light were first discovered by Endre Mester in the late 1960s [4, 5]. Since then, laser therapy has gained attention across nearly all fields of medicine [6], initially through low level lasers and, in recent decades, also through high-intensity laser therapy (HILT) as an electrophysical agent for noninvasive treatment of multiple pathologies.

Laser light is characterized by its *monochromaticity*, *coherence*, and *high collimation* [7]. Within the electromagnetic spectrum, laser emissions range approximately from 100 nm to 1 mm, encompassing ultraviolet (UV), visible, and infrared (IR) radiation [1]. In medical applications, wavelengths span from 193 nm (ArF laser) to 10,600 nm (surgical CO_2 laser) [6]. Therapeutic laser applications typically use wavelengths between 400 and 1064 nm [8]. Several authors have reported that

J. Aceituno-Gómez (✉)
University General Hospital "Nuestra Señora del Prado" – SESCAM,
Talavera de la Reina (Toledo), Spain

Faculty of Health Sciences, Medical Science Department, University of Castilla-La Mancha (UCLM), Talavera de la Reina, Spain
e-mail: Javier.aceituno@uclm.es

D. Stasinopoulos (ed.), *Application of Electrophysical Agents in Physiotherapy*,
https://doi.org/10.1007/978-3-032-32144-2_5

the most effective wavelengths for laser therapy fall within the visible red (RL) and near-infrared (NIR) regions of the spectrum (approximately 390–1600 nm), due to their high absorption by biological tissues [6].

Low-level laser therapy (LLLT), also referred to as *soft laser therapy* or *cold laser therapy*, is the term used in the field of physical therapy to describe laser systems operating at powers below 500 mW, producing intensities insufficient to generate heat in the irradiated tissues [2]. In 2016, a new MeSH term, *photobiomodulation therapy*, was introduced, defined as a "non-thermal form of light therapy that utilizes non-ionizing light sources—including lasers, LEDs, and broadband light—in the visible and infrared spectrum" [9]. RL (600–700 nm) and NIR light (780–1100 nm) are the most commonly used wavelengths in photobiomodulation (PBM) [10].

In the first decade of the twenty-first century, *high-intensity laser therapy (HILT)* emerged as a new therapeutic modality [11], developed through the adaptation of a surgical Nd:YAG laser for therapeutic use by defocusing its emission [12]. This approach employs powers exceeding 0.5 W at a specific wavelength (1064 nm in the case of Nd:YAG), producing a controlled thermal effect within the irradiated tissues.

To the best of our knowledge, this is one of the first clinical manuals on electrophysical agents to include high-intensity laser therapy; until now, only low-level laser therapy has been addressed. The aim is to provide clinicians with evidence-based guidance for the therapeutic use of laser technology in clinical practice.

5.2 Biophysics

5.2.1 Light, Lasers, and the Electromagnetic Spectrum

Light is electromagnetic radiation (Fig. 5.1). Visible light corresponds to electromagnetic energy within or near the visible region of the spectrum (400–700 nm). Radiation with shorter wavelengths lies in the ultraviolet region, whereas

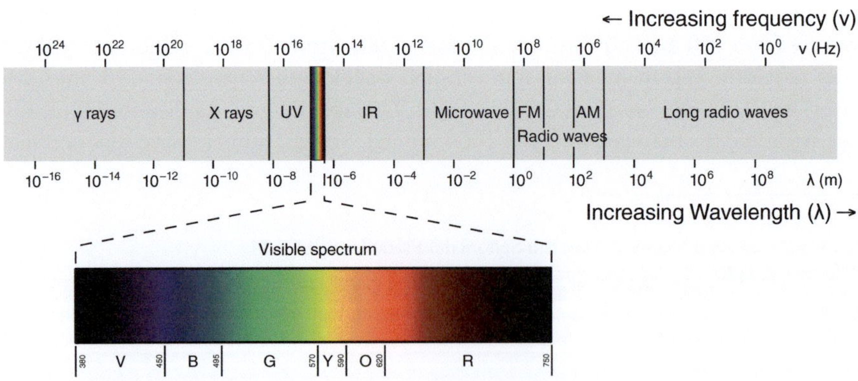

Fig. 5.1 Electromagnetic spectrum. (By User:Zedh and User:Gringer—and, CC BY-SA 3.0, https://commons.wikimedia.org/w/index.php?curid=144957951)

radiation with longer wavelengths corresponds to infrared radiation. Light consists of waves and discrete packets of energy known as photons [13]. Consequently, light exhibits a dual nature: it behaves both as a wave—demonstrated by Young's double-slit experiment—and as a particle, as evidenced by the photoelectric effect [14].

A laser is therefore a specific type of light characterized by being monochromatic, intense, unidirectional, and coherent. Its wavelength determines its precise position within the electromagnetic spectrum.

5.2.2 Stimulated Emission of Radiation

According to Planck's model, the atom consists of a nucleus surrounded by electrons that move in discrete orbits. When an electron occupies the lowest possible energy level, the atom is said to be in its ground state. When the electron is located at a higher energy level, the atom is considered to be in an excited state.

Through the processes of absorption and emission, light can induce transitions between atomic energy levels.

Absorption Light absorption occurs most efficiently when the energy of the incident photons matches the energy difference between two atomic energy levels. This results in an increased number of electrons transitioning to excited states within the atom or molecule.

Spontaneous emission An electron in an excited state is unstable and will eventually return to a lower energy level, emitting a photon whose energy corresponds to the difference between the two levels.

Stimulated emission When a photon interacts with an atom that is already in an excited state, it induces the atom to return to its ground state while emitting a second photon. This emitted photon is identical to the incident photon in energy, phase, direction, and polarization. Stimulated emission occurs only in the presence of an electromagnetic field. As the number of photons increases, further stimulated emissions are induced in other excited atoms, resulting in an amplification effect.

In general, a medium contains a mixture of atoms in the ground state (which absorb radiation) and atoms in excited states (which amplify radiation through stimulated emission). For laser operation to occur, the balance between absorption and amplification must favor stimulated emission. This condition is known as population inversion [1, 14] (Fig. 5.2).

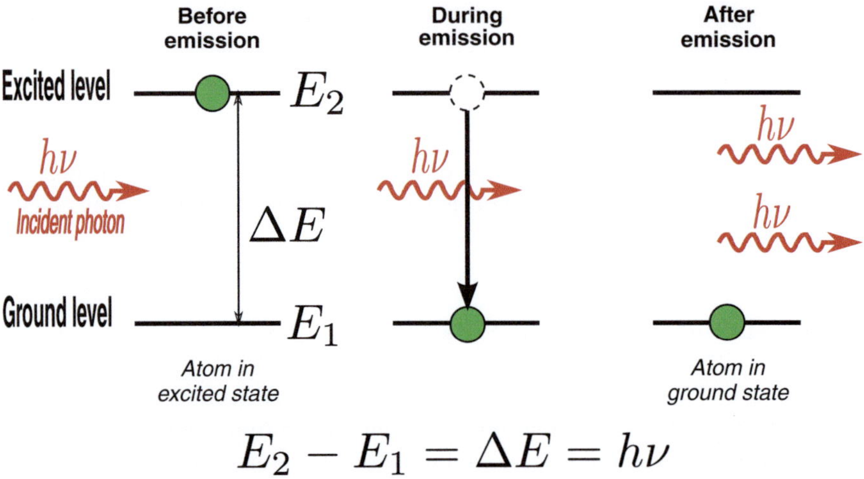

Fig. 5.2 Stimulated emission. (By V1adis1av (talk·contribs)—Own work, CC BY-SA 4.0, https://commons.wikimedia.org/w/index.php?curid=3983414)

5.2.3 Elements of a Laser

A laser system consists essentially of three fundamental components (Fig. 5.3):

Active medium A solid, liquid, or gaseous material that emits a specific radiation after being stimulated.

Activation source or pump system This component supplies energy to the active medium, enabling and sustaining stimulated emission over time by producing population inversion within the medium.

Optical resonator or resonant cavity This consists of a closed cavity with two opposing reflective surfaces that amplify electromagnetic waves traveling along the cavity axis. One of the mirrors is partially reflective, allowing a fraction of the radiation to exit the cavity as the laser beam. The resulting emission is coherent, with a constant phase relationship, directional, as only photons aligned with the cavity axis are amplified, and monochromatic, since all photons have the same wavelength [1, 14].

5.2.4 Laser Classification

Lasers can be classified according to several parameters:

(a) *According to emission power (Watts)*

Low-power lasers (Low-Level Laser Therapy, LLLT; cold laser or soft laser): emission power below 0.5 W.

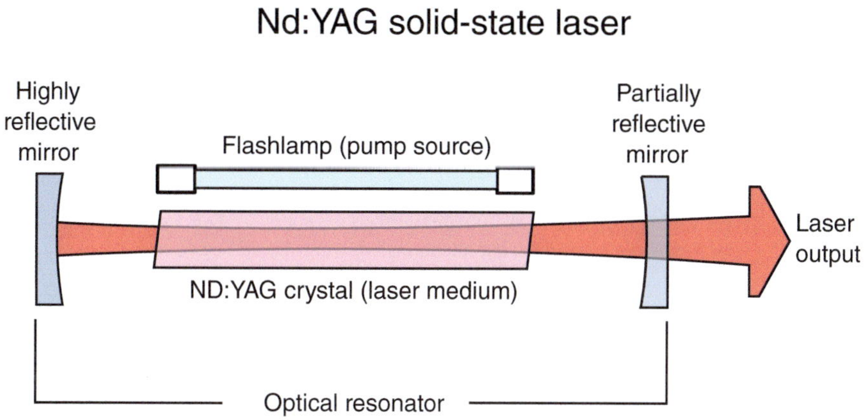

Fig. 5.3 Schematic diagram of a Nd:YAG laser. (By Lakkasuo—Own work, CC BY-SA 3.0, https://commons.wikimedia.org/w/index.php?curid=11446767)

High-power lasers (High-Intensity Laser Therapy, HILT; High-Power Laser Therapy, HPLT or Class IV): emission power above 0.5 W, typically exceeding 1 W.

(b) *According to the active medium*

Gas lasers: The active medium consists of a gas or gas mixture. Examples include He–Ne lasers, CO_2 lasers, and excimer (excited dimer) lasers.

Solid-state lasers: The active medium is a solid material (crystal or glass) doped with a small concentration of ions that emit laser radiation. Examples include Nd:YAG, Alexandrite, and Ruby lasers.

Liquid lasers: The active medium consists of organic dye solutions dissolved in liquids such as methyl alcohol.

Semiconductor lasers: Also known as diode lasers, in which the active medium is a semiconductor material or a semiconductor junction.

(c) *According to wavelength*

Wavelength is a key parameter, as it determines tissue penetration depth and absorption characteristics. Examples include: He–Ne (633 nm), dye lasers (450–900 nm), Nd:YAG (1064 nm), and ArF (194 nm).

(d) *According to emission mode*

Continuous wave (CW): Constant energy output over time.

Pulsed emission: Energy is delivered in pulses. Superpulsed: Very short and frequent pulses.

Q-switched: High-intensity pulses of very short duration (nanoseconds) [15].

(e) *According to IEC 60825–1 classification*

This classification is based on the potential hazards posed by laser radiation to the eyes and skin [16]. In physical therapy, Class 3R and 3B (low power) and Class 4 (high power) devices are commonly used (Table 5.1).

Table 5.1 Laser classification according to UNE EN 60825-1/A2-2002 and IEC 60825-1:07-2015

Class 1	Laser products that are safe under normal operating conditions
Class 1M	Emit radiation in the wavelength range of 302.5–4000 nm; may be hazardous when viewed with optical instruments
Class 1C	Introduced in IEC 60825–1:2015; includes lasers designed for direct contact with the target (e.g., skin). Protective measures ensure emissions do not exceed Class 1 limits.
Class 2	Emit visible radiation (400–700 nm) with power not exceeding 1 mW. Accidental exposure is not hazardous, but intentional viewing should be avoided
Class 2M	Emit visible radiation; hazardous when viewed with optical instruments
Class 3R	Emit radiation between 302.5 and 106 nm. Direct viewing is potentially hazardous. Safety requirements are less stringent than for classes 3B and 4. The accessible emission limit (AEL) is less than five times that of class 2 (400–700 nm) or class 1 at other wavelengths
Class 3B	Direct viewing is hazardous; maximum continuous wave output of 500 mW
Class 4	Direct and diffuse reflections are hazardous and can cause eye and skin injury. Their use requires extreme caution

Prepared by the author based on data from the National Institute for Occupational Safety and Health (www.insht.es) and laserworld.com. Accessed on 12/01/2026

5.2.5 Glossary of Laser Terminology

(a) *Characteristics of laser light*

Monochromaticity: The emitted light consists of a single wavelength with a very narrow spectral bandwidth.

Coherence: The emitted waves maintain a constant phase relationship in both time and space.

Directionality: The ability of laser radiation to propagate with minimal divergence, allowing it to be focused onto a very small spot.

Nondivergence: Photons propagate in parallel trajectories.

Brightness: The power emitted per unit area along a single spectral line [14, 17].

(b) *Laws governing laser emission*

Laser emission used in phototherapy is governed by the following physical laws:

Inverse Square Law: Radiation intensity is inversely proportional to the square of the distance between the source and the receiving surface.

Lambert's Cosine Law: Maximum radiation intensity on a surface is achieved when the beam is incident perpendicular to that surface.

Bunsen–Roscoe Law: The product of radiation intensity and exposure time raised to a power remains constant.

Grotthuss–Draper Law: Only radiation that is absorbed by tissues produces a biological effect [18].

5.3 Dosology and Parameters

The vast majority of studies analyzing the effectiveness of laser therapy in different pathologies tend to refer to the establishment of treatment protocols, dosages according to the pathology, etc., to mitigate the high heterogeneity present. Much of this may stem from a lack of minimum data or essential information to provide about the treatment protocol performed, whether in case series, clinical trials, etc., both to make effective comparisons and derive evidence-based dosages to guide treatment, and for the replicability of these protocols in other clinical populations.

Shurrab proposes standardized guidelines for reporting parameters and procedures of HLLT and LLLT in medical research articles, aiming to improve clarity, reproducibility, and scientific rigor in clinical reporting, because frequent omissions of essential data have been demonstrated [19].

5.3.1 What, Therefore, Would Be the Essential Information for This Purpose?

There are nine fundamental parameters for replicating the clinical application of a laser procedure, eleven if we consider irradiance and fluence separately: wavelength, operating mode, power and power density, energy and energy density, spot size, pulse parameters, irradiation time, number of treatments, and cooling (mainly relevant in HILT) [19]. Some authors consider the five essential parameters for maximizing the benefits of the laser device to be wavelength, power, spot size, pulse width, and cooling, although in this case the focus is on dermatological procedures [20], hence the inclusion of cooling. The duty cycle [21], the application mode of the technique, and the body site of application also provide relevant information [22], although these last two are external to the laser device. Recent research has introduced a new parameter in HILT therapy, the Pulse Energy Dose (PED). This parameter is used to assess laser-induced pressure waves and ensure that HILT systems operate safely within the thermoelastic window [23]. Without forgetting the patient's own data regarding the area to be treated: cross-sectional area, depth and volume of the area, skin type [24]. Indeed, sex-related data may help anticipate penetration depth, as some studies suggest that tissue penetration is greater in women than in men [25].

According to the World Association for Photobiomodulation Therapy (WALT), the number of sessions and the weekly frequency must be included, in addition to the data applied in each session: application procedure, wavelength, treatment time in seconds, energy in Joules, spot size in cm^2, power density in W/cm^2, and accumulated energy delivered from all sessions in Joules [26]. These guidelines must contain at least four types of parameters: (I) device manufacturer, (II) irradiation parameters, (III) treatment dosages and intervals, and (IV) protocol [19].

5.3.2 Parameters

Wavelength The distance between two subsequent peaks or troughs of a light wave. Usually, it is expressed in nm. Influencing tissue penetration depth and biological effects on target cells depends on the absorption of photons by chromophores (hemoglobin, melanin, exogenous pigments, water, and fat) and the part of the electromagnetic spectrum where they are located; shorter wavelengths (higher frequency) result in less tissue penetration, while longer wavelengths (lower frequency) result in greater tissue penetration [7, 19]. In this regard, simulation models corroborate an increase in tissue penetration depth as wavelength increases [27]. The choice of wavelength is fundamental to its relationship with the optical properties of the tissues (reflection and refraction) and the absorption by surface chromophores within the therapeutic window between 600 and 1100 nm. The wavelength of 1064 nm achieves greater penetration compared to 810 and 970 nm [8].

Operating mode Continuous wave (CW) emits constantly, while pulsed wave (PW) allows for higher peak intensities. In this respect, CW has been the gold standard for LLLT, although pulsed wave (PW) can be superior to CW, especially in wound healing and stroke. CW as a single treatment is more effective than PW in nerve regeneration [28].

Power Describes the amount of energy delivered, measured in watts (W) or milliwatts (mW). We can talk about *Peak Power*: which is the maximum energy output of a laser in short pulses, and *Average Power*: which is calculated by dividing the total energy emitted by the total emission time; it is used to determine whether or not to minimize the thermal effect. *Power Density, or irradiance*, is the average power divided by a unit of surface area (W/cm^2), useful for calculating tissue penetration.

Energy density The amount of energy deposited per unit area (J/cm^2), is the most frequently used measure of therapeutic dose in most devices, both LLLT and HILT, and allows for selecting the appropriate dose. Energy (J) or Fluence (J/cm^2).

Spot size This refers to the cross-sectional area of the laser beam and is expressed in cm^2. In clinical practice, it affects fluence (energy density) [19] and irradiance (power density) [29]. Decreasing the spot size decreases the depth of penetration [20, 30].

Pulse width Pulse width is the delivery time or exposure time of the selected energy delivered to the target tissue [20]. It is the duration of a light spot expressed in a unit of time.

Pulse repetition rate This is the number of times the pulse is repeated per unit of time, measured in Hertz (Hz).

Duty cycle (%) This is the fraction of time the laser is emitting pulses within a given time period, the time it is active. It is expressed as a percentage. The duty cycle in a pulsed laser system refers to the proportion of time the laser is actively emitting light compared to the total time period of the laser's operation. It's usually expressed as a percentage and is calculated by dividing the pulse duration by the pulse period, then multiplying by 100. This simple formula helps in understanding how long the laser is on versus off during each cycle.

A difference is established based on the duty cycle between high-intensity lasers (HILT) and high-power lasers (HPLT), where HILT has very low duty cycles (0.01–1%) with microsecond pulse durations and a low repetition rate with high power peaks. HPLT, on the other hand, operates with higher duty cycles (10–100%) with quasi-continuous pulses and medium-high power levels; however, the peak power is not as high. Photoacoustic effects are obtained with the former but not with the latter [31].

Cooling In order to lower the temperature of the compartments [19], cooling devices ensure the maintenance of a lower temperature at the epidermal level, yet reach the required higher temperature at the target level [32].

Pulse Energy Dose Equation (PED) Evaluates fluence in relation to penetration depth and emission time. In essence, if we know the spot size, peak power, and pulse repetition frequency, we can calculate the Pulse Energy Dose (PED) in J/cm^3 [23] (Table 5.2).

Table 5.2 Clinical laser parameters and their practical significance

Parameter	Unit	Typical clinical range	Clinical meaning/ practical significance	Common clinical mistake
Wavelength	Nm	~600–1100 nm (PBM range)	Determines depth of penetration and chromophore absorption; shorter wavelengths act more superficially, longer wavelengths penetrate deeper tissues	Assuming all wavelengths produce identical effects regardless of tissue depth
Power output	mW or W	Device-dependent	Influences energy delivery rate and treatment time	Power changes without adjusting treatment time or dose
Irradiance (power density)	mW or W/ cm^2	Variable (protocol dependent)	Power supplied to the tissue per unit area. Determines how quickly energy is delivered	Do not adjust irradiance according to target depth. Forget that high irradiance (HILT) in static application can burn the patient

(continued)

Table 5.2 (continued)

Parameter	Unit	Typical clinical range	Clinical meaning/ practical significance	Common clinical mistake
Energy density (fluence)	J/cm^2	Variable (condition dependent)	Total energy delivered per unit area; primary dosing parameter in photobiomodulation	Using excessively high fluence expecting stronger effects (ignoring biphasic response)
Spot size/ beam area	cm^2	Device-specific	Determines treatment precision and influences actual delivered dose	Ignoring spot size when calculating dose, leading to under- or overdosing
Treatment time	Seconds/ minutes	Calculated according to dose	Depends on power and target energy density	Using fixed time protocols instead of dose-based calculations
Emission mode	Continuous/ pulsed	Protocol dependent	Influences thermal accumulation and biological response	Assuming pulsed mode is always superior regardless of treatment goals
Duty cycle	%	10–100%	Defines percentage of active emission in pulsed mode; lower duty cycles reduce thermal effects	Ignoring duty cycle when calculating average energy delivery
Total energy delivered	Joules (J)	Calculated per session	Useful for documentation and treatment reproducibility	Reporting only power settings without total energy delivered
Treatment frequency	Sessions/ week	Typically 2–5 (condition dependent)	Determines cumulative biological dose across treatment course	Using identical frequency for acute and chronic conditions

5.3.3 Dosage

When determining laser dosage, the concept of "hormesis" must be taken into account. Hormesis explains the biphasic dose–response relationship observed in photobiomodulation, whereby LLLT administered at low doses tends to be more effective than the same wavelength delivered at higher doses [33, 34]. This phenomenon is grounded in the Arndt–Schulz law, a cornerstone of photobiomodulation, which describes a two-phase response curve dependent on the applied dose

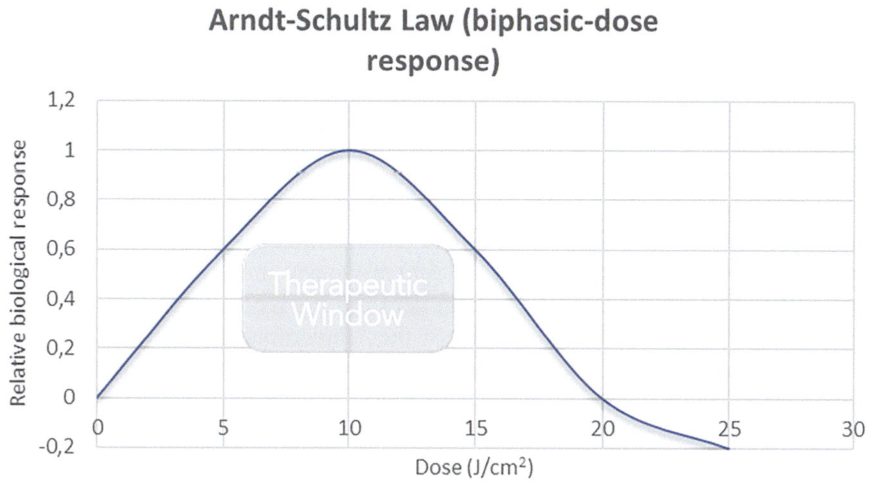

Fig. 5.4 Example of biphasic dose-response curve. Increased effectiveness up to a maximum point (≈10 J/cm^2), beyond which increasing the dose is less effective and even harmful

(Fig. 5.4). This principle suggests that there is an optimal therapeutic window for stimulation, while lower doses effectively promote cellular repair and anti-inflammatory processes, but excessively high doses (over-dosing) can reach an inhibitory threshold, potentially suppressing the desired biological response or leading to cellular stress [33]. Precise calibration of energy density is therefore essential to remain within the stimulatory range.

In photobiomodulation, increasing stimulus intensity is primarily achieved through longer exposure times and/or higher irradiance levels. This biphasic behavior challenges the Bunsen–Roscoe law of reciprocity, which posits that photochemical reactions in biological tissues are proportional to the total energy dose, irrespective of how that dose is distributed over time [34]. Supporting the hormetic model, experimental evidence indicates that red or near-infrared fluences as low as 3–5 J/cm^2 produce beneficial "in vivo" effects, whereas substantially higher doses, such as 50–100 J/cm^2, do not enhance therapeutic outcomes and may even induce adverse effects [33]. It is widely accepted that low fluences are associated with stimulatory effects, while high fluences are linked to inhibitory effects [10].

5.3.3.1 Dosage in Low-Level Laser Therapy

Low-level laser therapy typically employs wavelengths ranging from 600 to 1000 nm [35], with output powers between 1 and 500 mW [36]. Commonly reported energy densities range from 1 to 9 J/cm^2, and treatment protocols may involve single-, dual-, or triple-wavelength light sources [35].

Despite the considerable heterogeneity among studies and the frequent absence of statistically significant differences between parameters associated with positive outcomes versus those yielding no clinical improvement, several attempts have been made to propose pathology-adjusted dosages. Based on aggregated findings, it has been estimated that a wavelength of approximately 810 nm, an average power of 116 mW, a pulse frequency of 2588 Hz, an application time of 5.6 minutes, and a total of 11.7 treatment sessions are associated with improved clinical outcomes [35].

Bjordal et al. proposed wavelength- and device-specific power density ranges, with the highest values reported for 632 nm HeNe red-light lasers (3–500 mW/cm^2), followed by near-infrared GaAlAs and continuous-wave Nd:YAG lasers operating at 820, 830, and 1060 nm (15–500 mW/cm^2), and pulsed GaAs lasers at 904 nm (6–210 mW/cm^2). Lower power densities are recommended for superficial structures, such as finger joints or the temporomandibular joint (TMJ), whereas higher values are required for deeper anatomical targets, including vertebral joints [37].

The World Association for Photobiomodulation Therapy provides wavelength-specific dosage recommendations for LLLT. For Class 3B GaAlAs lasers operating at 780–860 nm, whether continuous or pulsed, with mean output powers ranging from 5 to 500 mW, irradiation times should range from 20 to 300 seconds. The recommended energy per point lies between 4 and 16 J, depending on the anatomical structure treated [38]. For Class 3B GaAs lasers at 904 nm (nanosecond pulsed lasers with peak output >5 mW or power density > 5 mW/cm^2), effective doses range from 1 to 4 J per point, with irradiation times between 30 and 600 seconds, depending on output characteristics [39].

In both cases, treatment is typically administered daily over a two-week period or on alternate days over 3–4 weeks, with a gradual reduction in intensity—up to 30% of the initial dose—as symptoms improve. Subsequent research has confirmed the continued suitability of these dosage ranges [38–40], while also highlighting the frequent absence of clear dose–response analyses in the published literature [41]. Accordingly, when LLLT is applied for pain management in musculoskeletal disorders, adherence to WALT-recommended dosages is associated with superior analgesic outcomes [42] and more favorable outcomes [43].

5.3.3.2 Dosage in High-Intensity Laser Therapy

In High-intensity laser therapy, wavelengths within the therapeutic window—generally between 800 and 1100 nm—are applied either individually or in combination. The most commonly used wavelength is 1064 nm, with systematic reviews indicating that approximately 73% of randomized controlled trials (RCTs) employ this wavelength [44, 45]. In more than 80% of studies using 1064 nm, Nd:YAG lasers serve as the active medium, whereas fewer studies utilize GdAl, GaAl, or unspecified laser media.

Combined-wavelength protocols reported in the literature include 830 + 1064 nm, 800 + 915 nm, 800 + 970 nm, 808 + 905 nm, 810 + 980 nm, and broadband ranges spanning 780–1100 nm. Single-wavelength applications at 808 nm, 940 nm, and 980 nm have also been documented [44, 45]. Overall, 1064 nm remains the most extensively studied and utilized wavelength in HILT, likely due to its superior tissue penetration capacity.

Meta-analyses examining the effects of HILT in musculoskeletal disorders consistently report substantial heterogeneity in both study populations and treatment protocols [44, 45]. A recurring limitation across systematic reviews is the absence of subgroup analyses that would allow inferences regarding optimal dosages for specific pathologies or anatomical regions. Only one study focusing on musculoskeletal disorders conducted a subgroup analysis based on applied energy density. No statistically significant differences were observed when comparing four dosage ranges (<10 J/cm^2, 10–50 J/cm^2, 50–100 J/cm^2, and 100–300 J/cm^2); however, analgesic effects tended to diminish as dosage increased. In terms of functional outcomes, intermediate dosage ranges demonstrated greater effect sizes than the extremes, despite the lack of statistical significance. Notably, energy densities between 10 and 50 J/cm^2 appeared to yield the most favorable results for both pain reduction and functional improvement [44]. Based on research and with the need for future observations, a mínimum cumulative dose of approximately 300 joules per session over 6–8 sessions may serve as a preliminary reference for HILT [21].

This tendency toward enhanced analgesic efficacy at lower energy densities in HILT is further supported by Ezzati et al., who reported superior outcomes with a dose of 8 J/cm^2 compared to 20 J/cm^2 [46]. Such findings may be partially explained by the modulation of the endogenous opioid system induced by laser irradiation [47].

5.4 Mechanism of Action

It should be noted that the optical properties of tissues can influence the results of the laser [48]. The interaction of light with body tissues is mediated by the physical properties of light: a small part is reflected [49], and another part is scattered within the tissues. This scattering is wavelength-dependent; the shorter the wavelength, the greater the degree of scattering [50]. This scattering is conditioned by refraction, or changes in direction as the light passes through different tissue elements [2]. Another part is absorbed by chromophores, which are endogenous molecules that absorb photons of a specific wavelength [48]. Examples include water, melanin, hemoglobin, and deoxyhemoglobin. This light energy can stimulate the chromophores to activate chemical reactions [7]. The presence of exogenous pigments, such as tattoo ink, medications, or other chromophore-containing substances, should also be taken into account, as they may absorb part of the incident laser energy, thereby decreasing tissue penetration and reducing the amount of energy reaching the target structure.

To achieve a broader cellular response, the concept of the optical window or therapeutic window must be considered. This is where optimal laser light penetration into tissues occurs and is found in the wavelength range between 600 nm and 1100 nm [51], due to low absorption by surface chromophores (water and hemoglobin), which allows for greater tissue penetration [12]. Optimizing penetration and absorption is key to achieving the therapeutic objectives in the target structure.

Utilizing wavelengths within this near-infrared spectrum allows the energy to reach deeper musculoskeletal structures—such as tendons, ligaments, and joint capsules—that would otherwise be inaccessible to shorter wavelengths.

5.4.1 Physiological Effects

According to the first law of photochemistry, also known as the Grotthuss–Draper law, photons must be absorbed by chromophores for any biological or cellular effect to occur [51]. Consequently, the primary—or direct—cellular effects of photobiomodulation are associated with the absorption of photon energy by mitochondrial chromophores [52], most notably cytochrome c oxidase (COX). COX is considered the main photoacceptor within mitochondria for red light (RL; 620–750 nm) [51].

For shorter wavelengths, different chromophores have been identified: in the blue spectrum (380–500 nm), cryptochromes, flavins, flavoproteins [5, 51, 53], and porphyrins [53] act as the primary photoacceptors. In the green wavelength range (500–570 nm), opsins [5] and potentially light-gated calcium (Ca^{2+}) channels [53] have been proposed as chromophores. In the near-infrared range (750–1100 nm), COX again appears to be the dominant chromophore [51, 53]. At wavelengths exceeding 1000 nm, water molecules may act as alternative chromophores through the activation of heat-sensitive ion channels [5].

Tissues with a high mitochondrial density—such as muscle, visceral organs, and nervous tissue—demonstrate a greater responsiveness to photobiomodulation compared to tissues with lower mitochondrial content, including tendons and bone [50]. Mitochondrial content may influence cellular responses to PBM [54]. At this stage, the therapeutic response is determined by the interplay between the optical properties of the tissue, the mitochondrial density of the irradiated cells, and the wavelength of the emitted laser radiation.

Secondary effects, also referred to as intracellular responses, are induced as a consequence of these primary photochemical events [52]. Specifically, stimulation of COX by red and near-infrared light leads to increased mitochondrial production of adenosine triphosphate (ATP), cyclic adenosine monophosphate (cAMP), the generation of reactive oxygen species (ROS), and elevated intracellular calcium (Ca^{2+}) levels (Maghfour). In addition, laser irradiation promotes the dissociation of nitric oxide (NO) from COX, resulting in an increased mitochondrial respiratory rate (Farivar) and the restoration of ATP synthesis [48].

These intracellular signaling events subsequently activate transcription factors such as nuclear factor kappa B (NF-κB) and activator protein 1 (AP-1), which regulate the expression of genes involved in key biological processes, including cell proliferation, migration, differentiation, apoptosis [55], wound healing, and pain modulation [51]. Photobiomodulation evokes intra- and extracellular redox mechanisms [56].

Tertiary effects have been described with some conceptual variability in the literature. Several authors include within this category the activation of a broad range of transcription factors leading to enhanced cell survival, increased proliferation and migration, and de novo protein synthesis [57]. These effects may align with the concept of indirect responses occurring in cells that were not directly exposed to photons but are influenced by signaling from irradiated cells. However, in the original definition proposed by Dyson, tertiary effects encompassed the systemic responses to phototherapy, extending beyond the local cellular environment [52, 58].

Ultimately, photobiomodulation induces a cascade of photochemical and photobiological reactions, beginning with photon absorption by surface or intracellular chromophores and culminating in clinically observable outcomes such as analgesic, anti-inflammatory, and biostimulatory effects.

5.4.2 Therapeutic Effects

Therapeutic effects are closely linked to the physiological mechanisms that generate them, as emphasized by Dyson through the introduction of the concept of tertiary effects, which encompass the systemic responses of the organism and ultimately correspond to therapeutic outcomes [52]. From a clinical perspective, Maya and Albornoz also proposed a classification in which laser emission produces primary or direct effects—including thermal, mechanical, biochemical, bioelectrical, and bioenergetic effects—which, through indirect effects such as microcirculatory stimulation and cellular trophic activation, lead to general therapeutic effects [59].

These general therapeutic effects include analgesic, anti-inflammatory, anti-edematous, and biostimulatory responses. Analgesic effects are attributed to an increased pain threshold secondary to neurometabolic activation and elevated endorphin levels [60]. Anti-inflammatory and anti-edematous effects result from enhanced microcirculation, modulation of prostaglandin levels, restoration of osmotic pressure balance [60], and a reduction in pro-inflammatory cytokine levels [48]. Cytokines play a fundamental role in regulating inflammation and immune responses [5, 51], and photobiomodulation has been shown to upregulate anti-inflammatory genes while downregulating pro-inflammatory gene expression [51].

Biostimulatory effects are mediated through modulation of gene expression and the release of growth factors [48], as well as alterations in messenger RNA (mRNA) levels [61]. In addition, Moshkovska and Mayberry describe further therapeutic outcomes, including stabilization of lipid peroxidation, stimulation of immune responses, and reflexogenic effects, which together contribute to the activation of physiological functions [62].

Consequently, laser irradiation within the red light and near-infrared ranges provides both analgesic benefits and stimulation of tissue repair processes [51]. The literature reports that RL and NIR have therapeutic effects in promoting tissue healing and alleviating inflammation [63]. Blue and green laser wavelengths have also been shown to stimulate osteoblastic differentiation [53] and act as antimicrobial and tissue-repair agents in superficial tissue layers. Blue light has demonstrated efficacy in superficial tissue repair and antimicrobial activity [51, 53, 63], whereas the therapeutic effects of green light require further investigation, although current evidence suggests potential roles in skin rejuvenation and inflammation reduction [51, 63].

5.4.3 Are There Additional Effects with High-Intensity Laser Therapy?

Photochemical, photomechanical, and photothermal biological effects collectively contribute to the analgesic, anti-inflammatory, and biostimulatory outcomes that are central to the patient's clinical response (Fig. 5.5). The photochemical effect—characterized by mitochondrial activation and redox modulation—is typical of low-level laser therapy (LLLT) [23], with photothermal responses largely confined to superficial tissues [31].

In contrast, high-power laser therapy (HPLT) combines photochemical and photothermal effects, including heat-induced vasodilation, collagen remodeling, and analgesia mediated by high average power output. High-intensity laser therapy (HILT) further incorporates a distinct mechanical component: mechanotransductive stimulation generated by short-duration, high–peak-power pulses that produce acoustic pressure waves. These waves arise from transient thermoelastic expansion following the emission of very high peak powers lasting microseconds, resulting in photoacoustic effects that are characteristic of HILT [23].

Some authors do not distinguish photoacoustic effects as a separate mechanism and instead group all such effects under the broader designation of HILT, considering mechanical effects to be secondary to thermal effects, as they induce changes in tissue morphology and structure [49].

HILT is capable of penetrating deeper into tissues, allowing for greater energy deposition at depth [29]. Accordingly, higher power outputs result in increased energy transmission with reduced dispersion in superficial tissues and enhanced therapeutic effects in deeper structures [3, 12], particularly in larger and/or deeper

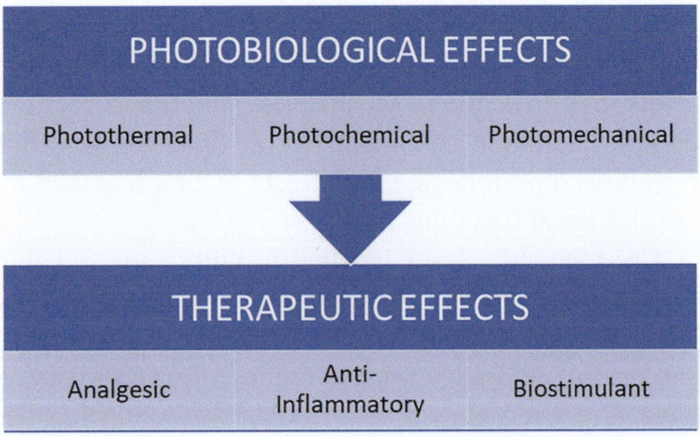

Fig. 5.5 Schematic representation of therapeutic effects

joints when compared with LLLT [64]. While LLLT primarily produces athermal and superficial effects (approximately 3–4 cm penetration), consistent with the Arndt–Schulz law, HILT can deliver therapeutic energy to deeper tissues (up to 10–12 cm), adding significant thermal effects to those achieved with LLLT [21].

Collectively, these mechanisms lead to enhanced tissue healing, increased collagen production, improved bone repair, modulation of inflammatory processes, optimized nerve regeneration, and enhanced muscle regeneration [65]. In addition to its increased thermal and mechanical therapeutic effects and improved access to deeper tissues, HILT offers a further clinical advantage over LLLT by significantly reducing the treatment time required to deliver an equivalent amount of energy to the tissues [43, 64, 66].

In conclusion, high-intensity laser therapy provides deeper tissue penetration, achieves therapeutic benefits through combined photothermal and photomechanical mechanisms, and reduces treatment duration compared with low-level laser therapy. These characteristics support the clinical utility of HILT in conditions requiring deeper tissue engagement and enhanced biological stimulation.

5.5 Indications, Contraindications, Precautions, and Side Effects

5.5.1 Indications

Due to the analgesic, anti-inflammatory, and biostimulatory effects of laser emission, it is generally indicated for soft tissue injuries, enhancement of ulcer and wound healing, arthritic and osteoarthritic conditions, and a variety of pain syndromes. This section will outline the main indications for both LLLT and HILT, which will be further detailed in the research evidence section.

5.5.1.1 Indications for Low-Level Laser Therapy

- *Pain relief*:
  LLLT has demonstrated effectiveness in reducing pain associated with musculoskeletal disorders, irrespective of the anatomical region (back, elbow, foot, hand, knee, neck, perineal region, shoulder, wrist) [42] among the nonpharmacological approaches to the temporomandibular joint, LLLT showed a high effect for treating this painful joint [67], LLLT is an approach with few side effects that reduces pain and morning stiffness in rheumatoid arthritis [68]. It offers a therapeutic option for alleviating acute and chronic pain in musculoskeletal conditions and in fibromyalgia [69]. Laser emission is effective both as an adjunct to therapeutic exercise and as a stand-alone intervention compared with placebo, reducing pain intensity, fatigue, and the number of tender points [70].
- *Wound healing*:
  Significant reductions in wound size and pain have been reported with 660 nm wavelengths [71]. Photobiomodulation at red wavelengths enhances healing in stage 2 and 3 pressure injuries compared with standard care [72]. Effective wave-

lengths typically range from 650 to 950 nm, with doses of 1–10 J/cm^2 [73]. Some authors suggest that 808 nm may be superior for promoting wound contraction and epithelialization compared with 830 nm and 980 nm [74]. When comparing LLLT with light-emitting diodes (LEDs), another PBM modality, both demonstrate similar preclinical efficacy; however, LLLT has shown greater increases in capillary density and type I collagen deposition [75].

- *Bone healing*:
  In the systematic review by Neto, no radiographic changes were observed after PBM, although improvements in pain and function were noted [76]. Compared with other electrophysical agents, LLLT demonstrated the greatest effect on pain reduction in fractures [77]. In subsequent studies with a larger number of trials, results were mixed: approximately half reported improvements in bone density and regeneration, while the remainder found no significant differences [78]. A recent animal-model meta-analysis concluded that although LLLT may enhance fracture healing, it does not affect maximum fracture force or hydroxyapatite Raman peaks [79]. A deeper understanding of the cellular mechanisms activated by LLLT is needed to optimize its clinical application [80].
- *Neurological disorders*:
  Preclinical and clinical studies have shown that PBM enhances central nervous system function and reduces peripheral nerve inflammation [81], offering considerable potential for neurological applications. High-power lasers with shorter wavelengths (below 760 nm) are indicated for deeper brain structures (e.g., brain injury, Parkinson's disease), whereas low-level lasers with wavelengths above 760 nm are better suited for superficial cortical applications such as cognitive disorders [82]. Transcranial PBM has shown improved outcomes in acute stroke [83]. Animal studies report positive effects in chronic stroke, traumatic brain injury, and neurodegenerative disorders [83]. Typical effective wavelengths include 665 and 810 nm [84]. Combining LLLT with other electrophysical agents—such as low-frequency electromagnetic fields [85], static magnetic fields [86], or neuromuscular electrical stimulation [87, 88]—may further enhance mobility and cognitive function [81]. PBM is applied both acutely as a neuroprotective/restorative therapy and chronically to improve symptoms or function [84].
- *Neuropathic pain*:
  Near-infrared wavelengths, particularly 800–900 nm with moderate energy densities, provide the most favorable outcomes [53]. In diabetic peripheral neuropathy, PBM has been shown to be effective and efficient in managing pain and altering plantar pressure in the diabetic foot [89].
  PBM Therapy in the Management of Orofacial Neuropathic Pain has been addressed by WALT through a position paper for developing WALT recommendations by delivering evidence-based Clinical Practical Guidelines for PBM in the management of neuropathic pain associated with various orofacial clinical conditions [90].
- *Peripheral nerve lesions*:
  LLLT benefits patients with peripheral nerve injury by reducing pain and improving sensory electromyography outcomes, though not motor outcomes [91].

- *Sport performance and muscle recovery*:
  Despite the low quality of evidence, the use of LLLT suggests improvements for exertion and recovery in athletes [92] and for improving recovery from sports-related injuries [93].
- *Lymphedema*:
  The use of LLLT for breast cancer–related lymphedema (BCRL), either as a standalone intervention or combined with other therapeutic approaches, has been shown to reduce swelling and pain in women with BCRL [94], alleviating symptoms by decreasing limb inflammation and improving quality of life. Greater therapeutic benefits have been reported with treatment protocols applying LLLT three times per week at a fluence of 1.5–2 J/cm^2 for inflammation reduction [95]. LLLT has demonstrated effectiveness in reducing arm volume and circumference, as well as improving shoulder mobility and pain [96].
  Nevertheless, some authors highlight that the overall low quality of evidence limits the certainty of these findings and complicates the formulation of strong clinical recommendations, underscoring the need for additional high-quality randomized controlled trials [97].

5.5.1.2 Indications for High-Intensity Laser Therapy

- *Musculoskeletal disorders*:
  Several systematic reviews with meta-analyses have shown that HILT is effective compared with placebo or other treatments for pain and functional improvement [44, 98, 99]. This remains the most extensively studied indication for HILT, encompassing disorders of the temporomandibular joint, cervical and lumbar spine, shoulder, elbow, wrist, knee, and foot. Specific systematic reviews on neck pain demonstrate improvements in pain and range of motion [100, 101]. HILT also reduces pain and disability in adhesive capsulitis [102], improves outcomes in spinal radiculopathy [103], and enhances pain and function in knee osteoarthritis [11]. It is additionally effective in reducing pain and disability and improving electrophysiological parameters in carpal tunnel syndrome (CTS) [104]
- *Wound healing*:
  Pulsed HILT has demonstrated effectiveness across several wound types, improving healing, reducing wound size, and decreasing pain and infection rates compared with standard care. Compared with LLLT, it offers greater depth of penetration and shorter session times, although care must be taken to avoid heat-related tissue damage [105]. A systematic review on foot ulcers (three RCTs: two diabetic, one neuropathic in children with spina bifida) showed improvements in wound surface area and appearance relative to placebo or standard care [106].
- *Osteopenia and osteoporosis*:
  Short-term evidence demonstrates that HILT combined with exercise is more effective than exercise alone or HILT alone for improving pain and quality of life [107]. After one year, HILT plus exercise is more effective than exercise alone in increasing lumbar bone mineral density in men with osteopenia [108]. In long-term osteoporotic hemiparetic patients, combining standard physiotherapy with

HILT or shockwave therapy improves outcomes, with HILT showing the greatest benefit [109].

- *Fibromyalgia and other pain syndromes*:
  A recent RCT evaluating HILT (1064 nm, mean power 10.5 W, fluence 610 mJ/cm^2) in women with fibromyalgia found significant improvements in pain, pressure pain threshold, health status, and quality of life compared with an exercise-only control [110].
  Positive effects have also been reported in complex regional pain syndrome type I of the hand using HILT (5 W; wavelengths 660, 800, 905, 970 nm; 20 J/cm^2) combined with mirror therapy, including reduction of pain and inflammation and improved muscle activity [111]. Several RCTs in hemiplegic shoulder pain post-stroke demonstrate significant improvements in pain, functional outcomes, ultrasound parameters [112], and grip strength [113].
  Laser therapy should be considered an adjunct intervention within a comprehensive rehabilitation program, supporting pain modulation and tissue healing while not replacing active therapeutic exercise and functional restoration strategies.

5.5.2 Contraindications and Precautions

Areas with active carcinoma, areas of infection, and the thoracoabdominal and pelvic regions in pregnant women [69] should be avoided, as well as direct irradiation of the retina, the use of photosensitive medications or drugs, epilepsy, and irradiation of the cervical region in cases of hyperthyroidism [114].

According to the Canadian Physiotherapy Association guidelines, regarding body structures, laser therapy is contraindicated over the eyes and gonads, and should be applied with caution over the carotid sinus and the anterior neck. With respect to specific conditions, it is contraindicated in hemorrhagic disorders and locally contraindicated in cases of active deep vein thrombosis or thrombophlebitis, malignancy, pregnancy, and tuberculosis. It should also be used cautiously in individuals with impaired cognition or communication, infection, photosensitivity, systemic lupus erythematosus, or recently irradiated tissues [115].

Over time, contraindications that were once considered absolute have evolved into relative or local contraindications—or even simple precautions—given current evidence suggesting that they may be safe and/or free of adverse effects [114]. In certain clinical situations, a thorough patient assessment and dose adjustments based on the patient's response are necessary [116].

Safety protocols are paramount. The primary risk associated with these laser devices is potential retinal damage from either direct or reflected beams (specular reflection). Consequently, the use of wavelength-specific safety goggles is mandatory for both the clinician and the patient throughout the treatment session.

Furthermore, particularly when utilizing Class 4 lasers (HILT), which deliver significantly higher power outputs than traditional LLLT for HILT, due to the rapid thermal accumulation associated with high irradiance, the laser handpiece must be kept in constant motion to prevent localized skin overheating or periosteal burns, especially over bony prominences, when working with thermal thresholds, particular caution is required in patients with impaired thermal sensitivity, as well as increased vigilance in individuals with higher skin phototypes (IV, V, and VI) and in areas containing exogenous pigments [3].

5.5.3 Adverse Effects

When PBM is applied by adequately trained personnel [117] and the appropriate preventive measures specific to each laser type are followed, the evidence indicates an absence of demonstrated adverse effects [69, 118], with reports describing an almost complete lack of side effects [24]. Only occasional cases of transient skin erythema or increased skin temperature have been documented [119] or mild sensations of pain/discomfort [10].

Regarding HILT, a systematic review including 48 clinical trials reported only a single case of photoallergy [120], although 62.5% of the RCTs did not specify this information [44]. Current evidence suggests that most complications are associated with thermal effects [117], underscoring the need to adjust the dose according to skin phototype [119]. Overall, HILT is considered a technique with a low incidence of adverse effects [98, 121].

5.6 Research Evidence

Laser therapy has been employed both conservatively and in surgical procedures by a wide range of healthcare professionals across various medical fields [122, 123], including dermatology [124], dentistry [125], podiatry [126], and physiotherapy. Photobiomodulation is applied in the management of numerous diseases and conditions beyond musculoskeletal disorders, as noted in the previous section, such as diabetes, traumatic brain injury, spinal cord damage, dermatological disorders, oral irritation, and in several dental specialties [127].

5.6.1 Musculoskeletal Conditions HILT Versus LLLT

The growing use of HILT as a therapeutic tool in the field of physical therapy has led to the development of studies comparing it with LLLT. Clinical trials in low back pain [128], dysmenorrhea [129], and plantar fasciitis [130] indicate that neither technique is superior to the other, nor do they show significant improvement over standard therapy [131], or that both lead to similarly satisfactory results in reducing pain [128–130] and disability [128]. The findings of these randomized controlled trials (RCTs) are further supported by systematic reviews on dysmenorrhea [132], tennis elbow [133], low back pain [134], and musculoskeletal disorders [135], which generally report no significant differences between the two modalities, or only slight advantages in favor of LLLT [132].

Evidence in favor of HILT over LLLT can be found in studies on knee osteoarthritis [64, 136, 137], where HILT has been shown to be either more effective [64], to produce more pronounced improvements in pain, functionality, and flexion range of motion than LLLT [136], or to achieve greater functional ability at one-month follow-up [137]. These significant improvements are confirmed in reviews and systematic reviews comparing both techniques, showing better outcomes in both pain reduction and functional improvement for the HILT group [138, 139]. Moreover, a 2022 network meta-analysis reported the superiority of HILT over other therapeutic modalities in terms of pain and self-reported function [140].

In shoulder disorders, when multimodal physiotherapy is applied, the addition of either LLLT or HILT to therapeutic exercise provides substantial benefits [141]. However, subsequent RCTs have indicated that the combination of HILT with therapeutic exercise is more effective than LLLT in terms of pain and functionality in subacromial impingement syndrome [142] and in adhesive capsulitis [143].

Regarding neck pain, Hao's 2024 network meta-analysis identified HILT as the primary physical agent to prioritize in treatment over other modalities (including LLLT) [144].

Finally, regarding plantar fasciitis, both techniques are safe and effective; however, HILT offers advantages in terms of its greater depth of tissue penetration and the need for fewer sessions to achieve therapeutic goals [145]. HILT may provide superior analgesic effects compared to LLLT, particularly when administered as a stand-alone intervention or in combination with exercise [21]. In comparison with LLLT, a network meta-analysis placed HILT combined with exercise among the top treatments for reducing musculoskeletal pain [43]. HILT may have potential in patients with chronic or refractory musculoskeletal pain due to the high energy delivered, in the context of a multimodal program [43].

5.6.2 Neurological and Pain Modulation Applications LLLT or HILT?

Photobiomodulation, delivered via low-level laser therapy (LLLT) or light-emitting diodes (LEDs), has been applied in the treatment of a wide range of central and peripheral nervous system disorders. Evidence suggests that combined PBM modalities may exert therapeutic effects and hold substantial potential for reducing adverse effects across various neurological conditions [81]. Nairuz et al. highlight the considerable promise of PBM—particularly through transcranial photobiomodulation—in the management of traumatic brain injuries, neurodegenerative diseases, neurodevelopmental disorders, and psychiatric conditions, underscoring the need for continued and rigorous research within the field of neuroscience [146]. Multiple sclerosis [147], incomplete spinal cord injury, and peripheral nerve injuries [148] represent additional pathological contexts in which, despite certain methodological limitations, clinical studies have reported symptom improvement with no major adverse effects.

Notably, some studies in the field of neurological pathology employ noncoherent light sources or LEDs, a form of photobiomodulation not covered in this chapter, for conditions including Parkinson's disease [149] and the treatment of cerebral palsy in children and adolescents [150].

However, better outcomes with HILT have been demonstrated in carpal tunnel syndrome, both in pain reduction and in electrophysiological parameters, compared to LLLT and therapeutic exercise alone [46], or demonstrate better outcomes, although without significant differences compared to LLLT [151].

5.6.3 Wound Healing and Tissue Repair—HILT or LLLT?

In this clinical indication, most of the available evidence supports the use of low-level laser therapy (LLLT), which has been shown to significantly reduce wound and ulcer size and to increase the proportion of complete wound healing compared with control interventions [71]. In contrast, high-intensity laser therapy (HILT) is supported by more limited evidence; a single narrative review suggests potential therapeutic benefits—particularly with pulsed emission modalities—in decreasing wound size, pain levels, and other clinically relevant outcomes [105]. To date, no studies have directly compared LLLT and HILT.

Regarding pressure ulcers, photobiomodulation (PBM) has demonstrated clinical utility in adult and older adult populations [72], showing effectiveness in the treatment and management of these lesions [152]. However, in the context of episiotomy healing, PBM has not yet shown superior effectiveness relative to control treatments [71].

5.6.4 Other/Emerging Applications

LLLT has also demonstrated beneficial effects in mitigating the side effects of cancer treatments, including acute oral mucositis, radiation dermatitis, lymphedema, neuropathic pain, and radiation enteropathy. Moreover, both preclinical and clinical evidence suggest its potential role as an adjunctive tool in cancer management [63]. Dermatitis, osteoradionecrosis, dysphagia, trismus, along with oral mucositis and head and neck lymphedema, had positive results after the application of different types of PBM, which included different devices with wavelengths between 630 and 1000 nm [153]. The WALT Working Group document, Photobiomodulation Therapy in the Management of Cancer Therapy–Induced Side Effects: WALT Position Paper 2022, provides evidence-based recommendations for the use of PBM in the prevention and/or management of complications related to cancer treatments. Specifically, it outlines therapeutic parameters and dosing guidelines for PBM in the management of oral mucositis and salivary gland dysfunction in patients undergoing cancer therapy [154]. PBM not only helps mitigate treatment-related side effects, but its potential as a complementary tool in tumor management is also suggested [63].

COVID-19, the first major pandemic of the twenty-first century, has also been investigated as a potential target for laser-based therapeutic interventions. The use of low-level laser therapy (LLLT) during the early stages of infection has demonstrated benefits in managing disease-related complications [155], as well as in improving neurosensory dysfunctions such as anosmia and ageusia [156]. Additionally, a randomized controlled trial employed HILT in the acute phase to evaluate its effects on respiratory function and key laboratory biomarkers. HILT + standard therapy resulted in superior improvements in oxygen saturation and greater reductions in C-reactive protein and interleukin-6 levels compared with standard therapy alone [157].

As demonstrated throughout this chapter, the application of laser therapy—whether through low-level laser therapy (LLLT) or high-intensity laser therapy (HILT)—extends beyond its traditional and well-established use in musculoskeletal disorders, encompassing neurological, pulmonary, oncological, and even genital conditions such as vulvodynia [99]. Although the use of laser therapy in individuals under 18 years of age remains controversial [10, 114], HILT has nevertheless been applied in children aged 9 to 13 years with hemophilic arthropathy, demonstrating improvements in functional capacity, gait parameters, and pain reduction [158]. A similar situation is observed in the context of cardiac pathology, where the potential application of PBM in conditions such as heart failure and myocardial infarction has been discussed, largely based on its proposed mechanisms of action [159]. Current evidence suggests that laser therapy achieves its greatest effectiveness when integrated into multimodal rehabilitation programs [21]. This synergistic effect has also been reported with high-intensity laser therapy (HILT) combined with invasive procedures—such as collagenase chemonucleolysis for the management of lumbar disc herniation—resulting in short-term improvements in both pain and functional outcomes [160].

5.6.5 Overall Interpretation

Overall, the research evidence for laser photobiomodulation is characterized by substantial methodological heterogeneity, including differences in wavelength, irradiance, energy density, treatment duration, and patient selection. Positive clinical outcomes are frequently reported in musculoskeletal pain and wound-healing applications; however, variability in treatment parameters limits direct comparison across studies and prevents universal clinical protocols. Current evidence suggests that therapeutic effectiveness is highly dependent on appropriate dosimetry and clinical reasoning. Therefore, laser therapy should be interpreted as an evidence-informed adjunct modality integrated within active rehabilitation rather than as a standalone intervention.

5.7 Laser Application

When working with LLLT or HILT, it is essential to follow a series of regulations to ensure safe application. Although these rules may vary by country or region [161, 162], they generally coincide in their fundamental principles.

5.7.1 Regarding the Treatment Room

- The laser must be operated in a dedicated room or in enclosed therapy modules, depending on the laser class and according to the classification established by current regulations of the competent legislative authority (European or other).
- Class 3B lasers and above must be used in isolated rooms within a restricted-access area equipped with a locking mechanism that prevents entry during laser emission, or with a warning light installed outside the room (Fig. 5.6).
- Warning signs must be placed in clearly visible areas near the laser treatment zone (Fig. 5.7).
- Room surfaces and equipment must be made of nonreflective, fire-retardant materials.

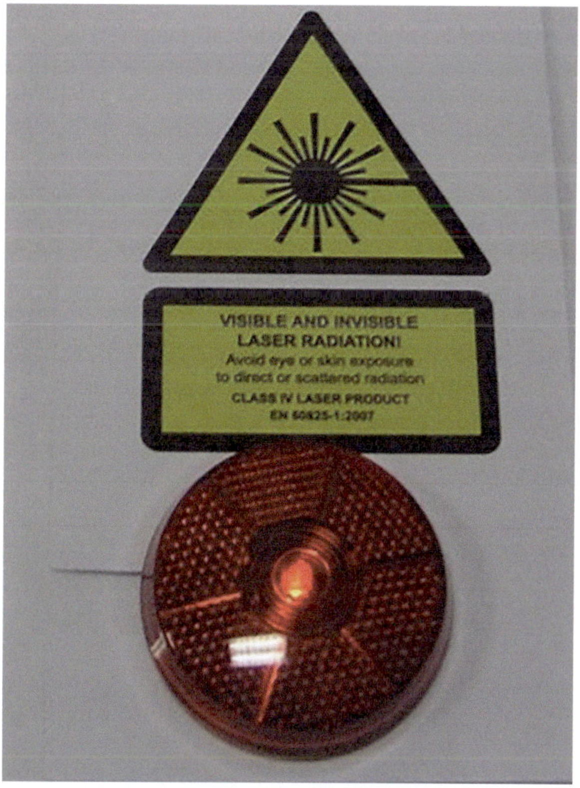

Fig. 5.6 Warning light

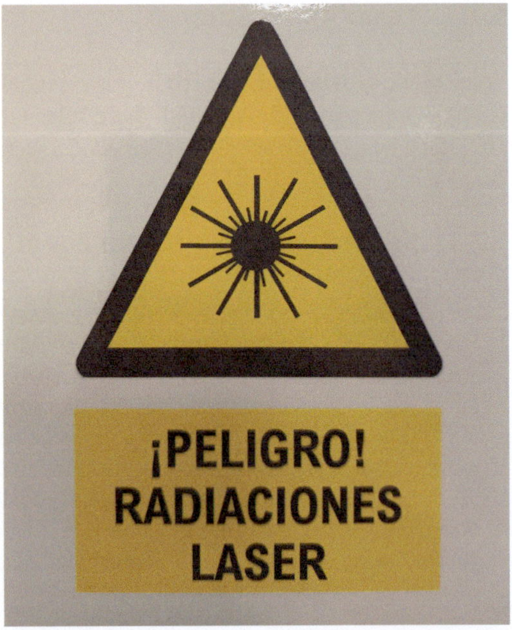

Fig. 5.7 Warning sign

- Adequate ventilation must be ensured.
- Transparent or nonopaque windows must be covered with material of appropriate optical density.

5.7.2 Regarding the Laser Device and Personal Protective Equipment

- A specific eye protection system must be used according to the type of laser and its wavelength, both for the patient and for healthcare personnel. It is important to note that when using devices with multiple wavelengths, protective goggles must provide coverage for all wavelengths emitted.
- The device must include a safety system that prevents accidental laser activation.
- An emergency stop system must be available.

5.7.3 HILT Application Technique (in 10 Steps)

1. Following a comprehensive clinical examination and review of the patient's medical history, the use of high-intensity laser therapy (HILT) is determined to be appropriate and indicated according to the current evidence.
2. It is advisable to employ a structured checklist of absolute and relative contra-indications, as well as safety precautions, to minimize errors and prevent adverse effects.
3. The procedure should be performed in a dedicated treatment room, with the laser emission warning sign displayed outside and the door kept closed through-out the session.
4. Ensure that the treatment area is free of creams, lotions, and dense hair that may interfere with superficial energy absorption. The skin should also be uncovered and free of clothing, jewelry, or reflective accessories.
5. Assess the patient's skin phototype in order to adjust the dose according to pigmentation. The Fitzpatrick scale classifies phototypes from I to VI. This assessment—distinguishing darker from lighter skin—is essential for laser therapy. In individuals with darker phototypes (V–VI), the use of longer wave-lengths, lower fluences, longer pulse durations, and reduced treatment densities is recommended to minimize the risk of thermal injury and adverse reactions [163]. Most HILT devices incorporate a specific setting to indicate the patient's phototype (Fig. 5.8).

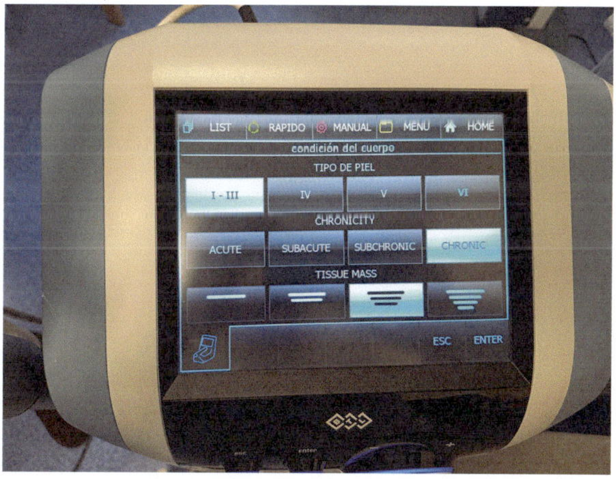

Fig. 5.8 Phototype selection screen

6. Device programming requires selecting the appropriate parameters according to the pathological condition and anatomical region to be treated. These parameters include average power (W), emission mode (continuous wave, pulsed wave, etc.), wavelength (in multi-wavelength devices, power distribution among wavelengths may vary depending on the system), treatment area (cm^2), energy density (J/cm^2) or total energy (J), and irradiance (W/cm^2). Spot size is generally predefined, and the degree of skin contact or separation is determined by the corresponding applicators. It is also necessary to consider the mode of delivery, such as scanning, manual technique, or spot application. Another possibility is the use of laser acupuncture, a modality that has been extensively investigated, particularly within the context of soft laser in musculoskeletal disorders [164–167] and, more recently, through studies involving high-intensity laser therapy (HILT) [168]. It is considered a safe technique with a low incidence of adverse effects [169], also employed, among other fields, in the dental context [170, 171].
7. Both the patient and the clinician must use protective eyewear that complies with laser safety standards.
8. Position the applicator either in contact with the skin or at a specified distance, depending on the type of tissue being treated. In all cases, the applicator should remain perpendicular to the treatment surface.
9. Inform the patient about the expected sensation of warmth and instruct them to immediately report any discomfort or unexpected reactions during the procedure.
10. Initiate the laser application (Fig. 5.9).

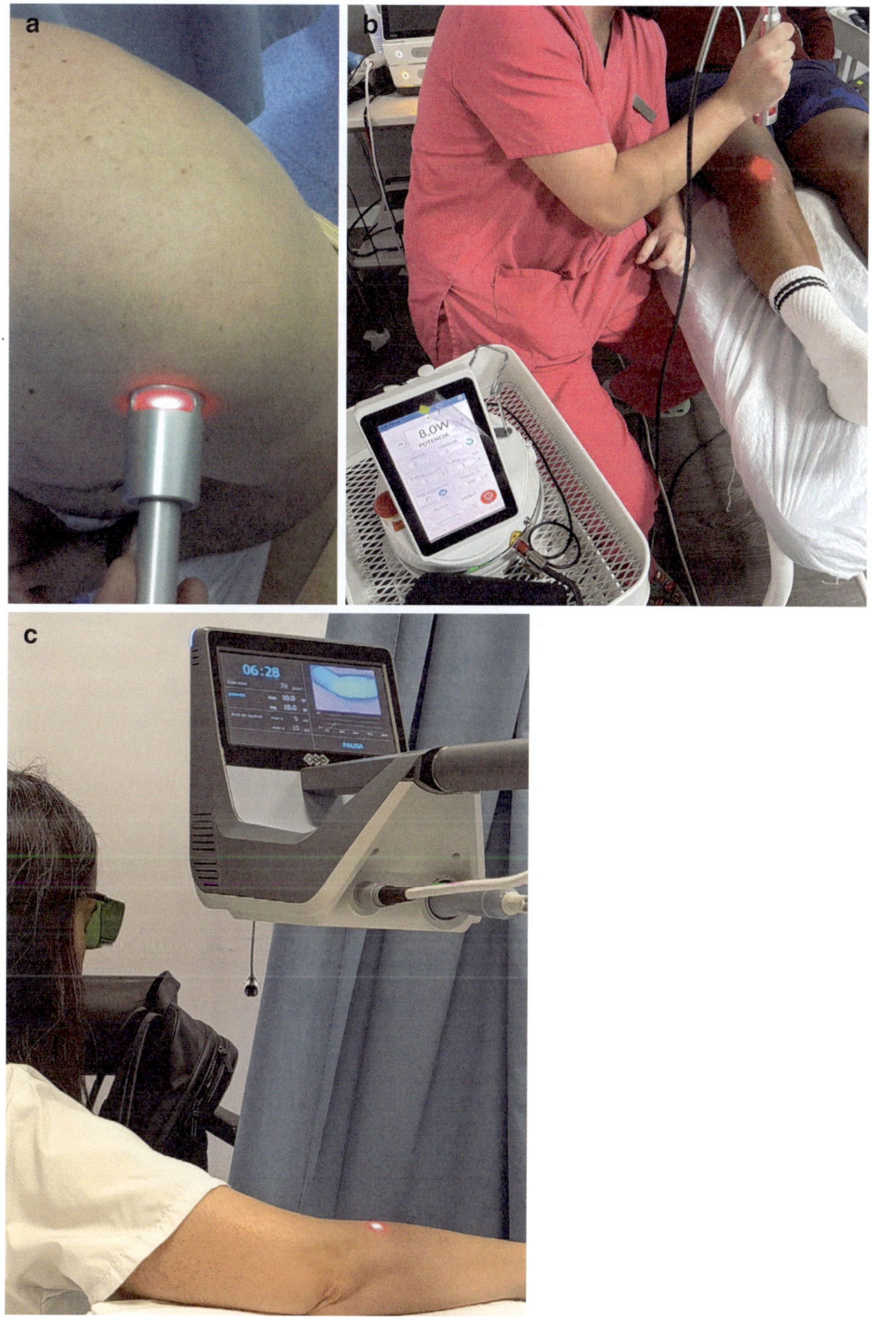

Fig. 5.9 Different HILT application approaches—(**a**) contact, (**b**) noncontact, and (**c**) scanning. ((**a**, **c**) Author; (**b**) Courtesy of Dr. Sánchez-Sierra)

5.8 Summary/Conclusion

Throughout this chapter, an evidence-based perspective on laser therapy has been presented. The discussion has followed a logical progression from the molecular mechanisms to the most effective clinical applications for each pathology or anatomical region, taking into account the parameter configuration and dose-management capabilities of different laser devices.

With respect to the molecular foundations, physiological effects, and therapeutic applications, recent research has been incorporated to further elucidate the modulatory pathways through which laser irradiation produces its intended biological effects. However, regarding dosage and therapeutic indications, the evidence frequently demonstrates considerable heterogeneity across studies and, in many cases, an insufficient description of dosage parameters. Consequently, the development of standardized research protocols—with precise and comprehensive reporting of all applied parameters—remains essential for generating more robust and clinically transferable recommendations.

Current trends indicate that the traditionally strict and narrowly focused application of laser therapy within musculoskeletal and rheumatological conditions is expanding. Emerging evidence supports its use in neurological disorders (both central and peripheral), oncological contexts—such as the management of cancer therapy–related side effects—and additional clinical domains. Both low-level laser therapy (LLLT) and high-intensity laser therapy (HILT) have demonstrated effectiveness in improving key outcome measures, including pain, functionality, and quality of life, across a wide range of conditions. Nevertheless, within the musculoskeletal field, HILT generally yields superior clinical outcomes compared with LLLT, offering greater tissue penetration and reducing overall treatment duration.

5.9 Clinical Cases

Two clinical cases are presented below. A nonexhaustive evidence search was conducted, as the aim is to simulate a rapid consultation scenario typical of routine clinical practice that can guide clinical decision-making—first, regarding the appropriateness of phototherapy, and second, the optimal dosing parameters.

5.9.1 Clinical Case 1: Low-Level Laser Therapy

A 67-year-old male patient presented with a stage II diabetic foot ulcer (Wagner–Merritt classification) located beneath the head of the first metatarsal of the left foot, with an approximate surface area of 6 cm^2 (3 cm × 2 cm).

Evidence Search
PICO Framework
P = Diabetic foot ulcer
I = Low-level laser therapy (LLLT)
C = No treatment or LLLT comparison
O = Complete healing, wound area reduction

Search Strategy
"Diabetic Foot" [Mesh] AND "Low-Level Light Therapy" [Mesh].

Of the 11 articles identified, 2 meta-analyses were selected—one specifically addressing stage I–II diabetic foot ulcers and another detailing the parameters used in LLLT applications. One umbrella review was also included.

1. Intervention effects of low-level laser therapy (LLLT) on grade I–II ulcers in diabetic foot patients: a meta-analysis [172].

   Chen B, Lin Z, Zou S, Huang C, Liu Y, Xu S. Wound Repair Regen. 2025;33(2):e70021. https://doi.org/10.1111/wrr.70021.

   This meta-analysis included 11 studies with a total of 657 patients (332 assigned to LLLT). Lasers employed wavelengths between 630 and 890 nm. The emission mode was typically a noncontact scanning technique across the ulcerated area, with fluence and irradiance values predominantly ranging from 3–10 J/cm^2 to 50 100 mW/cm^2, respectively. The authors concluded that LLLT is an effective adjunct therapy that accelerates wound healing in stage I–II diabetic foot ulcers.
2. Photobiomodulation: systematic review and meta-analysis of the most used parameters in the resolution of diabetic foot ulcers [173].

   Dos Santos Mendes-Costa L, de Lima VG, Barbosa MPR, Dos Santos LE, de Siqueira Rodrigues Fleury Rosa S, Tatmatsu-Rocha JC. Lasers Med Sci. 2021;36(6):1129–1138. https://doi.org/10.1007/s10103-020-03192-y.

   Seven studies met the inclusion criteria; only three scored >3 on the Jadad scale (0–5). The most frequently used parameters included wavelengths between 632.8 and 830 nm, continuous emission delivered via non-contact point application, mean power of 30 mW, and fluence of 4 J/cm^2.
3. Effects and parameterization of low-level laser therapy in diabetic ulcers: an umbrella review of systematic reviews and meta-analyses [75].

   Miranda MB, Alves RF, da Rocha RB, Cardoso VS. Lasers Med Sci. 2025;40(1):109. https://doi.org/10.1007/s10103-025-04366-2.

This umbrella review reported that, compared with standard care or no irradiation, photobiomodulation with a range of parameter combinations was effective in promoting healing of diabetic foot ulcers.

Treatment Plan
LLLT was incorporated as an adjunct intervention with the objectives of reducing wound area, promoting complete closure, and shortening time to healing. Parameters

were selected within the ranges most commonly associated with positive outcomes in the literature. For this case, a fluence of 6 J/cm^2 and an average power of 50 mW were applied.

Alternatively, when feasible, treatment parameters may be aligned with those used in RCTs employing lasers with similar wavelengths to the device available in the physiotherapy clinic. For example, using a 685-nm laser, the parameters and session durations described by Kaviani [174] (referenced in the first meta-analysis) could be replicated to mirror effective protocols reported in the literature.

5.9.2 Clinical Case 2: High-Intensity Laser Therapy

A 45-year-old woman employed as a supermarket cashier is currently on medical leave with a diagnosis of carpal tunnel syndrome (CTS). In her clinical history, she reports the onset of nocturnal paresthesia involving the thumb, index, and middle fingers, accompanied by morning hand numbness and the urge to shake her hands to relieve symptoms. She now experiences daytime tingling, pain, and loss of grip strength, which prevent her from continuing her job duties.

On physical examination, Phalen's test—performed following the procedure described by Fert et al. (Sensitivity = 0.79; Specificity = 0.92)—was positive. The Carpal Compression Test—following González et al. (Sensitivity = 0.87; Specificity = 0.95)—was also positive [175]. The patient is currently awaiting median nerve electromyography and wrist ultrasonography.

Evidence Search

PICO Framework

P = Carpal tunnel syndrome
I = High-intensity laser therapy (HILT)
C = No treatment or LLLT
O = Pain, disability, electrophysiological parameters

Search Strategy

("carpal tunnel syndrome" OR "median nerve entrapment") AND ("high-intensity laser therapy" OR "high-power laser therapy" OR HILT)

From the nine articles retrieved, the most recent systematic review with meta-analysis and one randomized controlled trial (RCT) specifically addressing dosage were selected.

1. Systematic review and meta-analysis: effectiveness of high-intensity laser therapy in patients with carpal tunnel syndrome [104].

   de la Barra Ortiz HA, Avila MA, Parizotto NA, Liebano RE. Physiotherapy. 2025;128:101780. https://doi.org/10.1016/j.physio.2025.101780.

This review included nine RCTs comprising 428 participants diagnosed with CTS (219 treated with HILT). Five studies used a wavelength of 1064 nm, two used 808 nm, and the remaining two applied combined wavelengths of 830–1064 nm and 810–910–1064 nm, respectively.

Despite the overall evidence being rated as moderate to low, the analysis concluded that HILT is effective in reducing pain and disability, and in improving electrophysiological sensorimotor parameters. The authors recommend applying a 1064 nm wavelength over 10 sessions, delivered within a 2–4-week period.

The RCT with the highest methodological quality applied a mean power of 7–8 W and a total energy dose of 2225 J [176].

2. Dose-dependent comparative study of LLLT and HILT on pain and electrophysiological parameters in carpal tunnel syndrome [46].

   Ezzati K, Laakso EL, Saberi A, Yousefzadeh Chabok S, Nasiri E, Bakhshayesh Eghbali B. Eur J Phys Rehabil Med. 2020;56(6):733–740. https://doi.org/10.23736/S1973-9087.19.05835-0.

   This RCT included 100 patients with CTS, divided into four intervention groups and one control group. The study compared the dose-dependent effects of both LLLT and HILT on pain intensity and electrophysiological outcomes, demonstrating that higher-dose HILT produced superior improvements, particularly in distal motor latency and sensory nerve conduction parameters.

LLLT	LLLT	HILT	HILT
8 J/cm^2	20 J/cm^2	8 J/cm^2	20 J/cm^2
50 mW	50 mW	1.6 W	1.6 W
860 nm	860 nm	808 nm	808 nm

Although clinical improvements were observed across different laser modalities and parameter settings, HILT delivered at 1.6 W with a fluence of 8 J/cm^2 demonstrated the greatest effects, showing superior reductions in pain and more pronounced improvements in electrophysiological measures of median nerve function compared with the other intervention groups.

Treatment Plan

Based on the current evidence, HILT was incorporated into the patient's treatment plan due to its analgesic and anti-inflammatory properties, as well as its potential to enhance nerve conduction. A 1064 nm Nd:YAG laser—the wavelength most frequently used in the literature—was selected. Treatment will be administered at 7 W, which allows for greater tissue penetration and shorter application times compared with lower-power devices such as the 1.6 W laser. The chosen parameters follow the protocol reported in the highest-quality RCT [176].

It is noteworthy that the energy density values provided by [46] align with the Arndt–Schulz principle, suggesting that beyond an optimal threshold, higher doses do not yield additional therapeutic benefits.

Clinical Case Tips

1. Confirm whether the selected PBM technique (LLLT or HILT) is effective for the specific pathology. Perform a rapid evidence search in databases such as PubMed or Scopus.
2. Prioritize recent systematic reviews with meta-analysis or network meta-analyses, as they provide an overview of the technique's effectiveness for the clinical outcomes of interest (e.g., pain, function, strength).
3. Select parameters supported by stronger evidence and associated with better clinical outcomes, ensuring reproducibility and therapeutic consistency.

5.10 Review Questions

5.10.1 Same Device, Different Wavelengths?

Some commercially available devices emit two or more wavelengths (e.g., 830–904 nm Multiwave locked system (MLS) laser therapy M6 Asa, 810–980–1064 nm The iLux-Triax® Mectronic, 660–800–905–970 nm Cube 4K-Laser). Employing multiple wavelengths enables therapeutic action at various tissue depths [177] and facilitates light absorption by different chromophores (Figure 5.10), thereby enhancing the photochemical response [178]. Working with different emission modes and power levels at each wavelength [179], all of these parameters act synergistically to enhance the resulting biological effects. Much of the published research on multi-wavelength laser therapy devices has been conducted in the fields of dermatology, aesthetics, and dentistry. In physical therapy, studies examining the use of these devices are increasingly being published, including both case series [180] and clinical trials [181, 182]. In a randomized controlled trial (RCT) comparing MLS 808–905 nm with 830 nm LLLT for neck pain, both groups showed improvements; however, the MLS group demonstrated greater clinical gains [179]. By answering the initial question, future research should explore whether the combination of two or more simultaneous wavelengths with other interventions—particularly single-wavelength laser therapy—can yield clinically meaningful outcomes (Fig. 5.10).

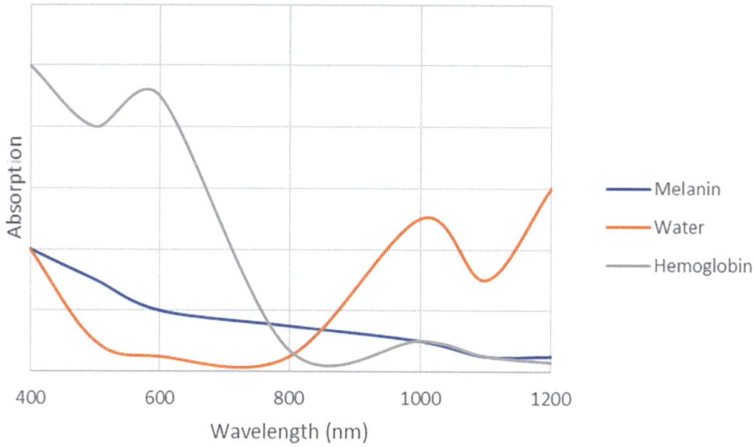

Fig. 5.10 Chromophore absorption level as a function of wavelength

5.10.2 Does Power Influence Treatment Time?

Yes. The energy delivered by a laser (*E*), expressed in joules (*J*), is calculated by multiplying the average power (*P*), in watts (*W*), by the irradiation time (*t*), in seconds.

$$E(J) = P(W) \times t(s)$$

In pulsed emission, the average power ($W_{average}$) is obtained by multiplying the peak power (W_{peak}) by the pulse duration (t_{pulse}) and the pulse frequency (*F*, in Hz) [183].

$$\text{Waverage} = W_{\text{peak}} \times t_{\text{pulse}} \times F$$

Consequently, for a given dose, the required treatment time decreases as power increases. In fact, this reduction in treatment time is one of the advantages highlighted in the scientific literature when comparing high-intensity laser therapy (HILT) with low-level laser therapy (LLLT) [66].

Example:

A total dose of 2000 J is to be delivered during a laser therapy session.

Using the formula

$$E(\text{J}) = P(\text{W}) \times t(\text{s})$$

$$t = \frac{E}{P}$$

LLLT (Class IIIb, 0.5 W): 2000/0.5 = 4000 s (66 min 40 s)
HILT (Class IV, 10 W): 2000/10 = 200 s (3 min 20 s)

Pulsed emission and surface-based calculations.

If the irradiation time must be calculated for pulsed emission over a defined treatment area, the following relationship applies:

$$t = \frac{E}{P} = \frac{J}{w_p \times t_i \times F}$$

where total energy (J) corresponds to: Fluence (J/cm^2) × Surface area (cm^2).

Here again, it becomes evident that higher power leads to shorter treatment times, regardless of whether continuous or pulsed emission is used.

And remember, 1 W is equivalent to 1 joule per second.

5.10.3 CW or PW?–Delivering Treatment Doses

Both laser devices and the scientific literature describe several emission modes, previously outlined in earlier sections. Continuous wave (CW) delivers energy in an uninterrupted manner, whereas pulsed wave (PW) alternates between ON and OFF phases according to the selected duty cycle (pulse duration × frequency). Within PW emissions, five main types are generally recognized as the most commonly employed: Q-switched, gain-switched, mode-locked, superpulsed, and chopped or gated [28].

PW emission offers a notable safety advantage over CW, as it permits the use of higher power levels while producing less cutaneous heating during treatment. By minimizing surface heating, PW enables higher peak power delivery compared with CW [184]. Superpulsed modes, characterized by very short pulse durations in the nanosecond range, operate with high peak power and low average power, with the aim of transferring energy to deeper tissues while avoiding excessive superficial heat accumulation. Current evidence indicates that deeper tissues can be reached when, among other parameters, very short pulses with high peak power are delivered [185].

In clinical practice, most published treatment protocols employ a combination of CW and PW modes. PW is generally used to achieve analgesic, antiinflammatory, and microcirculatory modulation effects, whereas CW is typically applied for biostimulation, thermal effects, and muscle relaxation. Additionally, manufacturers often include preconfigured pulsed programs, as well as custom-designed sequences specific to each device.

With regard to the choice between modes, the majority of recent evidence tends to support the use of PW over CW, although some studies report differing results in favor of CW [186], or in a specific pathology such as nerve repair [28, 187]. Nevertheless, there is broad consensus on the need for rigorous and comprehensive reporting of all dosimetric and technical parameters in scientific publications to enable meaningful comparison and facilitate the development of clinical guidelines [28, 187].

5.10.4 Test Your Knowledge

Laser Therapy Quiz (LLLT & HILT)

1. Which wavelength range is most commonly used in LLLT devices?
   A. 200–400 nm
   B. 600–1100 nm
   C. 1200–1500 nm
   D. 50–200 nm
   Commented answer:
   LLLT typically uses red and near-infrared light between 600 and 1100 nm, allowing deeper penetration into tissues while remaining nonthermal.
2. What is the main characteristic that differentiates HILT from LLLT?
   A. HILT uses continuous low-power emission
   B. HILT uses high-intensity pulsed laser energy
   C. HILT only works on superficial tissues
   D. HILT cannot stimulate cellular activity
   Commented answer:
   HILT uses high-intensity pulsed emissions (often >1 W peak power) that allow greater tissue penetration while controlling thermal effects—unlike LLLT's low-power continuous or pulsed light.
3. Which physiological effect is most associated with LLLT?
   A. Immediate thermal coagulation
   B. Photobiomodulation of mitochondrial activity
   C. Destruction of bacterial membranes through high heat
   D. Bone ablation
   Commented answer:
   LLLT produces photobiomodulation, enhancing mitochondrial function (e.g., increased ATP), improving tissue repair, and reducing inflammation without heat damage.
4. In laser dosage, which parameter indicates the total energy delivered to the tissue?
   A. Wavelength
   B. Spot size
   C. Power density
   D. Energy (Joules)
   Commented answer:
   Energy, expressed in Joules (J), represents the total amount of energy delivered and is critical for determining therapeutic effect, regardless of device type.

5. Which clinical condition is commonly treated with HILT due to its deeper tissue penetration?
   A. Mild skin abrasions
   B. Superficial fungal infections
   C. Deep musculoskeletal pain (e.g., low back pain)
   D. Acute conjunctivitis

   Commented answer:

   HILT can reach deep musculoskeletal structures, making it effective for conditions like low back pain, tendinopathies, or joint dysfunctions.
6. Which parameter most strongly influences tissue penetration during laser therapy?
   A. Beam coherence
   B. Wavelength
   C. Spot color
   D. Device brand

   Commented answer:

   Wavelength is the key factor affecting tissue penetration: longer wavelengths (near-infrared) reach deeper tissues, while shorter wavelengths are absorbed more superficially.
7. What is a typical power output range for LLLT devices used in clinical settings?
   A. 50–100 W
   B. 10–20 W
   C. 5–500 mW
   D. 2–4 kW

   Commented answer:

   LLLT operates at low power levels (5–500 mW) to create photobiomodulation without causing thermal damage.
8. Which type of laser emission is most characteristic of HILT?
   A. Low-power continuous emission
   B. High-intensity pulsed emission with short pulse durations
   C. Noncoherent blue light emission
   D. Constant thermal output

   Commented answer:

   HILT uses high-intensity pulsed emissions, allowing strong peak power while keeping average thermal load low.
9. Which of the following is a contraindication for both LLLT and HILT?
   A. Chronic tendinopathy
   B. Peripheral neuropathy
   C. Overactive cancerous lesions
   D. Delayed-onset muscle soreness

   Commented answer:

   Laser therapy should not be applied over malignant or suspicious cancerous tissues, regardless of power level.

10. What tissue type absorbs laser energy more efficiently at longer wavelengths (e.g., near-infrared)?
    A. Bone cortex
    B. Water
    C. Hemoglobin
    D. Deeper soft tissues (e.g., muscles, fascia)

    Commented answer:

    Near-infrared wavelengths penetrate deeper, making muscles and fascia the primary structures that benefit from longer-wavelength laser therapy.

Declaration

Competing Interests The author has no competing interests to declare that are relevant to the content of this manuscript.

References

1. Steiner R. Basic laser physics. In: Raulin C, Karsai S, editors. Laser and IPL technology in dermatology and aesthetic medicine. Berlin: Springer; 2011.
2. David Baxter G. Tratamiento con láser de baja intensidad. In: Watson T, editor. Electroterapia Práctica basada en la evidencia. 12th ed. Elsevier España; 2009. p. 161–78.
3. Aceituno-Gómez J. Abordaje del Síndrome Subacromial mediante la Terapia Láser de Alta Potencia. Talavera de la Reima: University of Castilla-La Mancha (UCLM); 2019.
4. Niemz MH. Laser-tissue interactions fundamentals and applications. 4th ed. Cham: Springer; 2019.
5. Hamblin MR. Mechanisms and applications of the anti-inflammatory effects of photobiomodulation. AIMS Biophys. 2017;4:337–61.
6. Arjmand B, Khodadost M, Sherafat SJ, Tavirani MR, Ahmadi N, Moghadam MH, et al. Low-level laser therapy: potential and complications. J Lasers Med Sci. 2021;12:e42. Available from: https://pmc.ncbi.nlm.nih.gov/articles/PMC8558713/.
7. Cameron MH. Láseres, luz y fotobiomodulación. In: Agentes físicos en rehabilitación Práctica basada en la evidencia. 6th ed. Elsevier España; 2023. p. 323–42.
8. Marshall RP, Vlkova K. Spectral dependence of laser light on light tissue interactions and its influence on laser therapy: an experimental study. Insights Biomed. 2020;5(1). https://doi.org/10.36648/2572-5610.4.4.66.
9. Anders JJ, Lanzafame RJ, Arany PR. Low-level light/laser therapy versus photobiomodulation therapy. Photomed Laser Surg. 2015;33(4):183–4.
10. Maghfour J, Mineroff J, Ozog DM, Jagdeo J, Lim HW, Kohli I, et al. Evidence-based consensus on the clinical application of photobiomodulation. J Am Acad Dermatol. 2025;93(2):429–43.
11. Wyszyńska J, Bal-Bocheńska M. Efficacy of high-intensity laser therapy in treating knee osteoarthritis: a first systematic review. Photomed Laser Surg. 2018:36. https://doi.org/10.1089/pho.2017.4425.
12. Clavel DH, Catalano M, López Isasi PH. Láser de alta potencia en kinesiología deportiva. Revista Iberoamericana de Fisioterapia y Kinesiologia. 2006;9:68–77.
13. Pérez-Bernal J, Castellanos-Angarita A, Cecilia-Valbuena M. Luz visible, una visión desde la dermatología. Dermatol Rev Mex. 2021;65(1):44–52.
14. Alonso B, Borrego R, Hernández C, Pérez J, Romero C. El láser, la luz de nuestro tiempo. Salamanca: Isabel Arias Tobalina – OSAL; 2010.
15. Banús Gassol JM. Física del láser. Arch Esp Urol. 2008;61:961–4.

16. Bargman H. Laser classification systems. J Clin Aesth Dermatol. 2010;3(10):19–20.
17. Patil U, Dhami L. Overview of lasers. Indian J Plast Surg. 2008;41(3 Suppl):S101–13.
18. Ulloa FJP. Agentes físicos superficiales y dolor. Análisis de su eficacia a la luz de la evidencia científica. Revista de la Sociedad Española del Dolor. 2009;16(3):182–9.
19. Shurrab K. Proposed guidelines for reporting parameters and procedures of high- and low-level laser therapy in medical research articles. Med Dev Evid Res. 2025;18:495–505.
20. Farkas JP, Hoopman JE, Kenkel JM. Five parameters you must understand to master control of your laser/light-based devices. Aesthet Surg J. 2013;33(7):1059–64.
21. de la Barra Ortiz HA. Laser therapy for musculoskeletal pain management: a preliminary network meta-analysis comparing High-intensity and low-level protocols. Sensors Transducers. 2025;269(2):40–52.
22. de la Barra Ortiz HA. Comments on "Dosage of high-intensity laser therapy for the management of musculoskeletal pain in physical therapy practice". Physiother Q. 2025;33:85–90.
23. Fortuna D, Margheri F, Parker S, Rossi F. A biophysical framework for high-intensity laser therapy based on photoacoustic pressure thresholds. Appl Sci. 2026;16(1):487. Available from: https://www.mdpi.com/2076-3417/16/1/487.
24. Gendron DJ, Hamblin MR. Applications of photobiomodulation therapy to musculoskeletal disorders and osteoarthritis with particular relevance to Canada. Photobiomodul Photomed Laser Surg. 2019;37(7):408–20. Available from: https://europepmc.org/articles/PMC6648198.
25. Hu D, van Zeyl M, Valter K, Potas JR. Sex, but not skin tone affects penetration of red-light (660 nm) through sites susceptible to sports injury in lean live and cadaveric tissues. J Biophotonics. 2019;12(7):e201900010.
26. World Association of Laser Therapy (WALT). Consensus agreement on the design and conduct of clinical studies with low-level laser therapy and light therapy for musculoskeletal pain and disorders. Photomed Laser Surg. 2006;24:761.
27. Ash C, Dubec M, Donne K, Bashford T. Effect of wavelength and beam width on penetration in light-tissue interaction using computational methods. Lasers Med Sci. 2017;32(8):1909–18.
28. Hashmi JT, Huang YY, Sharma SK, Kurup DB, De Taboada L, Carroll JD, et al. Effect of pulsing in low-level light therapy. Lasers Surg Med. 2010;42:450–66.
29. Penberthy WT, Vorwaller CE. The importance of power in photobiomodulation, a systematic review and meta-analysis of high intensity laser therapy. 2024. https://doi.org/10.21203/rs.3.rs-4813995/v1.
30. Lanzafame R. Light dosing and tissue penetration: it Is complicated. Photobiomodul Photomed Laser Surg. 2020;38(7):393–4.
31. Fortuna D, Margheri F, Parker S, Rossi F. High-intensity vs. high-power laser therapy: biophysical implications of a semantic ambiguity and the distinct role of photoacoustic effects. Appl Sci. 2025;16(1):67.
32. Das A, Sarda A, De A. Cooling devices in laser therapy. J Cutan Aesthet Surg. 2016;9:215.
33. Huang YY, Chen ACH, Carroll JD, Hamblin MR. Biphasic dose response in low level light therapy. Dose-Response. 2009;7(4):358–83.
34. Nie F, Hao S, Ji Y, Zhang Y, Sun H, Will M, et al. Biphasic dose response in the anti-inflammation experiment of PBM. Lasers Med Sci. 2023;38:66.
35. Taylor DN, Winfield T, Wynd S. Low-level laser light therapy dosage variables vs treatment efficacy of neuromusculoskeletal conditions: a scoping review. J Chiropr Med. 2020;19(2):119. Available from: https://pmc.ncbi.nlm.nih.gov/articles/PMC7729198/.
36. Chow RT, Barnsley L. Systematic review of the literature of low-level laser therapy (LLLT) in the management of neck pain. Lasers Surg Med. 2005;37:46–52.
37. Bjordal JM, Couppé C, Chow RT, Tunér J, Ljunggren EA. A systematic review of low level laser therapy with location-specific doses for pain from chronic joint disorders. Aust J Physiother. 2003;49(2):107–16.
38. Word Association for Photobiomodulation Therapy (WALT). Recommended treatment doses for Low Level Laser Therapy Laser class 3 B, 780–860 nm GaAlAs Lasers.

39. World Association for Photobiomodulation Therapy (WALT). Recommended treatment doses for Low Level Laser Therapy Laser class 3 B, 904 nm GaAs Lasers.
40. Bjordal JM. Low level laser therapy (LLLT) and world association for laser therapy (WALT) dosage recommendations. Photomed Laser Surg. 2012;30(2):61–2.
41. Lopes-Martins RAB, Marcos RL, ECP L-J, Bjordal JM. Low-level laser therapy and World Association for Laser Therapy dosage recommendations in musculoskeletal disorders and injuries. Photomed Laser Surg. 2018;36(9):457–9. Available from: https://pubmed.ncbi.nlm.nih.gov/30188251/.
42. Clijsen R, Brunner A, Barbero M, Clarys P, Taeymans J. Effects of low-level laser therapy on pain in patients with musculoskeletal disorders: a systematic review and meta-analysis. Eur J Phys Rehabil Med. 2017;53(4):603–10. Available from: https://www.minervamedica.it/en/journals/europa-medicophysica/article.php?cod=R33Y2017N04A0603.
43. de la Barra Ortiz HA, Parizotto NA, Liebano RE. Comparison of the effectiveness of high-intensity laser therapy versus low-level laser therapy in musculoskeletal disorders: a systematic review and network meta-analysis. Lasers Med Sci. 2026;41(1):30.
44. Arroyo-Fernández R, Aceituno-Gómez J, Serrano-Muñoz D, Avendaño-Coy J. High-intensity laser therapy for musculoskeletal disorders: a systematic review and meta-analysis of randomized clinical trials. J Clin Med. 2023;12(4). Available from: https://pubmed.ncbi.nlm.nih.gov/36836014/.
45. Song HJ, Seo HJ, Lee Y, Kim SK. Effectiveness of high-intensity laser therapy in the treatment of musculoskeletal disorders: a systematic review and meta-analysis of randomized controlled trials. Medicine (United States). 2018;97(51):e14274.
46. Ezzati K, Laakso EL, Saberi A, Chabok SY, Nasiri E, Eghbali BB. A comparative study of the dose-dependent effects of low level and high intensity photobiomodulation (laser) therapy on pain and electrophysiological parameters in patients with carpal tunnel syndrome. Eur J Phys Rehabil Med. 2020;56(6):733–40. Available from: https://pubmed.ncbi.nlm.nih.gov/31742366/
47. Pereira FC, Parisi JR, Maglioni CB, Machado GB, Barragán-Iglesias P, Silva JRT, et al. Antinociceptive effects of low-level laser therapy at 3 and 8 j/cm2 in a rat model of postoperative pain: possible role of endogenous opioids. Lasers Surg Med. 2017;49(9):844–51.
48. Maghfour J, Ozog DM, Mineroff J, Jagdeo J, Kohli I, Lim HW. Photobiomodulation CME part I: overview and mechanism of action. J Am Acad Dermatol. 2024;91:793–802.
49. Cialdai F, Monici M. Relationship between cellular and systemic effects of pulsed Nd:YAG laser. Energy Health. 2010;5:4–9.
50. Zein R, Selting W, Hamblin MR. Review of light parameters and photobiomodulation efficacy: dive into complexity. J Biomed Opt. 2018;23(12):120901.
51. Tamimi R, Benisi SZ, Boroujeni ME, Torkamani MJ. Review on the molecular mechanisms of low-level laser therapy: gene expression and signaling pathways. Lasers Med Sci. 2025;40(1). Available from: https://pubmed.ncbi.nlm.nih.gov/40131476/.
52. Dyson M. Primary, secondary, and tertiary effects of phototherapy: a review. In: Hamblin MR, Waynant RW, Anders J, editors. Proceedings of SPIE – the international society for optical engineering. SPIE; 2006. p. 614005.
53. Martins DO, Rocha IRC, Watkins LR, Chacur M. Photobiomodulation therapy in neuropathic pain: mechanisms, evidence, and future directions. Front Photon. 2025;6. https://doi.org/10.3389/fphot.2025.1730347.
54. Serrage HJ, Joanisse S, Cooper PR, Palin W, Hadis M, Darch O, et al. Differential responses of myoblasts and myotubes to photobiomodulation are associated with mitochondrial number. J Biophotonics. 2019;12(6):e201800411.
55. da Silva TG, Ribeiro RS, Mencalha AL, de Souza Fonseca A. Photobiomodulation at molecular, cellular, and systemic levels. Lasers Med Sci. 2023;38(1):136.
56. Ponnusamy S, Amin M, Bhat A, Garczynski S, Rahman SU, Rasam S, et al. Photobiomodulation activates coordinated signaling networks to modulate inflammation, adaptive stress, and tissue healing via redox-mediated NFκB–TGF-β1–ATF-4 axis. Cells. 2026;15(1):88.

57. Antonio PN, Cleber F. Enhancing physiotherapy outcomes with photobiomodulation: a comprehensive review. J Nov Physiother Rehabil. 2024;8(2):31.
58. Harrington P, Vickers J. Class IV therapy lasers maximize primary biostimulative effects. Pain Pract Manag. 2012;8(7):1–6.
59. Maya J, Albornoz M. Laserterapia. In: Albornoz M, Maya J, Toledo J, editors. Electroterapia práctica Avances en investigación clínica. Elsevier España; 2016. p. 239–51.
60. Awotidebe AW, Inglis-Jassiem G, Young T. Low-level laser therapy and exercise for patients with shoulder disorders in physiotherapy practice (a systematic review protocol). Syst Rev. 2015;4(1):60.
61. de Souza da Fonseca A, de Souza Alves E, de Paoli F, Mencalha AL. Low-power therapeutic lasers on mRNA levels. Lasers Med Sci. 2022;37(5):2353–62. Available from: https://pubmed.ncbi.nlm.nih.gov/35288806/
62. Moshkovska T, Mayberry J. It is time to test low level laser therapy in Great Britain. Postgrad Med J. 2005;81:436–41.
63. Wang Q, Oh PS, Jeong HJ. From molecular mechanisms to clinical applications: a comprehensive review of photobiomodulation in cancer treatment. Photochem Photobiol. 2026;102(1):27–42.
64. Kheshie AR, Alayat MSM, Ali MME. High-intensity versus low-level laser therapy in the treatment of patients with knee osteoarthritis: a randomized controlled trial. Lasers Med Sci. 2014;29(4):1371–6.
65. Berčič T, Bracic M. Effectiveness of high-intensity laser therapy on pain in tendinopathy. J Health Rehabil Sci. 2024;3(2):1–11.
66. Prouza O, Jeníček J, Procházka M. Class 4. Non-invasive laser therapy in clinical rehabilitation. Rehabil Fyz Lék. 2013;20:113–9.
67. Argueta-Figueroa L, Flores-Mejía LA, Ávila-Curiel BX, Flores-Ferreyra BI, Torres-Rosas R. Nonpharmacological interventions for pain in patients with temporomandibular joint disorders: a systematic review. Eur J Dent. 2022;16(03):500–13.
68. Brosseau L, Welch V, Wells GA, de Bie R, Gam A, Harman K, et al. Low level laser therapy (Classes I, II and III) for treating rheumatoid arthritis. Cochrane Database Syst Rev. 2005;2010(7). https://doi.org/10.1002/14651858.CD002049.pub2.
69. De Oliveira MF, Johnson DS, Demchak T, Tomazoni SS, Leal-Junior EC. Low-intensity LASER and LED (photobiomodulation therapy) for pain control of the most common musculoskeletal conditions. Eur J Phys Rehabil Med. 2022;58(2):282–9.
70. Yeh SW, Hong CH, Shih MC, Tam KW, Huang YH, Kuan YC. Low-level laser therapy for fibromyalgia: a systematic review and meta-analysis. Pain Physician. 2019;22(3):241–54.
71. Taha N, Daoud H, Malik T, Shettysowkoor J, Rahman S. The effects of low-level laser therapy on wound healing and pain management in skin wounds: a systematic review and meta-analysis. Cureus. 2024. https://doi.org/10.7759/cureus.72542.
72. Vieceli AS, Martins JC, Hendler KG, Santos APT, das Neves LMS, Barbosa RI, et al. Effectiveness of electrophysical agents for treating pressure injuries: a systematic review. Lasers Med Sci. 2022;37(9):3363–77.
73. Al Balah OF, Rafie M, Osama AR. Immunomodulatory effects of photobiomodulation: a comprehensive review. Lasers Med Sci. 2025;40. https://doi.org/10.1007/s10103-025-04417-8.
74. Imani M. Therapeutic mechanisms and applications of 808 nm laser irradiation: from wound healing to neurological recovery—a review. Lasers Med Sci. 2025;40(1):526.
75. Miranda MB, Alves RF, da Rocha RB, Cardoso VS. Effects and parameterization of low-level laser therapy in diabetic ulcers: an umbrella review of systematic reviews and meta-umbrella. Lasers Med Sci. 2025;40(1):109.
76. Neto FCJ, Martimbianco ALC, de Andrade RP, Bussadori SK, Mesquita-Ferrari RA, Fernandes KPS. Effects of photobiomodulation in the treatment of fractures: a systematic review and meta-analysis of randomized clinical trials. Lasers Med Sci. 2020;35(3):513–22.
77. Li L, Yang L, Yang Y, Zhu J, Shi R, Deng Q, et al. Evaluation of the efficacy of physical agent modalities in patients with fractures: a systematic review and network meta-analysis. Front Med (Lausanne). 2025;12:1646903.

78. Sadeghian A, Rohani B, Salehi-Marzijarani M, Fekrazad R. Radiographical impact of photobiomodulation therapy on bone regeneration in clinical studies: a systematic review. Lasers Med Sci. 2025;40(1):23.
79. Hazrati P, Azadi A, Fekrazad S, Wang HL, Fekrazad R. The effect of photobiomodulation therapy on fracture healing: a systematic review and meta-analysis of animal studies. Lasers Med Sci. 2025;40(1):121.
80. Berni M, Brancato AM, Torriani C, Bina V, Annunziata S, Cornella E, et al. The role of low-level laser therapy in bone healing: systematic review. Int J Mol Sci. 2023;24(8). Available from: https://pubmed.ncbi.nlm.nih.gov/37108257/.
81. Farazi N, Salehi-Pourmehr H, Farajdokht F, Mahmoudi J, Sadigh-Eteghad S. Photobiomodulation combination therapy as a new insight in neurological disorders: a comprehensive systematic review. BMC Neurol. 2024;24(1):101.
82. Zhang Z, Xue X, Liu P, Zhang C, Li J, Liu Y, et al. The role of photobiomodulation in modulating neural activity and brain function: a systematic bibliometric analysis. Photodiagn Photodyn Ther. 2025;55:104712.
83. Hashmi JT, Huang YY, Osmani BZ, Sharma SK, Naeser MA, Hamblin MR. Role of low-level laser therapy in neurorehabilitation. PM&R. 2010;2(12 Suppl):S292–305.
84. Stevens AR, Hadis M, Milward M, Ahmed Z, Belli A, Palin W, et al. Photobiomodulation in acute traumatic brain injury: a systematic review and meta-analysis. J Neurotrauma. 2023;40:210–27.
85. Ashrafi F, Rezaei A, Azhideh A, Tabeie F, Gachkar L, Arab-Ahmadi M, et al. Effectiveness of extremely low frequency electromagnetic field and pulsed low-level laser therapy in acute stroke treatment. Int Clin Neurosci J. 2020;7(3):127–31.
86. Casalechi HL, Dumont AJL, Ferreira LAB, de Paiva PRV, dos Santos Monteiro Machado C, de Carvalho PTC, et al. Acute effects of photobiomodulation therapy and magnetic field on functional mobility in stroke survivors: a randomized, sham-controlled, triple-blind, crossover, clinical trial. Lasers Med Sci. 2020;35(6):1253–62.
87. Paolillo FR, Luccas GAA, Parizotto NA, Paolillo AR, de Castro Neto JC, Bagnato VS. The effects of transcranial laser photobiomodulation and neuromuscular electrical stimulation in the treatment of post-stroke dysfunctions. J Biophotonics. 2023;16(4). https://doi.org/10.1002/jbio.202200260.
88. Dumont AJL, Casalechi HL, Tomazoni SS, Grecco LC, Galli M, Oliveira CS, et al. Photobiomodulation therapy combined with static magnetic field (PBMT–SMF) on spatiotemporal and kinematics gait parameters in post-stroke: a pilot study. Life. 2022;12(2):186.
89. Korada HY, Arora E, Maiya GA, Rao S, Hande M, Shetty S, et al. Effectiveness of photobiomodulation therapy on neuropathic pain, nerve conduction and plantar pressure distribution in diabetic peripheral neuropathy – a systematic review. Curr Diabetes Rev. 2023;19(9):e290422204244.
90. Hanna R, Chow R, Dalvi S, Arany PR, Bensadoun RJ, Santos-Silva AR, et al. Photobiomodulation therapy in the management of orofacial neuropathic pain—WALT position paper 2026. J Clin Med. 2026;15(3):1304.
91. Rashad UM, Sadik Badawy M, Abdelkader Fahmy A, El Fakharany MS, Abdelaziz EA. The effect of low-level laser therapy on peripheral nerve lesions: a systematic review. Physiother Q. 2025;33:26–33.
92. Lawrence J, Sorra K. Photobiomodulation as medicine: Low-Level Laser Therapy (LLLT) for acute tissue injury or sport performance recovery. J Funct Morphol Kinesiol. 2024;9(4):181.
93. Gadah AM, Khiyami AT, Almalki RS, Otaif BM, Khayame NT, Al-Moalad OM, et al. A review of low-level laser therapy application in sports physical therapy. Saudi J Sports Med. 2025;25(2):39–46.
94. Smoot B, Chiavola-Larson L, Lee J, Manibusan H, Allen DD. Effect of low-level laser therapy on pain and swelling in women with breast cancer-related lymphedema: a systematic review and meta-analysis. J Cancer Surviv. 2015;9(2):287–304.

95. Chiu ST, Lai UH, Huang YC, Leong CP, Chen PC. Effect of various photobiomodulation regimens on breast cancer-related lymphedema: a systematic review and meta-analysis. Lasers Med Sci. 2023;39(1):11.
96. Mahmood D, Ahmad A, Sharif F, Arslan SA. Clinical application of low-level laser therapy (Photo-biomodulation therapy) in the management of breast cancer-related lymphedema: a systematic review. BMC Cancer. 2022;22(1):937.
97. Wang Y, Ge Y, Xing W, Liu J, Wu J, Lin H, et al. The effectiveness and safety of low-level laser therapy on breast cancer–related lymphedema: an overview and update of systematic reviews. Lasers Med Sci. 2022;37(3):1389–413.
98. Song HJ, Seo HJ, Kim D. Effectiveness of high-intensity laser therapy in the management of patients with knee osteoarthritis: a systematic review and meta-analysis of randomized controlled trials. J Back Musculoskelet Rehabil. 2020;33(6):875–84.
99. Starzec-Proserpio M, Bardin MG, Fradette J, Tu LM, Bérubè-Lauzière Y, Paré J, et al. High-Intensity Laser Therapy (HILT) as an emerging treatment for vulvodynia and chronic musculoskeletal pain disorders: a systematic review of treatment efficacy. J Clin Med. 2022;11:3701.
100. Xie YH, Liao MX, Lam FMH, Gu YM, Hewith A, Fernando WC, Liao LR, et al. The effectiveness of high-intensity laser therapy in individuals with neck pain: a systematic review and meta-analysis. Physiotherapy (United Kingdom). 2023;121:23–36.
101. de la Barra Ortiz HA, Arias M, Liebano RE. A systematic review and meta-analysis of randomized controlled trials on the effectiveness of high-intensity laser therapy in the management of neck pain. Lasers Med Sci. 2024;39(1):124.
102. de la Barra Ortiz HA, Parizotto N, Arias M, Liebano R. Effectiveness of high-intensity laser therapy in the treatment of patients with frozen shoulder: a systematic review and meta-analysis. Lasers Med Sci. 2023;38:266.
103. de la Barra Ortiz HA, Parizotto NA, Liebano RE. Effectiveness of high-intensity laser therapy in patients with spinal radiculopathy: a systematic review with meta-analysis. Lasers Med Sci. 2025;40:328.
104. de la Barra Ortiz HA, Avila MA, Parizotto NA, Liebano RE. A systematic review and meta-analysis of the effectiveness of high-intensity laser therapy in patients with carpal tunnel syndrome. Physiotherapy (United Kingdom). 2025;128:101780.
105. Yoon SH, Huh BK, Abdi S, Javed S. The efficacy of high-intensity laser therapy in wound healing: a narrative review. Lasers Med Sci. 2024;39:208.
106. Alayat MS, El-Sodany AM, Ebid AA, Shousha TM, Abdelgalil AA, Alhasan H, et al. Efficacy of high intensity laser therapy in the management of foot ulcers: a systematic review. J Phys Ther Sci. 2018;30(10):1341–5.
107. Alayat MSM, Abdel-Kafy EM, Elsoudany AM, Helal OF, Alshehri MA. Efficacy of high intensity laser therapy in the treatment of male with osteopenia or osteoporosis: a randomized placebo-controlled trial. J Phys Ther Sci. 2017;29(9):1675–9.
108. Alayat MSM, Abdel-Kafy EM, Thabet AAM, Abdel-Malek AS, Ali TH, Header EA. Long-term effect of pulsed Nd-YAG laser combined with exercise on bone mineral density in men with osteopenia or osteoporosis: 1 year of follow-up. Photomed Laser Surg. 2018;36(2):105–11.
109. Abo Elyazed TI, Al-Azab IM, Abd El-Hakim AAEM, Elkady SM, Afifi RMM, Obaya HE. Effect of high-intensity laser therapy versus shockwave therapy on selected outcome measures in osteoporotic long-term hemiparetic patients: a randomized control trial. J Orthop Surg Res. 2023;18(1):653.
110. Kelini KIS, Saleh MSM, Abbas MAM, Bayoumi MBI, Ahmed SM. High-intensity laser therapy can improve pain, health status and quality of life in women with fibromyalgia: a single blinded-randomized controlled trial. Lasers Med Sci. 2025;40(1):123.
111. Khoramdel F, Ravanbod R, Akbari H. Effect of high-intensity laser therapy and mirror therapy on complex regional pain syndrome type I in the hand area: a randomized controlled trial. J Hand Ther. 2025;38(4):791–8.

112. Korkmaz N, Gurcay E, Demir Y, Tezen Ö, Korkmaz İ, Atar MÖ, et al. The effectiveness of high-intensity laser therapy in the treatment of post-stroke patients with hemiplegic shoulder pain: a prospective randomized controlled study. Lasers Med Sci. 2022;37(51):1–9.
113. Abdelhakiem NM, Mustafa Saleh MS, Shabana MMA, Abd EL Wahaab HA, Saleh HM. Effectiveness of a high-intensity laser for improving hemiplegic shoulder dysfunction: a randomized controlled trial. Sci Rep. 2024;14(1):7346.
114. Navratil L, Kymplova J. Contraindications in noninvasive laser therapy: truth and fiction. J Clin Laser Med Surg. 2002;20(6):341–3.
115. Rennie S. ELECTROPHYSICAL AGENTS – Contraindications and precautions: an evidence-based approach to clinical decision making in physical therapy. Physiother Can. 2010;62(5):1–80.
116. Arany PR. Photobiomodulation therapy. JADA Found Sci. 2025;4:100045.
117. Al-Niaimi F. Laser and energy-based devices' complications in dermatology. J Cosmet Laser Ther. 2015;18:1–7.
118. Jang H, Lee H. Meta-analysis of pain relief effects by laser irradiation on joint areas. Photomed Laser Surg. 2012;30(8):405–17.
119. Hernández-Bule ML, Naharro-Rodríguez J, Bacci S, Fernández-Guarino M. Unlocking the power of light on the skin: a comprehensive review on Photobiomodulation. Int J Mol Sci. 2024;25(8):4483.
120. Atan T, Bahar-Ozdemir Y. Efficacy of high-intensity laser therapy in patients with adhesive capsulitis: a sham-controlled randomized controlled trial. Lasers Med Sci. 2021;36(1):207–17.
121. Alayat MSM, Alshehri MA, Shousha TM, Abdelgalil AA, Alhasan H, Khayyat OK, et al. The effectiveness of high intensity laser therapy in the management of spinal disorders: a systematic review and meta-analysis. J Back Musculoskelet Rehabil. 2019;32(6):869–84.
122. Wen D, McAlinden C, Flitcroft I, Tu R, Wang Q, Alió J, et al. Postoperative efficacy, predictability, safety, and visual quality of laser corneal refractive surgery: a network meta-analysis Am J Ophthalmol. 2017;178:65–78.
123. Shivappa P, Basha S, Biswas S, Prabhu V, Prabhu SS, Pai AR, et al. From light to healing: photobiomodulation therapy in medical disciplines. J Transl Med. 2025;23(1):1430.
124. Zhai Q, Cheng S, Liu R, Xie J, Han X, Yu Z. Meta-analysis of the efficacy of intense pulsed light and pulsed-dye laser therapy in the management of Rosacea. J Cosmet Dermatol. 2024;23(12):3821–7.
125. Sarangi P, Suman S, Satapathy SK, Meher R, Das A, Pradeep DM. The pros and cons of dental laser therapy in conservative dentistry and endodontics—a systematic review. J Pharm Bioallied Sci. 2024;16(Suppl 4):S3083–5.
126. de Oliveira Alves R, Urzedo LOR, de Toledo PTA, Ferreira-Baptista C, Ragghianti MHF, Pereira TC, et al. Antimicrobial photodynamic therapy in onychomycosis management: a systematic review of clinical trials. Photodiagn Photodyn Ther. 2025;54:104640.
127. Dompe C, Moncrieff L, Matys J, Grzech-Leśniak K, Kocherova I, Bryja A, et al. Photobiomodulation—underlying mechanism and clinical applications. J Clin Med. 2020;9(6):1–17.
128. Abdelbasset WK, Nambi G, Alsubaie SF, Abodonya AM, Saleh AK, Ataalla NN, et al. A randomized comparative study between high-intensity and low-level laser therapy in the treatment of chronic nonspecific low back pain. Evid Based Complement Alternat Med. 2020;2020:1350281.
129. Thabet AA, Ebid AA, El-Boshy ME, Almuwallad AO, Hudaimoor EA, Alsaeedi FE, et al. Pulsed high-intensity laser therapy versus low level laser therapy in the management of primary dysmenorrhea. J Phys Ther Sci. 2021;33(9):695–9. Available from: http://www.ncbi.nlm.nih.gov/pubmed/34539076.
130. Naruseviciute D, Kubilius R. The effect of high-intensity versus low-level laser therapy in the management of plantar fasciitis: randomized participant blind controlled trial. Clin Rehabil. 2020;34(8):1072–82.

131. Taradaj J, Rajfur K, Rajfur J, Ptaszkowski K, Ptaszkowska L, Sopel M, et al. Effect of laser treatment on postural control parameters in patients with chronic nonspecific low back pain: a randomized placebo-controlled trial. Braz J Med Biol Res. 2019;52(12):e8474.
132. Ang L, Song E, Choi S, Kim J. Effectiveness and safety of light therapy for treating primary dysmenorrhea: a systematic review and meta-analysis of randomized controlled trials. Complement Ther Med. 2025;93:103232.
133. Zhang M, Zhao Z, Wu Z, Li F. Is there any difference between high-intensity laser and low-level laser in the treatment of tennis elbow? A meta-analysis of randomized controlled trials. Am J Phys Med Rehabil. 2025. Available from: https://pubmed.ncbi.nlm.nih.gov/40856482/.
134. Chauhan D, Sharma S. Adjunctive approach to therapeutic laser and exercise therapies in alleviating pain and disability in patients with low back pain: a systematic review. J Lifestyle Med. 2024;14(2):69–79. Available from: https://pubmed.ncbi.nlm.nih.gov/39280939/.
135. Saleh MS, Shahien M, Mortada H, Elaraby A, Hammad YS, Hamed M, et al. High-intensity versus low-level laser in musculoskeletal disorders. Lasers Med Sci. 2024;39(1):179. Available from: https://pmc.ncbi.nlm.nih.gov/articles/PMC11239763/.
136. Şen SB, Koçyiğit BF, Ortaç EA, Kösehasanoğulları M, Bilecik NA. Comparison of the effects of high-intensity laser therapy and low-level laser therapy in knee osteoarthritis. Clin Rheumatol. 2025. Available from: https://pubmed.ncbi.nlm.nih.gov/41042410/.
137. Ezzati K, Esmaili K, Reihanian Z, Hasannejad A, Soleymanha M, Keshavarz S, et al. The effects of high-intensity laser therapy vs. low-level laser therapy on functional ability and quadriceps architecture in patients with knee osteoarthritis: a single-blinded randomized clinical trial. J Lasers Med Sci. 2024;15:e66. Available from: http://www.ncbi.nlm.nih.gov/pubmed/39949479.
138. Poenaru D, Sandulescu MI, Potcovaru CG, Cinteza D. High-intensity laser therapy in pain management of knee osteoarthritis. Biomedicines. 2024;12(8). Available from: https://pubmed.ncbi.nlm.nih.gov/39200144/.
139. Khalilizad M, Hosseinzade D, Marzban Abbas Abadi M. Efficacy of high-intensity and low-level laser therapy combined with exercise therapy on pain and function in knee osteoarthritis: a systematic review and network meta-analysis. J Lasers Med Sci. 2024;15:e34. Available from: http://www.ncbi.nlm.nih.gov/pubmed/39193110.
140. Wu M, Luan L, Pranata A, Witchalls J, Adams R, Bousie J, et al. Is high intensity laser therapy more effective than other physical therapy modalities for treating knee osteoarthritis? A systematic review and network meta-analysis. Front Med (Lausanne). 2022;9:956188. Available from: http://www.ncbi.nlm.nih.gov/pubmed/36186780.
141. Aguilar García M, González Muñoz A, Pérez Montilla JJ, Aguilar Nuñez D, Hamed Hamed D, Pruimboom L, et al. Which multimodal physiotherapy treatment is the most effective in people with shoulder pain? A systematic review and meta-analyses. Healthcare (Basel). 2024;12(12). Available from: https://pubmed.ncbi.nlm.nih.gov/38921347/.
142. Saleh MS, Galal DOS, Ali MS, Ibrahim DI. High-intensity versus low-level laser therapy in treatment of patients with subacromial impingement syndrome: a randomized, double-blind, controlled trial. Lasers Med Sci. 2025;40(1). Available from: https://pubmed.ncbi.nlm.nih.gov/39757334/.
143. Ordahan B, Yigit F, Mülkoglu C. Efficacy of low-level laser versus high-intensity laser therapy in the management of adhesive capsulitis: a randomized clinical trial. Saudi J Med Med Sci. 2023;11(3):201–7.
144. Hao J, He Z, Huang B, Li Y, Remis A, Yao Z, et al. Comparative effectiveness of six biophysical agents on neck pain rehabilitation: a systematic review and network meta-analysis. Eur Spine J. 2025;34(6):2183–200.
145. Yadav S, Sharma S, Chatterjee S, Sharma A, Thakur S. Effect of LASER therapy on plantar fasciitis pain: illuminating a promising treatment approach – a systematic review. Lasers Med Sci. 2025;40(1):18.
146. Nairuz T, Sangwoo-Cho LJH. Photobiomodulation therapy on brain: pioneering an innovative approach to revolutionize cognitive dynamics. Cells. 2024;13(11):966.

147. Oliveira de Andrade Filho V, Amarante MOC, Gonzalez-Lima F, Gomes da Silva S, dos Santos Cardoso F. Systematic review of photobiomodulation for multiple sclerosis. Front Neurol. 2024;15:1465621.
148. Weimer GH, Kolling da Rocha CF. Photobiomodulation treatment in incomplete spinal cord injuries or peripheral nerve injuries: a comprehensive systematic review of randomized clinical trials. Lasers Med Sci. 2025;40(1):286.
149. Liebert A, Bicknell B, Laakso EL, Tilley S, Heller G, Kiat H, et al. Improvements in clinical signs and symptoms of Parkinson's disease using photobiomodulation: a five-year follow-up. BMC Neurol. 2024;24(1):381.
150. Zöll AC, Amorim ACFG, Shimozato IAD, de Moraes FLB, Rodrigues MFSD, Mesquita-Ferrari RA, et al. Photobiomodulation in the treatment of spasticity in children and adolescents with cerebral palsy: a controlled, single-blinded, pilot randomized trial. Disabilities. 2025;5(4):112.
151. Hojjati F, Mohammad Hosein A, Ismail Ebrahimi T, Seyed Mansour R, Sarrafzadeh J, Seyed Ahmad R, et al. The effect of high-power and low-power lasers on symptoms and the nerve conduction study in patients with carpal tunnel syndrome. A prospective randomized single-blind clinical trial. J Lasers Med Sci. 2020;11(4):73–9.
152. da Silva AM, Silva GM, Martins JC, Bavaresco T, Echevarría-Guanilo ME. Photobiomodulation and photodynamic therapy in the treatment of pressure injuries: a scoping review. Rev Lat Am Enfermagem. 2025;33:e4488.
153. Mansouri V, Arjmand B, Tavirani MR, Razzaghi M, Rostami-Nejad M, Hamdieh M. Evaluation of efficacy of low-level laser therapy. J Lasers Med Sci. 2020;11(4):369–80.
154. Robijns J, Nair RG, Lodewijckx J, Arany P, Barasch A, Bjordal JM, et al. Photobiomodulation therapy in management of cancer therapy-induced side effects: WALT position paper 2022. Front Oncol. 2022;12:927685.
155. de Matos BTL, Buchaim DV, Pomini KT, Barbalho SM, Guiguer EL, Reis CHB, et al. Photobiomodulation therapy as a possible new approach in COVID-19: a systematic. Review. 2021;11(6):580.
156. de Toledo Telles-Araujo G, da Cruz KM, Preto KA, Araujo-Silva G, Kraychete DC, da Silva Santos PS, et al. Photobiomodulation in the management of persistent olfactory and gustatory dysfunction post-COVID-19: a systematic review. Lasers Med Sci. 2025;40(1):283.
157. Ehsani F, Bagheri R, Darban M, Hemati M, Bahrami M, Sharafieh F. Effects of photobiomodulation therapy on lung function and inflammatory factors in patients with COVID-19 during acute stage. Photobiomodul Photomed Laser Surg. 2023;41(9):483–9.
158. El-Shamy SM, Abdelaal AAM. Efficacy of pulsed high-intensity laser therapy on pain, functional capacity, and gait in children with haemophilic arthropathy. Disabil Rehabil. 2018;40(4):462–8.
159. Ganipineni VDP, Gutlapalli SD, Ajay Sai Krishna Kumar I, Monica P, Vagdevi M, Samuel Sowrab T. Exploring the potential of energy-based therapeutics (photobiomodulation/low-level laser light therapy) in cardiovascular disorders: a review and perspective. Cureus. 2023;15(4):e37880.
160. Song P, Ma C, Xu C, Zhang Y, Yuan Y. Efficacy of combined high-intensity laser therapy and collagenase chemonucleolysis in lumbar disc herniation management: a prospective randomized controlled trial. Pain Ther. 2025;14(4):1379–98.
161. MHRA. Lasers, intense light source systems and LEDs—guidance for safe use in medical, surgical, dental and aesthetic practices. MHRA; 2015.
162. Orden 132/2025, de 16 de septiembre, de la Consejería de Sanidad, de los requisitos técnico-sanitarios de los centros y servicios de fisioterapia. Diario Oficial de Castilla La Mancha (DOCM). 24 Sept 2025. https://docm.jccm.es/docm/eli/es-cm/o/2025/09/16/132.
163. Sharma AN, Patel BC. Laser Fitzpatrick skin type recommendations. In: StatPearls [Internet]. Treasure Island: StatPearls Publishing; 2025.
164. Law D, McDonough S, Bleakley C, Baxter GD, Tumilty S. Laser acupuncture for treating musculoskeletal pain: a systematic review with meta-analysis. J Acupunct Meridian Stud. 2015;8(1):2–16.

165. Zeng DH, Yuan DN, Zhou QQ, Liu YY, Ma WB, Lan L. Laser acupuncture for the pain of knee osteoarthritis: a systematic review and meta-analysis of randomized controlled trials. J Pain Res. 2025;18:3833–41.
166. Mao X, He H, Ding J. Efficacy of laser acupuncture for treatment of chronic low back pain: a systematic review and meta-analysis. Pain Manag Nurs. 2024;25(5):529–37.
167. da Silva Mira PC, Biagini ACSCF, Gomes MG, Galo R, Corona SAM, Borsatto MC. Laser acupuncture to reduce temporomandibular disorder (TMD) symptoms: systematic review and meta-analysis. Lasers Med Sci. 2024;39(1):66.
168. Wu D, Lan X, Litscher G, Zhao YL, Wu YQ, Dai RJ, et al. Laser acupuncture and photobiomodulation therapy in bell's palsy with a duration of greater than 8 weeks: a randomized controlled trial. Lasers Med Sci. 2024;39(1):29.
169. Yang J, Mallory MJ, Wu Q, Bublitz SE, Do A, Xiong D, et al. The safety of laser acupuncture: a systematic review. Med Acupunct. 2020;32(4):209–17.
170. Manente R, Pedroso GL, Gomes e Moura AP, Borsatto MC, Corona SAM. Laser acupuncture in the treatment of neuropathies in dentistry: a systematic review. Lasers Med Sci. 2023;38(1):92.
171. da Silva Mira PC, Vilela LD, Corona SAM, Borsatto MC. Effect of low-level laser stimulation of acupuncture points in pediatric dentistry: a systematic review. Lasers Med Sci. 2023;38(1):52.
172. Chen B, Lin Z, Zou S, Huang C, Liu Y, Xu S. Intervention effects of low-level laser therapy (LLLT) on grade I–II ulcers in diabetic foot patients: a meta-analysis. Wound Repair Regen. 2025;33(2):e70021.
173. dos Santos Mendes-Costa L, de Lima VG, Barbosa MPR, dos Santos LE, de Siqueira Rodrigues Fleury Rosa S, Tatmatsu-Rocha JC. Photobiomodulation: systematic review and meta-analysis of the most used parameters in the resolution diabetic foot ulcers. Lasers Med Sci. 2021;36(6):1129–38.
174. Kaviani A, Djavid GE, Ataie-Fashtami L, Fateh M, Ghodsi M, Salami M, et al. A randomized clinical trial on the effect of low-level laser therapy on chronic diabetic foot wound healing: a preliminary report. Photomed Laser Surg. 2011;29(2):109–14.
175. Joshua C, Netter FH. Netter. Exploración clínica en ortopedia: un enfoque para fisioterapeutas basado en la evidencia. Masson; 2006. 510 p.
176. Ashour AA, Yehia RM, ElMeligie MM, Hanafy AF. Effectiveness of high intensity laser therapy on pain, grip strength and median nerve conductivity in pregnant women with carpal tunnel syndrome: a randomized controlled trial. J Hand Ther. 2023;36(3):536–45.
177. Alayat MS, Elsodany AM, AlMatrafi NA, El FAAR. Effectiveness of multiwave locked system laser on the treatment of patients with idiopathic bell's palsy: a randomized double-blind placebo controlled trial. Lasers Med Sci. 2022;37(9):3495–502.
178. Thomé Lima AMC, da Silva Sergio LP, da Silva Neto Trajano LA, de Souza BP, da Motta Mendes JP, Cardoso AFR, et al. Photobiomodulation by dual-wavelength low-power laser effects on infected pressure ulcers. Lasers Med Sci. 2020;35(3):651–60.
179. Alayat MS, Elsoudany AM, Ali ME. Efficacy of multiwave locked system laser on pain and function in patients with chronic neck pain: a randomized placebo-controlled trial. Photomed Laser Surg. 2017;35(8):450–5.
180. Nair HKR, Kee PC. The use of photo biomodulation as an adjunct therapy to aid wound healing: a case series. Wounds Asia. 2023;6(2):44–52.
181. Labanca L, Platano D, Tedeschi R, Cappelli E, Benedetti MG, Berti L. Multi-wave locked system laser therapy in chronic non-specific neck pain: a double-blind placebo randomized-controlled trial. Eur J Phys Rehabil Med. 2025;61(4):645–54.
182. Osti R, Pari C, Salvatori G, Massari L. Tri-length laser therapy associated to tecar therapy in the treatment of low-back pain in adults: a preliminary report of a prospective case series. Lasers Med Sci. 2015;30(1):407–12.
183. Rodríguez Martín JM. Electroterapia en fisioterapia. Editorial Médica Panamericana; 2000. 624 p.

184. Chaki C, De Taboada L, Tse KM. Comparative analysis of pulsed and continuous wave modes in high-intensity laser light therapy: implications for deep tissue treatment. J Biophotonics. 2025;18(7):e202400164.
185. Kaub L, Schmitz C. More than ninety percent of the light energy emitted by near-infrared laser therapy devices used to treat musculoskeletal disorders is absorbed within the first ten millimeters of biological tissue. Biomedicine. 2022;10(12):3204.
186. Mantineo M, Pinheiro JP, Morgado AM. Low-level laser therapy on skeletal muscle inflammation: evaluation of irradiation parameters. J Biomed Opt. 2014;19(9):098002.
187. Al-Timimi Z. The function and value of laser pulsing operation mode in wound healing therapy. J Blood Lymph. 2023;13(1):1–6.

Polarised Polychromatic Non-coherent Light

6

Sara Valencia Garcia

6.1 Introduction

Polarized polychromatic noncoherent light (PPNCL) has emerged as a tool in modern physiotherapy, rehabilitation, dermatology, and wound management, offering a noninvasive approach to biostimulation.

Photobiomodulation refers to the capacity of specific wavelengths of light to influence biological processes through the absorption of photons by endogenous chromophores and molecules. In polarized polychromatic systems, light is delivered across a broad spectral range, typically spanning visible and near-infrared wavelengths (350–3400 nm).

Another important characteristic of PPNCL is its polarization, to an extent of >95%. This allows the light waves to penetrate the tissue with minimal scattering, reaching the underlying microcirculation and trigger points effectively. The polarization of light waves is thought to influence photon tissue interactions, although its clinical relevance remains an area of ongoing investigation.

In contrast to coherent laser systems, noncoherent polychromatic light does not exhibit phase alignment between photons, allowing an effective and soft light dosage. Both coherent and noncoherent light can induce photochemical and photobiological responses, provided that appropriate wavelengths and energy densities are delivered.

Clinically, polarized polychromatic light has been used as an adjunctive modality in the management of acute and chronic wounds, musculoskeletal pain, inflammatory conditions, and soft-tissue injuries. However, the strength of evidence varies by indication, and treatment protocols are not yet fully standardized across studies.

S. Valencia Garcia (✉)
Bioptron AG, Wollerau, Switzerland
e-mail: valencia@bioptron.com

D. Stasinopoulos (ed.), *Application of Electrophysical Agents in Physiotherapy*,
https://doi.org/10.1007/978-3-032-32144-2_6

The purpose of this chapter is to present a structured analysis of polarized polychromatic non-coherent light within the framework of rehabilitation and healing. The mechanisms of action, clinical indication, and research evidence will be discussed. Emphasis will be placed on integrating polarized light therapy within comprehensive, exercise-based, and function-oriented rehabilitation programs rather than considering it as a standalone intervention.

6.2 Biophysics of Polarized Polychromatic Noncoherent Light (PPNCL)

6.2.1 Polarization

Electromagnetic radiation consists of oscillating electric and magnetic fields propagating perpendicular to each other and to the direction of wave travel.

Polarization refers to the orientation of the electric field vector. In polarized light, the electric field oscillates predominantly in a single plane rather than randomly in multiple directions. Theoretically, polarization may influence photon–tissue interaction by promoting more organized electromagnetic field interaction at biological interfaces. However, the clinical significance of polarization remains under investigation. Current literature does not conclusively isolate polarization as an independent therapeutic variable when wavelength and dosimetry are controlled.

6.2.2 Coherence

Coherence refers to phase alignment between photons. Laser systems produce coherent light, whereas polychromatic systems emit noncoherent light with random phase distribution. Importantly, biological tissues respond primarily to photon absorption rather than coherence per se. Therefore, noncoherent light can still produce photobiomodulatory effects provided appropriate parameters are used.

6.2.3 Wavelengths and Penetration Depth

Wavelength refers to the distance between successive peaks of a light wave, measured in nanometers (nm), which determines the light's color and depth of penetration into biological tissue. Different wavelengths target specific chromophores within the body to trigger distinct physiological responses. Unlike lasers, which are monochromatic (emitting a single, narrow wavelength), PPNCL technology utilizes polychromacy, emitting a broad spectrum of wavelengths simultaneously.

Penetration depth depends primarily on wavelength and tissue optical properties.

- Shorter wavelengths (blue–green) are absorbed more superficially due to higher scattering and melanin absorption.

- Red and near-infrared wavelengths (600–1000 nm) demonstrate greater penetration into soft tissues due to lower absorption by superficial chromophores.

Penetration depth in soft tissues is generally limited to a few millimeters to several centimeters, depending on wavelength and tissue composition. Scattering plays a dominant role in limiting deep penetration, particularly in highly hydrated or collagen-rich tissues.

This polychromatic approach ensures a combined effect, in which a wide range of wavelengths—spanning from visible light to near-infrared—collectively stimulate various cellular processes at different tissue depths, potentially enabling interactions with multiple chromophores, although comparative superiority over single-wavelength sources has not been conclusively established.

Therapeutic systems in this category typically emit light across a broad spectral range, typically between 480 and 3400 nm. However, the biologically active range in rehabilitation practice is usually limited to 600–1000 nm.

6.2.4 Irradiance and Energy Density

In photomedicine, "dosimetry" refers to the measurement and calculation of the light dose delivered to biological tissue. Understanding the relationship between irradiance and energy density is critical for ensuring clinical efficacy and patient safety.

Irradiance (power density; measured in Watts per square centimeter (W/cm^2) represents the "intensity" of the light at a specific moment. It is defined as the amount of electromagnetic power (flux) delivered per unit area of the treatment surface. Irradiance determines the rate at which photons are delivered to the tissue. High irradiance can lead to thermal effects (heat), whereas lower irradiance is typically used for nonthermal biostimulation (photobiomodulation). It is influenced by the device's output and the distance between the device and the patient's skin.

Energy density (measured in Joules per square centimeter (J/cm^2) represents the total "dose" of light delivered over the entire duration of a treatment session. This is the most important parameter for clinical protocols. Medical guidelines (such as those for wound healing or pain management) specify a target energy density required to trigger a biological response. If the energy density is too low, the treatment may be sub-therapeutic; if it is too high, it may inhibit cellular repair or cause tissue damage (the biphasic dose-response).

6.2.5 Light–Tissue Interaction

When light reaches biological tissue, four primary processes occur:

1. Reflection—a portion of incident light is reflected at the skin surface.
2. Absorption—photons are absorbed by chromophores within tissues.

3. Scattering—photons change direction within tissue, reducing penetration depth but increasing interaction volume.
4. Transmission—a small fraction may pass through superficial layers.

A fundamental principle governing these interactions is the Grotthuss–Draper Law, which states that chromophores—specifically, molecular chromophores—must absorb light to produce a biological effect. If a receptor does not capture the light energy, no physiological change can occur. In PPNCL therapy, this law is practically applied by delivering a broad spectrum of wavelengths to ensure optimal absorption by key cellular targets.

PPNCL is considered a nonthermal modality primarily when applied within therapeutic irradiance levels. Although minimal superficial warming may occur, the therapeutic mechanism is attributed predominantly to photochemical and photobiological modulation rather than to heat transfer.

This distinction sets polarized light therapy apart from thermotherapy and infrared heating modalities.

6.2.6 Dosology/Parameters

In clinical applications, effective dosimetry is governed by four primary parameters: wavelength (nm), irradiance (mW/cm^2), energy density (J/cm^2), and treatment duration. A standard therapeutic dose usually ranges from 2 to 10 J/cm^2 per session, depending on whether the target is superficial wound tissue or deeper musculoskeletal structures. Irradiance is generally maintained at a nonthermal level—typically between 40 and 100 mW/cm^2 to trigger photobiomodulation without inducing tissue hyperthermia. Precise adherence to these parameters is essential, as the biological response follows a biphasic dose-response curve: insufficient energy fails to trigger repair, while excessive exposure may lead to bio-inhibition.

6.2.7 Differences Between Polarized Polychromatic Noncoherent Light and Low-Level Laser Therapy (LLLT)

PPNCL and low-level laser therapy (LLLT), both belong to the broader category of light-based therapeutic modalities. However, they differ significantly in their physical properties, beam characteristics, and clinical delivery.

6.2.7.1 Coherence

LLLT uses coherent light, meaning the emitted photons are phase-locked and travel in synchrony. In contrast, PPNCL emits noncoherent light, in which photons have random phase relationships.

Current evidence suggests that biological tissues respond primarily to photon absorption rather than coherence itself. Therefore, both coherent and noncoherent light may produce photobiomodulatory effects, provided appropriate wavelengths and dosimetric parameters are used.

6.2.8 Monochromatic Versus Polychromatic Emission

LLLT typically emits monochromatic light, meaning a single, narrow wavelength (e.g., 630 nm, 810 nm, 904 nm). This allows precise targeting of specific chromophores and deeper tissue penetration, depending on the selected wavelength. In contrast, PPNCL emits polychromatic light, spanning a broader wavelength range. This may allow interaction with multiple chromophores simultaneously but reduces spectral specificity.

6.2.9 Power Density

Laser beams of LLLT can achieve higher power densities in small, focused areas. This allows for precise application and deeper tissue energy delivery when appropriate wavelengths are used.

PPNCL systems produce lower power density over larger treatment areas. As a result, energy delivery is typically more diffuse, penetration depth may be more limited, and treatment areas can be larger without repositioning.

6.2.10 Penetration Characteristics

Laser systems operating at near-infrared wavelengths (e.g., 800–1000 nm) may achieve deeper tissue penetration due to their narrow spectral emission and higher power density.

PPNCL systems rely on wavelength distribution and irradiance rather than coherence for penetration. Although near-infrared components contribute to tissue penetration, energy attenuation due to scattering remains significant.

6.2.11 Dosimetry and Standardization

LLLT has more extensively standardized dosimetry protocols in the literature, including specific recommendations for energy density and treatment points.

PPNCL dosimetry is less standardized across studies, and treatment parameters may vary depending on device design and spectral output.

Table 6.1 Comparison of LLLT and PPNCL characteristics

Parameter	LLLT	PPNCL
Coherence	Coherent	Noncoherent
Wavelength	Monochromatic	Polychromatic
Polarization	No	Yes, varied
Dosimetry	Typically between 40 and 100 mW/cm^2	Typically between 40 and 100 mW/cm^2
Power density	Higher, focused	Lower, diffuse
Spectral specificity	High	Moderate
Treatment area	Localized	Larger areas

6.2.12 Clinical Implications

From a clinical perspective, both modalities aim to induce photobiomodulation through similar mechanisms (see below). Importantly, current evidence does not conclusively demonstrate the superiority of coherence over noncoherence in producing biological effects. The therapeutic response appears to depend primarily on wavelength, irradiance, energy density, and total dose rather than on coherence alone (Table 6.1).

6.3 Practical Implementation: How to Use

Appropriate dosing is critical for achieving therapeutic photobiomodulation effects. As with other electro-physical agents, clinical outcomes depend not only on the modality itself but primarily on the correct selection of parameters, including wavelength distribution, irradiance, energy density, exposure time, and treatment frequency. To achieve the analgesic and functional outcomes, users should adhere to the following evidence-based guidelines:

1. *Spectral range*

   Polarized polychromatic non-coherent light systems emit a broad wavelength spectrum, typically covering visible and near-infrared regions.

   - Visible range (≈ 480–700 nm): More superficial tissue interaction
   - Red and near-infrared range (≈ 600–1000 nm): Deeper soft-tissue penetration
   - The red and near-infrared components are considered most relevant for musculoskeletal and wound-healing applications due to improved tissue penetration and mitochondrial absorption.

2. *Irradiance (power density)*

   Typical therapeutic irradiance values for PPNCL systems range approximately between 20 and 100 mW/cm^2, depending on device specifications and treatment distance.

   Higher irradiance does not necessarily produce better results. Excessive irradiance may reduce therapeutic efficiency due to the biphasic dose–response phenomenon.

3. *Energy density*

   Energy density is one of the most important parameters in photobiomodulation and is expressed in J/cm^2.

   Typical therapeutic ranges reported in clinical photobiomodulation literature:

   - 2–10 J/cm^2 for superficial wounds
   - 4–12 J/cm^2 for musculoskeletal conditions
   - Higher doses may be used cautiously in chronic conditions, depending on tissue depth.

   It is important to note that energy density delivered at the skin surface does not equal the energy reaching deeper tissues due to attenuation and scattering.

4. *Treatment duration, distance and angle:*

   The clinical efficacy of PPNCL is critically dependent on the spatial relationship between the light source and the target tissue, specifically the distance and the angle of incidence. To maximize energy delivery, the light source should ideally be positioned at a 90-degree angle (perpendicular) to the skin surface. This "normal incidence" minimizes photon reflection, thereby ensuring that the maximum number of polarized photons penetrate the dermal layers rather than scatter off the stratum corneum. As the angle deviates from the perpendicular (oblique incidence), the effective power density (irradiance) decreases, requiring longer treatment times to achieve the same therapeutic dose. Similarly, the distance between the emitter and the tissue must be carefully controlled; while LLLT is often applied in contact or near-contact to reduce beam divergence and bypass the inverse square law, noncoherent polarized sources are typically held at a fixed distance (usually 5–10 cm) to allow for uniform coverage of a specific area. Maintaining a consistent distance is essential for dosage reproducibility, as even minor increases in separation can lead to a significant drop in energy density, potentially falling below the threshold required for biostimulation.

   Treatment duration is determined by desired energy density and irradiance. Common clinical application times range from 4 to 10 min/treatment zone.

   A longer duration increases the total energy delivered, but it must remain within therapeutic windows (Fig. 6.1).

5. *Treatment areas*

   The light should be applied directly to the affected region (e.g., the dorsum of the hand or the lumbar region for back pain). The area must be clean and free of creams, moisturizers, or serums to avoid any interaction between light and these products.

6. *Treatment frequency*

   For chronic conditions, three to five sessions per week for 2–4 weeks are recommended to ensure sustained therapeutic effects. Ideally, for home-based users, a once- or twice-daily application protocol is recommended to maintain consistent biostimulatory effects throughout a 24-h cycle.

7. *Application*

   Therapy should be initiated at the earliest possible stage of injury or diagnosis to maximize early-stage mobility gains and pain reduction.

   Treatment sessions typically last between 4 and 10 min/zone, once or twice daily. To accommodate diverse therapeutic needs, PPNCL technology is avail-

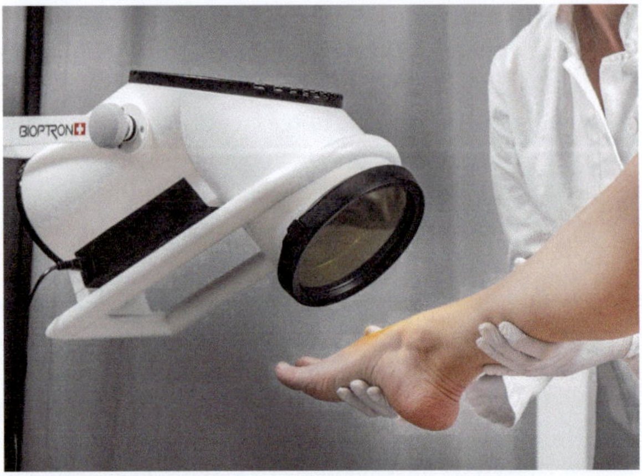

Fig. 6.1 Illustration of a typical PPNCL session: device positioned at around 10 cm with the light beam accurately directed to the treatment area

able in various models tailored for both professional clinical environments and private home use. The flexibility of these delivery systems allows for optimized dosing schedules based on the patient's setting. Ideally, for home-based users, a once- or twice-daily application protocol is recommended to maintain consistent biostimulatory effects throughout a 24-h cycle.

While such high-frequency administration is often impractical in a clinical or outpatient setting, therapeutic efficacy is by no means compromised by a professional schedule. Peer-reviewed literature confirms that three sessions per week remain clinically impactful, yielding significant reductions in pain and improvements in functional recovery. Thus, for chronic conditions, 3 to 5 sessions per week for 2 to 4 weeks are recommended to ensure sustained therapeutic effects. This adaptability ensures that, whether used as an intensive home regimen or a structured clinical intervention, the treatment remains a solution for managing chronic pathology.

8. *Adjuvant use*

While PPNCL can be used as monotherapy, it is more commonly used as an adjunct; integrating it with standard protocols—such as kinesiotherapy, cryotherapy, or LFMF—yields a combined effect. Significantly enhancing the outcomes of these traditional treatments is associated with analgesic relief and the concurrent optimization of joint function and mobility. This multimodal approach ensures that the biological benefits of light therapy work in tandem with physical interventions to produce positive clinical results.

9. *Practical clinical considerations*

- Clean the skin surface before application, and apply without creams or serums.
- Avoid ocular exposure.
- Do not apply over an active malignancy.
- Monitor patient feedback for warmth or discomfort.
- Follow the instructions provided by the manufacturer.

Polarized polychromatic light should be integrated into a broader rehabilitation program rather than used as a standalone intervention.

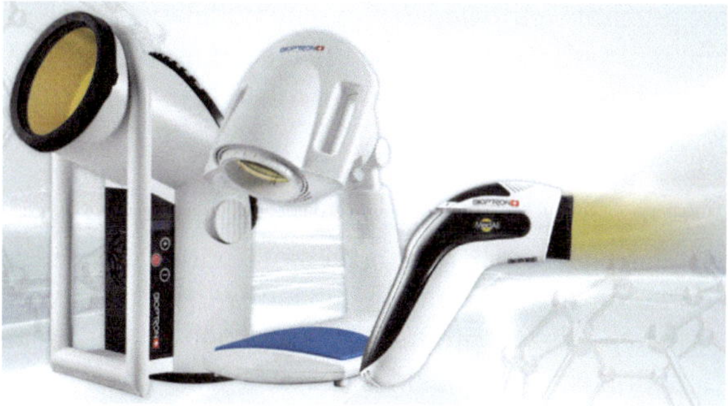

Fig. 6.2 Some examples of PPNCL devices

Table 6.2 Summary of core dosological parameters

Parameter	Typical clinical range
Wavelength	480–3400 nm (active: 600–1000 nm)
Irradiance	20–100 mW/cm²
Energy density	2–12 J/cm²
Duration	4–10 min per zone
Frequency	3–5 times/week

10. *PPNCL devices*

Devices that provide PPNCL are engineered to emit a unique form of light that combines the properties of broad-spectrum (polychromatic) light with a specific spatial orientation (polarization), while remaining noncoherent and low-energy.

The defining feature of these devices is a multilayer polarizing filter. This component ensures that the light waves are oriented in parallel planes. In most clinical PPNCL devices, the degree of polarization exceeds 95%. It has been hypothesized that polarization may influence lipid bilayer organization and the dipole orientation of water molecules in blood and interstitial fluid; however, these mechanisms remain theoretical and require further experimental validation (Fig. 6.2, Table 6.2).

6.4 Mechanism of Action

Over three decades ago, it was proposed that when the cell membrane phospholipid bilayer is exposed to a laser or polarized light, the random distribution of polar-headed phospholipids is replaced by a more structured configuration, possibly redistributing the biologically active proteins and enabling more efficient function. Additionally, it has been suggested that PPNCL could improve cellular processes such as active and passive transport, recognition of antibodies and hormones, release and reception of neurotransmitters, and energy transmission and conversion, all of which may contribute to improved healing. More recently, it was proposed that different wavelengths cause different rates of cellular apoptosis; however, the underlying physiological mechanisms remain unclear. The therapeutic effects of PPNCL are primarily attributed to photobiomodulation mechanisms occurring at the cellular and molecular levels. These effects are mediated by photon absorption by endogenous chromophores, which subsequently modulate intracellular signaling pathways.

Key chromophores include the following:

- Cytochrome c oxidase (mitochondrial respiratory chain): It is considered one of the principal photoacceptors within the red and near-infrared spectrum. Photon absorption may enhance mitochondrial electron transport, leading to increased ATP production and modulation of reactive oxygen species (ROS) within physiological ranges.
- Hemoglobin
- Melanin
- Water (particularly at higher infrared wavelengths)

Importantly, the biological response is wavelength-dependent and dose-dependent, and does not rely on tissue heating or mechanical stimulation.

6.4.1 Mitochondrial Activation and ATP Production [13, 33, 35]

One of the most widely accepted mechanisms in photobiomodulation involves the absorption of red and near-infrared photons by cytochrome c oxidase (Complex IV) in the mitochondrial respiratory chain.

Photon absorption may:

- Enhance electron transport chain activity
- Increase mitochondrial membrane potential
- Improve ATP synthesis

Increased ATP availability supports cellular repair processes, protein synthesis, and ion pump regulation. This mechanism is considered central to tissue regeneration and functional recovery.

6.4.2 Nitric Oxide (NO) Modulation [4, 12, 26]

Light exposure may promote the dissociation of nitric oxide (NO) from cytochrome c oxidase, facilitating improved mitochondrial respiration. In addition, increased nitric oxide availability contributes to:

- Vasodilation
- Improved microcirculation
- Enhanced oxygen delivery
- Modulation of inflammatory responses

The NO-mediated pathway may partly explain the improved perfusion observed in wound healing and inflammatory conditions.

6.4.3 Reactive Oxygen Species (ROS) Signaling [14, 34]

Photobiomodulation may induce controlled increases in reactive oxygen species (ROS) within physiological limits. These transient increases act as signaling molecules that activate transcription factors that can lead to upregulation of genes involved in:

- Cellular proliferation
- Growth factor production
- Tissue repair

Importantly, excessive irradiation may produce inhibitory or oxidative stress effects, reinforcing the biphasic dose–response principle.

6.4.4 Inflammatory Modulation [6, 7, 20, 35, 36]

PPNCL has been associated with the modulation of inflammatory mediators, including the following:

- Reduction of proinflammatory cytokines (e.g., TNF-α, IL-1β)
- Upregulation of anti-inflammatory pathways

This regulatory effect may contribute to:

- Decreased pain
- Reduced edema
- Accelerated resolution of inflammation

These effects are particularly relevant to soft-tissue injuries and chronic inflammatory disorders.

6.4.5 Angiogenesis and Tissue Repair [2, 5, 8, 18, 25, 26, 32, 36]

Photobiomodulation may stimulate angiogenic factors such as vascular endothelial growth factor (VEGF), promoting neovascularization in damaged tissues and promoting the elongation of preexisting capillaries.

In wound healing contexts, reported effects include the following:

- Enhanced fibroblast proliferation
- Increased collagen synthesis
- Improved epithelialization

These processes support tissue remodeling and structural recovery.

6.4.6 Neural and Analgesic Effects [9, 10, 11, 15–17]

Light therapy may influence neural tissue through:

- Modulation of nerve conduction
- Reduction in inflammatory sensitization
- Altered nociceptor activity

Analgesic effects are likely multifactorial, involving:

- Decreased inflammatory mediators
- Improved local circulation
- Modulation of peripheral nerve excitability

However, the precise neural mechanisms remain under investigation.

The intricate cascade of cellular events triggered by light therapy serves as the biological foundation for systemic healing. These microscopic interactions are not merely isolated physiological events; they translate directly into measurable therapeutic benefits for the patient. By optimizing cellular metabolism and regulating the inflammatory response, the technology achieves profound effects across a spectrum of medical disciplines. In the following sections, we will detail the specific clinical implications of these mechanisms, demonstrating how they manifest in accelerated wound repair, significant pain reduction, and the successful management of diverse dermatological and musculoskeletal conditions.

The therapeutic efficacy is rooted in the principles of photobiomodulation, wherein incoherent, polarized, and polychromatic light interacts with cells and biomolecules and triggers specific cellular mechanisms (Fig. 6.3).

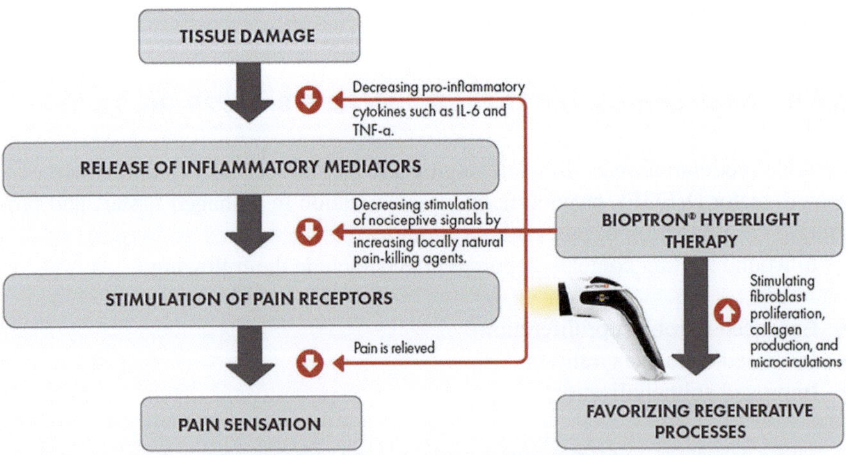

Fig. 6.3 Graphical representation of cellular actions of PPNCL devices in pain management

6.4.7 Pain Relief Action

PPNCL helps to mitigate inflammation, a key contributor to pain and delayed healing. It increases the release of local nitric oxide (NO) and decreases IL-6 release. This dual action, targeting both inflammatory and pain-signaling pathways, contributes to efficacy by providing significant pain relief throughout the rehabilitation and healing processes.

6.4.8 Increased Fibroblast Proliferation and Migration

Fibroblasts play an important role in providing structural support to muscles by synthesizing collagen, forming granulation tissue, and remodeling the extracellular matrix. PPNCL increases the proliferation of newly formed fibroblasts, promoting tissue regeneration, extracellular matrix production, and remodeling.

6.4.9 Boosted Collagen Production

PPNCL stimulates the production of endogenous collagen, providing the structural framework and scaffolding necessary for tissue repair. Collagen deposition helps to repair the damage, providing tensile strength and elasticity.

6.4.10 Improved Microcirculation

Impaired microcirculation can significantly delay tissue repair. PPNCL increases blood flow in capillaries, creating an environment conducive to regenerative cellular mechanisms by ensuring adequate delivery of oxygen and nutrients, removal of waste, immune response, and tissue regeneration. PPNCL stimulates the reparative processes.

The clinical efficacy of PPNCL in physiotherapy and rehabilitation is fundamentally rooted in the orchestration of multiple, simultaneous cellular responses. By integrating an analgesic effect with the mitigation of inflammatory processes, the therapy creates a biological environment conducive to recovery. This is further supported at the structural level by stimulating fibroblast proliferation and migration, which, together with increased collagen production, facilitate the restoration of soft tissue integrity. When coupled with significantly improved microcirculation, these mechanisms act together to produce a statistically significant reduction in localized pain (see Sect. 6.6). Consequently, this multimodal biological stimulation leads to a measurable increase in mobility and functional range in the affected region.

Clinical Effects of Polarized Polychromatic Noncoherent Light

Polarized polychromatic non-coherent light is associated with several clinically relevant effects, including pain reduction, modulation of inflammatory processes, and enhancement of tissue repair. Analgesic effects are likely mediated through combined peripheral and central mechanisms, including modulation of nociceptive signaling and improved microcirculation.

In addition, photobiomodulation may support tissue regeneration through increased fibroblast activity, collagen synthesis, and angiogenesis. These effects contribute to improved tissue quality and functional recovery.

Clinically, these responses may enhance tolerance to therapeutic loading and facilitate integration within rehabilitation programs.

6.5 Indications, Contraindications, Precautions, and Side Effects

6.5.1 Indications

Polarized polychromatic non-coherent light (PPNCL) is primarily used as an adjunct modality within rehabilitation and wound management. The strength of evidence varies depending on the clinical indication.

Wound Healing

- Acute and chronic wounds
- Pressure ulcers
- Diabetic ulcers
- Postsurgical wounds
- Burns (superficial to partial thickness)

Photobiomodulation may support epithelialization, angiogenesis, and collagen synthesis.

Musculoskeletal Conditions

- Tendinopathies
- Muscle strains
- Ligament sprains
- Myofascial pain
- Osteoarthritis (adjunct use)

Potential benefits include reducing inflammation, relieving pain, and supporting tissue repair.

Inflammatory and Soft Tissue Disorders

- Bursitis
- Mild synovitis
- Localized inflammatory conditions

Dermatological Applications

- Acne vulgaris
- Psoriasis
- Dermatitis
- Scar management

Pain Management

- Localized acute or chronic pain
- Neuropathic pain (adjunctive)

It should be emphasized that PPNCL is not considered a standalone treatment but rather a supportive intervention within comprehensive rehabilitation programs.

6.5.2 Contraindications

PPNCL should not be applied in the following situations:

- Active malignancy in the treatment area.
- Direct irradiation of the eyes (risk of retinal injury).
- Active hemorrhage or uncontrolled bleeding.
- Photosensitive epilepsy (when applied near the head/face).
- Specific photosensitive pathologies/disorders of the eyes and/or skin.
- Use of photosensitizing medications.

Direct ocular exposure must always be avoided, and appropriate eye protection is recommended for both patient and therapist.

Caution is advised in:

- Pregnancy (avoid direct application over the abdomen or lumbar region)
- Autoimmune inflammatory conditions
- Endocrine glands (e.g., thyroid region)

Clinical judgment by a healthcare professional should guide application in these cases.

6.5.3 Precautions

- Maintain appropriate treatment distance as per device specifications.
- Avoid prolonged exposure beyond the recommended energy density.
- Use protective eyewear when indicated.
- Monitor patient response during initial sessions.

6.5.4 Side Effects

When used at therapeutic doses, PPNCL is generally considered safe and well-tolerated.

Reported side effects are rare and typically mild:

- Transient erythema
- Mild warmth
- Temporary increase in local sensitivity

No significant systemic adverse effects have been consistently reported in the literature when appropriate dosimetry is respected.

6.5.5 Safety Considerations

PPNCL is a nonionizing modality and does not produce DNA-damaging radiation when applied within therapeutic ranges. However, adherence to recommended dosing parameters remains essential to avoid overexposure and diminished therapeutic response.

6.6 Research Evidence: Clinical Scope of Polarized Polychromatic Noncoherent Light (PPNCL)

The clinical application of polarized polychromatic non-coherent light (PPNCL) is rooted in its unique ability to trigger multilayered biological responses, and it is supported by a growing but heterogeneous body of literature. Evidence varies depending on the indication, treatment protocol, wavelength distribution, and study design. As with other photobiomodulation modalities, methodological variability limits direct comparison between studies.

PPNCL is primarily indicated for the acceleration of wound healing—including chronic ulcers, postsurgical incisions, and thermal burns—by enhancing microcirculation and stimulating fibroblast proliferation for tissue regeneration. In rheumatology and pain management, it is utilized to reduce inflammation and alleviate discomfort associated with osteoarthritis, rheumatoid arthritis, and acute musculoskeletal injuries (such as sprains and strains). Furthermore, its dermatological indications include inflammatory conditions such as acne, dermatitis, and psoriasis. The efficacy of PPNCL across these diverse indications is attributed to the combined action of its polychromatic wavelengths, which ensure deeper, more comprehensive penetration than monochromatic sources, thereby modulating cellular metabolism at varying depths within the integumentary and musculoskeletal systems.

6.6.1 Clinical Applications in Physiotherapy and Rehabilitation

Studies investigating light-based photobiomodulation for:

- Tendinopathies
- Osteoarthritis
- Muscle injuries
- Myofascial pain

have reported improvements in pain scores and functional outcomes when used alongside exercise-based rehabilitation or other treatments, such as low-frequency magnetic fields (LFMF).

However, many studies combine different modalities, sample sizes are often small to moderate, and the treatment parameters differ substantially.

Therefore, for musculoskeletal disorders, the level of evidence may be considered moderate due to the diverse protocols and pathologies.

6.6.2 Clinical Applications in Wound Healing

The strongest body of evidence for light-based therapies relates to wound healing.

Several randomized and controlled studies investigating photobiomodulation in acute and chronic wounds have reported:

- Accelerated epithelialization
- Increased granulation tissue formation
- Improved microcirculation
- Reduced healing time

However, heterogeneity in:

- Energy density
- Treatment frequency
- Wound type
- Outcome measures

makes definitive protocol standardization difficult.

Overall, evidence for the adjunctive use in wound healing is moderate, with stronger support for superficial and chronic wounds than for deep tissue lesions.

6.6.3 Inflammatory and Dermatological Conditions

In dermatology and inflammatory disorders, photobiomodulation has demonstrated:

- Anti-inflammatory effects
- Improved collagen remodeling
- Reduction in acne lesion count (in some studies)
- Repair and skin regeneration

While promising, these findings are not consistent across studies, and long-term comparative trials are limited.

Evidence in this domain may be classified as low and emerging.

6.6.4 Analgesic Effects

The proposed and proven mechanisms were explained in the previous Sects. 6.4.7, 6.4.8, 6.4.9 and 6.4.10, which include the following:

- Pain relief action
- Increased fibroblast proliferation and migration
- Boosted collagen production
- Improved microcirculation

Clinical trials suggest short-term pain reduction in selected conditions. However, variability in dosing and patient populations limits generalizability.

Analgesic evidence is therefore considered supportive but condition-specific.

6.6.5 Limitations of Current Literature

Several methodological limitations should be acknowledged:

- Lack of standardized dosimetry
- Variable spectral output across devices
- Limited long-term follow-up
- Small sample sizes in many studies

6.6.6 Overall Interpretation

Based on available literature:

- The most consistent support exists for adjunctive wound healing applications.
- Evidence in musculoskeletal conditions is moderate but variable.
- Evidence in dermatological and inflammatory conditions is promising but heterogeneous.

Polarized polychromatic non-coherent light should therefore be considered an adjunct modality within comprehensive rehabilitation or wound care protocols, rather than a primary standalone treatment.

Further high-quality randomized controlled trials with standardized dosimetry are required to clarify optimal treatment parameters.

6.6.7 Summary and Conclusions

Polarized polychromatic non-coherent light (PPNCL) represents a nonthermal photobiomodulation modality operating within the visible and near-infrared spectrum. Its biological effects are primarily mediated by photon absorption by endogenous chromophores, which modulate mitochondrial activity, nitric oxide signaling, controlled production of reactive oxygen species, and inflammatory pathways.

From a biophysical perspective, therapeutic response depends on wavelength distribution, irradiance, energy density, and total dose rather than on coherence alone. While polarization may influence the orientation of the electromagnetic field at tissue interfaces, current evidence suggests that wavelength and dosimetry remain the primary determinants of clinical outcome.

Clinically, PPNCL is most consistently supported as an adjunct modality for wound healing, with evidence suggesting potential benefits in epithelialization, angiogenesis, and tissue repair. In musculoskeletal and inflammatory conditions, findings are more heterogeneous, and treatment effects appear to be condition-specific.

The modality demonstrates a favorable safety profile when applied within recommended dosimetric parameters, provided that appropriate precautions are observed, particularly regarding ocular exposure and application over malignancy.

Given the variability in protocols and study designs, further high-quality randomized controlled trials with standardized dosing parameters are required. Until such standardization is achieved, PPNCL should be integrated into comprehensive, function-oriented rehabilitation programs rather than used as a standalone intervention.

In conclusion, polarized, polychromatic, noncoherent light is a potentially useful adjunct in rehabilitation and wound management, provided that its application is guided by sound biophysical principles, appropriate dosing, and careful interpretation of current evidence.

Key Messages

- Polarized polychromatic non-coherent light is a nonthermal photobiomodulation modality.
- Therapeutic effects are mediated primarily through cellular photochemical mechanisms rather than heat.
- Clinical outcomes depend on appropriate dosing, wavelength distribution, and treatment consistency.
- The strongest evidence supports its use in wound healing applications.
- Evidence in musculoskeletal and dermatological conditions is variable and condition-specific.
- PPNCL should be used as an adjunct to active rehabilitation rather than as a standalone treatment.

6.7 Clinical Trials and Case Studies

6.7.1 Rheumatology: Managing Pain and Joint Functionality

In the field of rheumatology, the primary therapeutic challenge lies in managing chronic pain and slowing the progression of degenerative joint diseases. PPNCL serves as a noninvasive intervention for conditions such as rheumatoid arthritis and osteoarthritis by reducing pain and improving mobility.

6.7.1.1 Clinical Trial 1: Osteoarthritis [1]

Osteoarthritis (OA) is the most common form of arthritis. It is a degeneration of joint cartilage and the underlying bone, most common from middle age onward. It causes pain and stiffness, especially in the hip, knee, and thumb joints.

Patients Profile

In the clinical trial by Abramovich et al. [1], patients aged between 40 and 69 years with primary deforming OA of the knee joints, Grade 1–3.

Treatment Parameters

They were divided into two groups (Fig. 6.4):

1. Treated only with naphtalan (anti-inflammatory, anti-pain properties) cream
2. Naphtalan in combination with PPNCL
   - Wavelength range: Visible and near-infrared spectrum
   - Irradiance: Approximately 40 mW/cm^2
   - Energy density: 2.4 J/cm^2
   - Duration: 6 min/reatment zone
   - Frequency: 5 sessions per session
   - Application distance: As per device specifications, perpendicular to the knee
   - Treatment duration: 2 weeks

The following parameters were measured before and after 2 weeks of treatment:

- Oxford Knee Score: A 12-item patient-reported PRO specifically designed and developed to assess function and pain after total knee replacement (TKR) surgery.

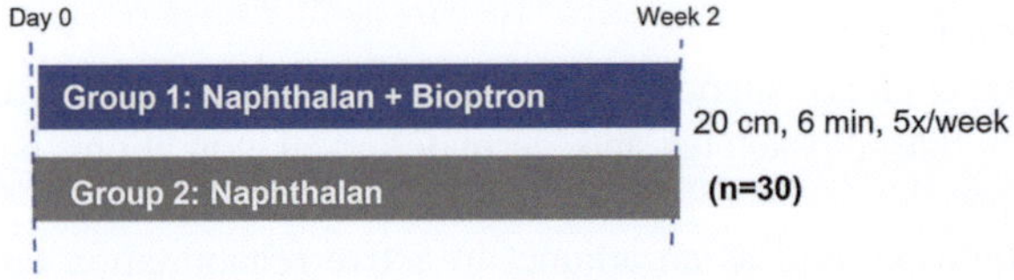

Fig. 6.4 Protocol followed by [1], to assess the effects of naphtalan and the combination naphtalan + PPNCL. For 2 weeks, PPNCL was used at a distance of 20 cm from the knees for 6 min, 5 times a week

- WOMAC arthritis Index: Is widely used in the evaluation of hip and knee osteoarthritis. It is a self-administered questionnaire consisting of 24 items.
- 15-meter walk test.
- Lequesne Index: Measuring the severity of OA.
- Visual Analog Scale (VAS) pain (0–100).
- Short Form-36 (QOL): To assess postsurgery quality of life in knee osteoarthritis.

Outcome

The clinical data indicate that treatment with PPNCL significantly improves the efficacy of standard naphtalan therapy for managing knee osteoarthritis symptoms. Following a two-week intervention, patients in the PPNCL group exhibited a marked reduction in pain, while those in the control group showed no change. This analgesic effect was accompanied by a substantial improvement in physical function; most notably, PPNCL patients demonstrated a 20% improvement on the 15-meter walk test, reducing their mean travel time from 25.22 s to 20.28 s (Fig. 6.5).

Interpretation

These objective findings were further corroborated by significant improvements in the Oxford Knee Score and the WOMAC index, reflecting both a recovery of joint mobility and a decrease in localized stiffness. Importantly, the therapeutic profile of PPNCL was characterized by excellent patient tolerance, with no adverse side effects reported during the study period.

Treating osteoarthritis and other chronic rheumatology pathologies often involves a precarious balance between pain management and systemic health risks. Conventional treatments typically rely on nonsteroidal anti-inflammatory drugs (NSAIDs), corticosteroids, and opioids. While these can provide temporary relief, they are frequently associated with significant side effects. In contrast, PPNCL has emerged as a noninvasive alternative for these patients. Clinical evidence, as the article above highlights, demonstrates that it can significantly reduce pain and stiffness while improving mobility—all with no known side effects.

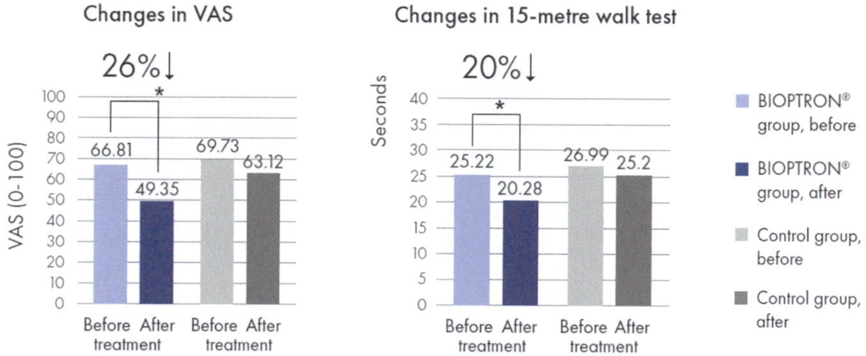

Fig. 6.5 Changes in the different tests performed in patients treated (n = 32) and not treated (n = 32) with PPNCL (*$p < 0.05$). (Modified from Abramovich et al. [1])

6.7.1.2 Clinical Trial 2: Total Knee Arthroplasty [3]

For patients whose condition has progressed to the point of requiring total knee arthroplasty, PPNCL remains a safe and reliable component of the postoperative recovery protocol. While surgery addresses the mechanical failure of the joint, the subsequent rehabilitation period is often plagued by acute pain, significant swelling, and a reliance on heavy analgesics (Fig. 6.6).

Patients profile

Patients who underwent a primary unilateral TKA for primary knee OA were divided into three groups:

Treatment parameters

1. Control: Exercise program
2. Exercise program + LLLT
   - Wavelength: 804 nm, Ga-Al-As semiconductor diodes
   - Power density of 500 mW
   - Dosage of 10 J per session in 2 points (5 J/Point), for 10 seconds
   - The intervention was applied during the first 3 days after the operation, with one session of laser therapy each day.
3. Exercise program + PPNCL
   - 10-min treatment
   - Wavelength 480–3400 nm
   - 95% polarization
   - 40 mW/cm^2; 2.4 J/cm^2
   - 10-cm distance from the device

Outcomes

This three-arm randomized clinical trial demonstrated that both LLLT and PPNCL effectively controlled immediate postoperative pain and swelling. Notably, the study found that patients utilizing these light-based modalities required significantly

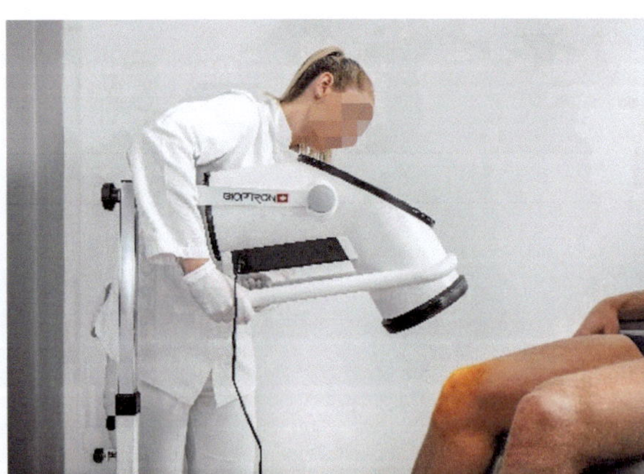

Fig. 6.6 Clinical application of PPNCL on the knee: the device is positioned at a distance of approximately 10 cm, with the light beam precisely targeted to the area of localized pain

lower amounts of opiate painkillers (specifically oxycodone) during the whole recovery compared to the control group. As illustrated in Fig. 6.7, the data regarding oxycodone consumption on the ninth postoperative day reveal a significant reduction in patient reliance on opioids. This decrease in medication intake serves as a clinical proxy for improved pain management, suggesting that the light therapy successfully mitigated acute discomfort. These results persisted until 3 months postoperative follow-up and were not statistically significant at 1-year follow-up, demonstrating a sustained analgesic effect throughout the recovery period.

Furthermore, the researchers observed better functional outcomes and a greater range of motion (ROM) in the early stages of recovery (starting on day 2 after surgery) and in the later stages. As shown in Fig. 6.8, a significant improvement in range of motion at 3 months is observed in the groups treated with LLLT and PPNCL compared with controls.

Interpretation

These studies show the roles of PPNCL and LLLT as noninvasive adjuvant therapies that could accelerate the transition from surgery back to daily activities. The successful integration of light therapies into the postsurgical continuum for total knee arthroplasty could improve the patient's overall quality of life. As patients regain the ability to perform activities of daily living with greater ease and reduced reliance on opioids, their subjective well-being and confidence in the surgical outcome may significantly increase. Nevertheless, the absence of long-term follow-up prevents drawing conclusions about long-term analgesic effects.

6.7.2 Physiotherapy: Restoring Mobility and Functional Range

The management of chronic musculoskeletal conditions represents a significant challenge in modern rehabilitative medicine and represents a staggering global health and economic burden worldwide. When combined with manual therapy,

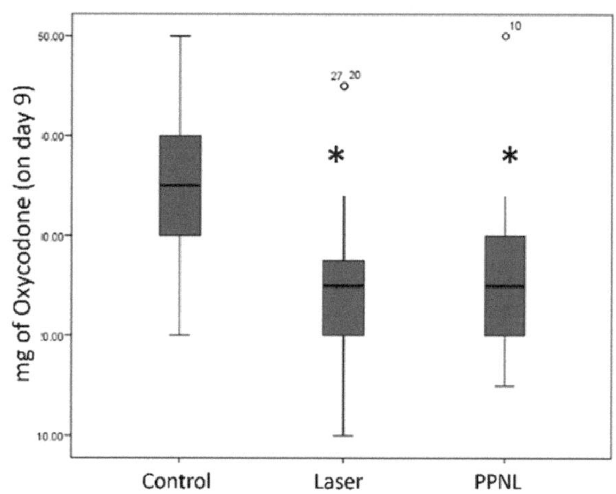

Fig. 6.7 Changes in the oxycodone intake for the three groups (control, LLLT, and PPNCL) on day 9 after surgery. (* $p < 0.05$), highlighting the decrease in pain in groups laser and PPNCL. (Modified from Bahrami et al. [3])

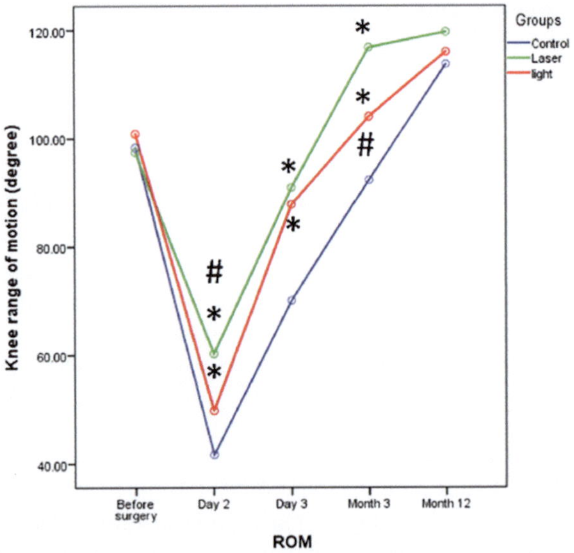

Fig. 6.8 Changes in the range of motion of the knee for the three groups (control, LLLT, and PPNCL) along the recovery period (*$p < 0.05$ group vs. control, #$p < 0.05$ between laser and PPNCL group). (Modified from Bahrami et al. [3])

kinesiology, or pharmacological interventions, PPNCL was associated with improved tissue repair, modulation of inflammatory pathways, and increased range of motion in the affected body part. PPNCL action is combined with the analgesic impact of concurrent treatments, leading to a more rapid restoration of patient mobility and mechanical function.

6.7.2.1 Clinical Trial 3: Low-Back Pain [19]

Low back pain describes pain between the lower edge of the ribs and the buttocks. It can last for a short time (acute), or a long time (chronic). It can affect anyone. Low back pain makes it hard to move and can affect quality of life and mental well-being, and is a major cause of absence from work.

Rehabilitation is essential to reduce the pain, support recovery, and improve function. Specialized care pathways are needed to treat low back pain.

Patient Profile

The clinical efficacy of PPNCL as an adjunctive treatment for lumbar pathology was rigorously evaluated in a study by Mihaylova et al. [19] involving 60 patients (aged 18–55) with chronic low back pain.

Treatment Parameters

All participants received a standardized regimen of LFMF and ultrasound therapy; however, the experimental group ($n = 30$) was additionally treated with 10 min of daily PPNCL:

- 10-min treatment
- Wavelength 480–3400 nm

- 95% polarization
- 40 mW/cm^2; 2.4 J/cm^2
- 10-cm distance from the device

The researchers utilized a comprehensive battery of assessments, including:

- The Visual Analog Scale (VAS) for subjective pain.
- The Roland-Morris questionnaire for quality of life.
- Schoeber test: Objective motor activity measuring lumbar flexion.
- Thomayer test: Objective motor activity measuring finger-to-floor distance.

Outcome

While both groups showed a statistically significant reduction in pain (*$p < 0.05$), the group receiving PPNCL in addition exhibited statistically better outcomes compared to the control group (#$p < 0.05$; VAS score: 3.83 vs. 2.6 after treatment and 2.53 vs. 1.4 at one-month follow-up). The significant reduction in clinical pain intensity has a direct and profound impact on the patients' overall quality of life. This improvement is clearly reflected in the results of the Roland-Morris Disability Questionnaire, where a lower score indicates a marked reduction in physical limitations. The group receiving PPNCL displayed a significant decrease in their Roland-Morris scores immediately following the treatment course (score 6.89 for control vs. 4.37 for treated group; #$p < 0.05$), a trend that was maintained at the one-month follow-up (score 6.29 for control vs. 3.84 for treated group; #$p < 0.05$). In contrast, the control group, which received only LFMF and ultrasound, showed no significant change in their disability scores over the same period. This divergence suggests that the biostimulatory effects of polarized light do not merely provide transient relief but are associated with sustained clinical improvement that stabilizes the patient's functional recovery well after the clinical sessions have concluded.

The assessment of spinal flexibility using the Schober test further corroborated the greater improvements observed in the PPNCL-treated group compared with the control group. Patients receiving the adjunctive PPNCL therapy demonstrated a notable improvement in lumbar mobility, with the mean Schober test measurement increasing by 1.82 cm from baseline. In comparison, the control group exhibited a more modest increase of 1.22 cm (*$p < 0.05$).

In the Thomayer test (finger-to-floor distance), a statistically significant improvement was observed in both groups (*$p < 0.05$). However, the magnitude of functional recovery was significantly more pronounced in the group treated with PPNCL. On average, patients in this group increased their trunk flexion by 10.68 cm, nearly doubling the 5.78 cm improvement observed in the control group (#$p < 0.05$).

Interpretation

These quantitative data suggest that adding PPNCL to standard rehabilitation protocols increases analgesic relief and significantly enhances restoration of spinal ROM and functional recovery.

Nevertheless, the absence of detailed procedural parameters—such as dosage, frequency, and application technique—obscures the treatment intervention and hinders a clear understanding of the established protocol.

6.7.2.2 Clinical Trial 4: Complex Regional Pain Syndrome (CRPS/Sudeck Atrophy) [23]

The use of PPNCL extends to complex recovery scenarios, such as preventing complex regional pain syndrome (CRPS/Sudeck atrophy). The management of distal radius fractures—one of the most common skeletal injuries in the geriatric population—is frequently complicated by the onset of CRPS, a form of chronic pain that usually affects an arm or a leg, developed after an injury.

Patients Profile

The study by Petrovic et al. [23] evaluated the prophylactic and therapeutic effects of PPNCL in 72 female patients with distal radius fractures.

Treatment Parameters

Participants were randomized into two groups: Group 1 (Control) received a standard protocol of NSAIDs, cryotherapy, and kinesiotherapy, while Group 2 (Experimental) received the same protocol plus daily 10-min sessions of PPNCL applied to the dorsal hand region.

- 10-min treatment
- Wavelength 480–3400 nm
- 95% polarization
- 40 mW/cm^2; 2.4 J/cm^2
- 10-cm distance from the device

Patients were monitored at 7 and 15 days for wrist pain using a Visual Analog Scale (VAS), wrist range of motion (supination, pronation), and hand ability to make a fist.

Outcome

The results indicated that while pain levels (VAS) were comparable between groups at day 7, the PPNCL group experienced a significant decline in pain by the end of the 15-day treatment period compared to the control group (#$p < 0.05$; Fig. 6.9).

The clinical intervention with PPNCL has demonstrated an earlier and significant improvement in wrist movement. While both groups underwent standard rehabilitation and showed improvement in motion (*$p < 0.05$), the group additionally treated with PPNCL exhibited significantly higher scores in both supination and pronation than the control group (#$p < 0.05$). Pronation improved more in the PPNCL group during the initial 7-day assessment (#$p < 0.05$). This early acceleration of mobility increases the likelihood that patients can move the wrist effectively in the crucial first stage of recovery. Such rapid gains in range of motion are instrumental in preventing joint stiffness and facilitating a faster transition toward complex manual tasks.

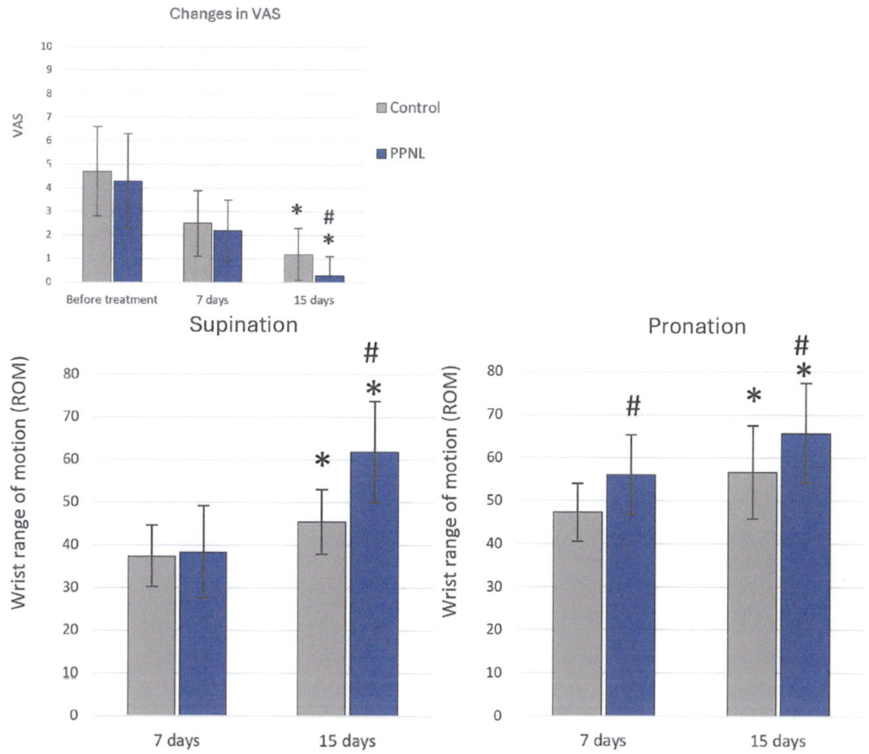

Fig. 6.9 Changes in the pain measured by VAS, and wrist ROM measured by supination and pronation in both groups (control and PPNCL) (*$p < 0.05$ 7 days vs. 15 days within the same group, #$p < 0.05$ control vs. PPNCL group). (Modified from Petrovic et al. [23])

Perhaps most striking was the recovery of fine motor control: 75.6% of patients in the PPNCL group were able to successfully form a fist by the end of the treatment period, compared to only 51.2% in the control group ($p = 0.022$).

Interpretation

The clinical data underscore that early-stage integration of adjuvant PPNCL therapy, initiated at the very onset of recovery, yields therapeutic outcomes. Within just the first week of treatment, patients demonstrated a statistically significant acceleration in functional recovery compared to the control group. Specifically, wrist mobility was greater in the PPNCL group. This rapid enhancement of joint flexibility is complemented by a significant analgesic effect. By addressing both pain and mobility simultaneously from the outset, this adjuvant approach ensures that the greater range of motion in the wrist is achieved sooner, effectively shortening the rehabilitation window and improving the patient's early-stage clinical profile.

The second most profound clinical implication of the study emerged during the six-month follow-up period. In the control group, 22% of patients (9 individuals) developed complex regional pain syndrome, a debilitating condition characterized by chronic pain and vasomotor instability. In contrast, only 4.9% (2 individuals) in the PPNCL group experienced CRPS symptoms. This statistically significant difference ($p = 0.023$) could underscore the role of polarized light as a preventive tool.

6.7.2.3 Clinical Trial 5: Carpal Tunnel Syndrome [27]

Carpal tunnel syndrome (CTS) is a prevalent entrapment neuropathy characterized by compression of the median nerve at the wrist, leading to significant sensory and motor deficits, with symptoms including numbness, paresthesia (tingling), and diminished strength in the thumb and adjacent fingers. While conservative management often involves splinting or corticosteroid injections, these interventions may be contraindicated or undesirable in specific populations, such as pregnant women.

Patients Profile

A pivotal clinical study by Stasinopoulos et al. [27] evaluated the therapeutic impact of PPNCL as a monotherapy for 46 pregnant women in their third trimester suffering from CTS.

Treatment Parameters

The treatment protocol consisted of:

- 10-min treatment
- Wavelength 480–3400 nm
- 95% polarization
- 40 mW/cm^2; 2.4 J/cm^2
- 10-cm distance from the device
- Twice-daily applications
- Five days a week
- Two-week duration.

The research focused on three clinical markers: Subjective pain intensity, paresthesia (tingling and numbness), and objective pinch strength (the force exerted by the thumb and fingers when pinching an object).

Outcomes

The study recorded clinically significant reductions ($*p < 0.05$) in both pain and paresthesia at both follow-up times (Fig. 6.10). Remarkably, the intervention reduced pain and discomfort by more than half.

Interpretation

These benefits were sustained for at least 4 weeks posttreatment, suggesting that PPNCL therapy induces a lasting therapeutic effect rather than a transient masking of symptoms. Beyond symptom relief, patients demonstrated marked improvements in hand function. The data on pinch strength showed a continuous increase over the study period ($*p < 0.05$).

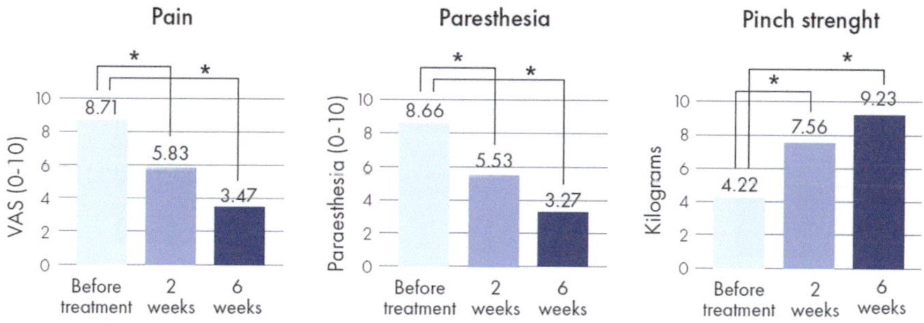

Fig. 6.10 Changes in pain (VAS), paresthesia, and pinch strength from baseline to 2 weeks post-treatment and a 4-week follow-up (*$p < 0.05$ before vs. days of treatment). (Modified from Stasinopoulos et al. [27])

The continued gain in strength posttreatment indicates a progressive restoration of motor nerve conduction and muscular efficiency.

6.7.2.4 Clinical Trial 6: Carpal Tunnel Syndrome [24]

Building on the established efficacy of PPNCL, a recent study by Safaa et al. [24] provides critical electrophysiological evidence of PPNCL's impact on pregnancy-related CTS. While previous research focused on subjective pain and physical strength, this study utilized nerve conduction studies (NCS) to objectively measure the physiological recovery of the median nerve.

Patients Profile

Sixty-two pregnant women were randomized into two groups.

Treatment Parameters

1. Group A received PPNCL therapy alongside wrist bracing and education
   - 10-min treatment
   - Wavelength 480–3400 nm
   - 95% polarization
   - 40 mW/cm^2; 2.4 J/cm^2
   - 10-cm distance from the device
   - Three days a week
   - Four-week duration
2. Group B served as the control, utilizing only the brace and education.

To assess clinical and electrophysiological effects, the researchers used NCS, which records sensory and motor nerve action potentials, to determine the severity of median nerve entrapment.

They measured:

- Motor conduction velocity (MCV), a key indicator of the speed at which electrical impulses travel through the nerve.

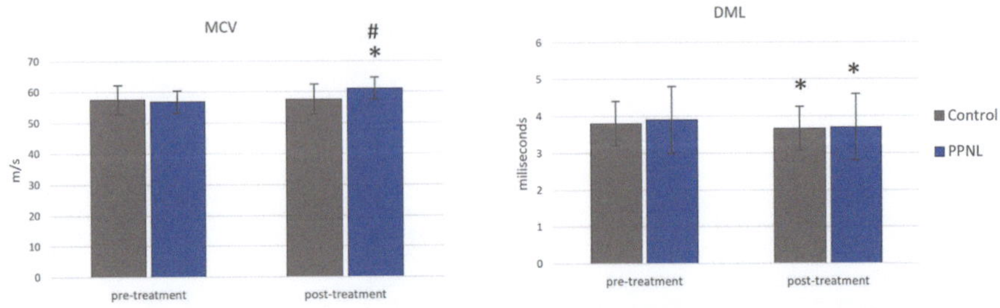

Fig. 6.11 Changes in motor conduction velocity (MCV) and distal motor latency (DML) pre- and posttreatment. (*$p < 0.05$ pre vs. posttreatment; #$p < 0.05$ control vs. PPNCL group). (Modified from Safaa et al. [24])

- Distal motor latency (DML), the time in milliseconds that it takes the impulse to travel from the abductor pollicis brevis muscle to the first metacarpal phalangeal joint.

Outcomes

MCV showed a statistically significant improvement in the PPNCL group ($p = 0.001$), whereas the control group showed no significant change ($p = 0.301$; Fig. 6.11). Furthermore, both groups experienced a decrease in DML, but the reduction was significantly more pronounced in favor of the PPNCL group ($p = 0.001$). These findings suggest that polarized light therapy not only alleviates symptoms but also enhances the conductivity and functional integrity of the compressed median nerve.

Interpretation

When viewed alongside the work of Stasinopoulos [28], a comprehensive picture of PPNCL utility in pregnancy-related CTS emerges. While Stasinopoulos highlighted the 50% reduction in pain and the amplified gains in pinch strength, Safaa provides the biological "why" by confirming the restoration of nerve conduction velocity. Together, these studies highlight PPNCL as a multidimensional tool that could address the sensory, motor, and electrophysiological aspects of entrapment neuropathies.

While the clinical evidence presented in this chapter focuses heavily on pregnant women—a particularly sensitive subpopulation requiring the highest standards of safety and noninvasive care—it is important to note that the therapeutic efficacy of PPNCL is not limited to this group. The positive outcomes regarding pain reduction, nerve conduction restoration, and functional recovery have been consistently validated across a broader demographic spectrum. Numerous peer-reviewed clinical trials, longitudinal case studies, and specialized case reports in the existing bibliography confirm that these results are reproducible in general populations with CTS.

6.7.3 Sports Medicine: Acute Injury and Performance Recovery

In sports medicine, the priority shifts toward the speed of recovery and the management of acute trauma. Whether dealing with professional athletes or active individuals, the goal is a safe and rapid "Return to Play."

PPNCL can be integrated into standard physiotherapy procedures in rehabilitation programs for common sports injuries, such as ankle and knee injuries, tendinitis, and muscle pain.

In the clinical setting, the overarching goals of treatment are to rapidly alleviate pain and inflammation, stimulate the biological healing of damaged ligamentous structures, and restore the full functional range of motion of the ankle. PPNCL devices are used to rehabilitate ankle sprains because they directly address critical recovery needs by reducing pain and localized inflammation. Simultaneously, it promotes the cellular regeneration and repair of ligament tissue, ultimately enhancing its tensile strength and structural integrity. This noninvasive approach could facilitate a more efficient recovery trajectory and may support earlier functional recovery in selected cases.

6.7.3.1 Clinical Trial 7: Ankle Sprains [27]

Patients Profile

The clinical utility of PPNCL in the acute phase of musculoskeletal injury was evaluated by Stasinopoulos et al. in a study involving 50 patients with ankle sprains.

Treatment Parameters

All participants received standard cryotherapy for 20 min every 2 h over a five-day period, while the experimental group ($n = 27$) was additionally treated with 10 min of daily PPNCL therapy.

1. Group 1 received PPNCL therapy alongside cryotherapy for 20 min every 2 h over a five-day period
   - 10-min treatment
   - Wavelength 480–3400 nm
   - 95% polarization
   - 40 mW/cm^2; 2.4 J/cm^2
   - 10-cm distance from the device
   - Once per day
   - Five days a week
2. Group B served as the control, utilizing only the cryotherapy.
   To quantify the therapeutic outcomes, the researchers assessed:

- Pain levels via VAS
- Ankle edema, via circumference measurements
- Ankle motility using goniometry to measure range of motion (Fig. 6.12)

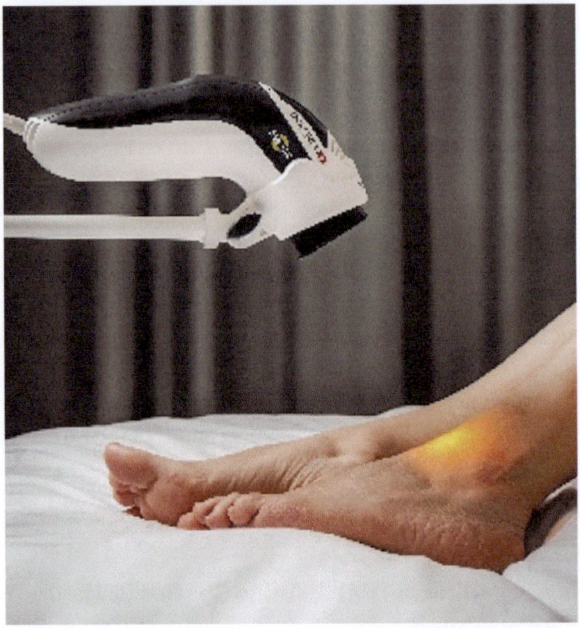

Fig. 6.12 Clinical application of PPNCL on the ankle: The device is positioned approximately 10 cm away, with the light beam precisely directed to the affected ankle

Outcomes

Both groups experienced a decrease in pain before and after the treatment (#p < 0.0005), but patients receiving adjunctive PPNCL reported significantly greater pain relief than those using only cryotherapy (*p < 0.0005; Fig. 6.13).

One of the most statistically significant findings of the study was the reduction in ankle swelling. While both groups experienced a decrease in edema, the PPNCL-treated group exhibited a significantly greater reduction in ankle circumference, averaging 2.67 cm compared with 1.52 cm in the control group (*p < 0.0005). This suggests that the polarized light therapy was associated with a greater reduction in posttraumatic edema in this study, and enhances localized microcirculation more effectively than cryotherapy alone (Fig. 6.13).

Interpretation

Although both groups demonstrated a notable increase in ankle motility—encompassing plantarflexion and dorsiflexion—the improvement in range of motion was significantly greater in patients treated with PPNCL (Fig. 6.14). These results highlight the therapy's ability to facilitate a more rapid return to joint mechanics by simultaneously targeting pain and structural stiffness.

Given its significant pain-relieving and anti-inflammatory properties, along with its ability to optimize regenerative and reparative processes, integrating PPNCL therapy into standard treatment protocols offers an opportunity to treat tendonitis more effectively. This is particularly important as it can enable the application of other necessary treatments that might otherwise be intolerable due to excessive pain.

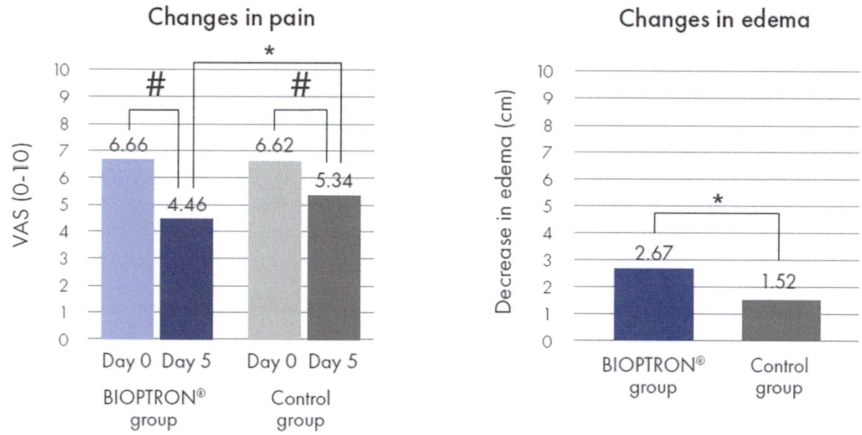

Fig. 6.13 Changes in VAS and edema pretreatment and after 5 days of treatment (#$p < 0.05$ pre vs. post treatment; *$p < 0.05$ control vs. PPNCL group). (Modified from Stasinopoulos et al. [27])

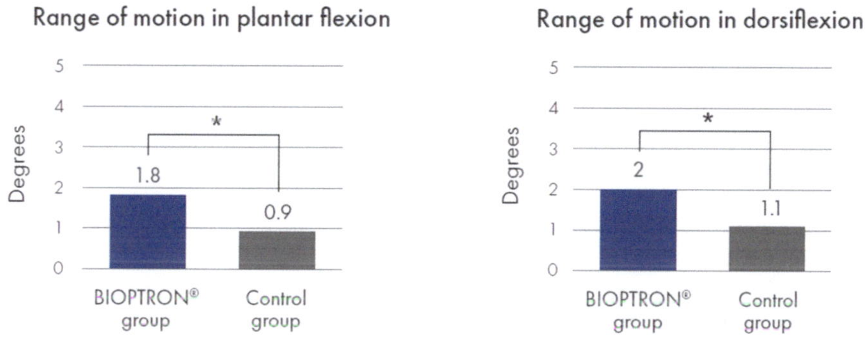

Fig. 6.14 Changes in range of motion via goniometer pretreatment and after 5 days of treatment (*$p < 0.05$ control vs. PPNCL group). (Modified from Stasinopoulos et al. [27])

Building on its established efficacy in acute joint injuries, PPNCL has also demonstrated significant therapeutic value in managing chronic conditions, such as tendinopathies.

6.7.3.2 Clinical Trial 8: Rotator Cuff Tendinopathy [30]

Patients Profile

In a 2020 study by Stasinopoulos et al., 50 patients with rotator cuff tendinopathy participated in a structured 4-week exercise program focused on pain reduction and improved mobility.

Treatment Parameters

1. Group 1 received PPNCL therapy alongside an exercise program
    - 10-min treatment
    - Wavelength 480–3400 nm

- 95% polarization
- 40 mW/cm^2; 2.4 J/cm^2
- 10-cm distance from the device
- Once per day
- Five days a week
- Four-week intervention

2. Group B served as the control, utilizing only the exercise program.
   To evaluate clinical progress, the researchers utilized:

- Shoulder Pain and Disability Index (SPADI) for subjective assessment of pain and disability due to pain.
- Muscular strength using a handheld dynamometer.

Outcome

While both study groups reported a reduction in pain, the group receiving PPNCL therapy demonstrated a significantly greater analgesic relief ($*p < 0.0005$). The PPNCL group also exhibited significantly greater grip strength ($*p < 0.0005$; Fig. 6.15). These findings suggest that polarized light therapy not only accelerates the reduction of discomfort but also optimizes the recovery of motor function and muscle force.

Interpretation

These findings reinforce that PPNCL effectively mitigates the inflammatory and painful barriers of chronic tendonitis, thereby increasing the outcomes of active rehabilitation protocols.

6.7.3.3 Case Report 1– Acute Elbow Tendinopathy [27]

Patient Profile

A 23-year-old female complained of acute pain (less than 48 h) in the lateral aspect of her right elbow, in her dominant hand. The pain was in the facet of the lateral epicondyle. She played tennis for about 4 h, 36 h ago. She experienced pain about 6 h after completing the tennis practice.

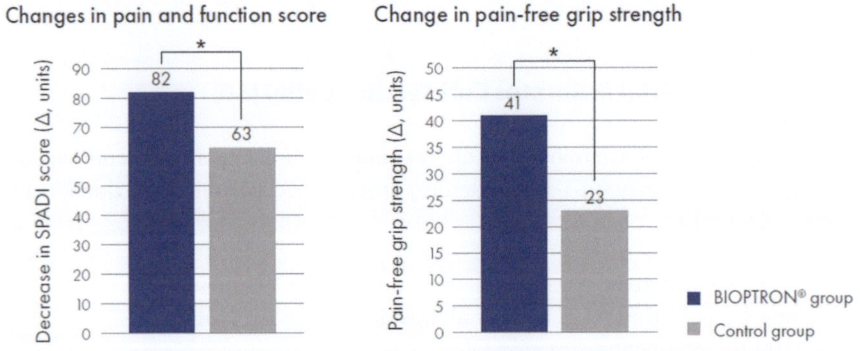

Fig. 6.15 Pre- and posttreatment changes in pain levels (SPADI score) and grip strength ($*p < 0.05$ control vs. PPNCL group). (Modified from Stasinopoulos et al. [30])

Treatment Parameters

- 10-min treatment
- Wavelength 480–3400 nm
- 95% polarization
- 40 mW/cm^2; 2.4 J/cm^2
- 10-cm distance from the device
- Twice a day
- Five days a week
- Five-day intervention

Pain and function were measured on a Visual Analog Scale (VAS), a valid and sensitive approach of the LET. In addition, pain-free grip strength was used to measure function. Pain and function were measured using the Patient-Rated Tennis Elbow Evaluation (PRTEE) (Fig. 6.16).

Outcome

At the end of the treatment (session 10), there was a decline in pain on the VAS of 6 units, a rise in function on the VAS of 6 units, a rise in pain-free grip strength of 35 units, and a decline in the PRTEE questionnaire score of 74 units.

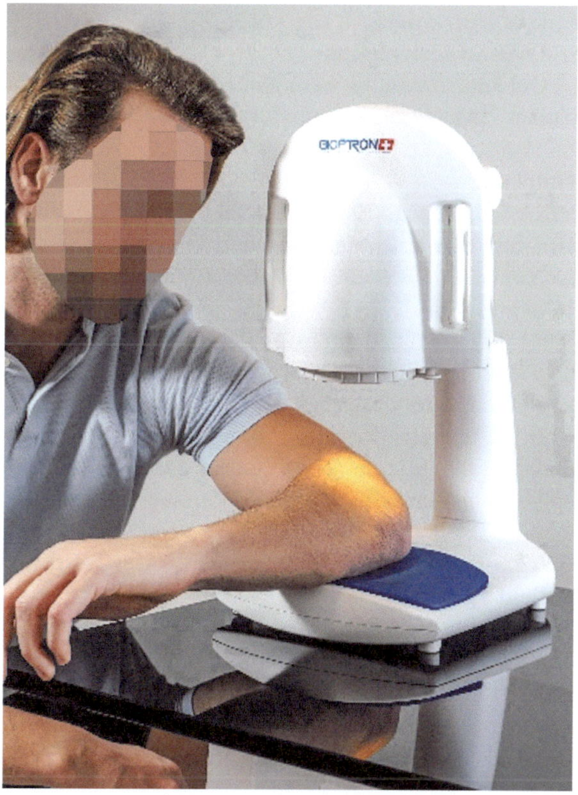

Fig. 6.16 Patient set up to treat the elbow; the PPNCL device is positioned approximately 10 cm away, with the light beam precisely targeted to the localized pain area

Interpretation
A course of PPNCL treatment reduced pain and improved function in a patient with acute LET by the end of treatment. Further well-designed trials are needed to confirm the results of the present case study.

6.7.3.4 Case Report 2: Acute Patellar Tendinopathy [30]

Patient Profile
A 24-year-old male basketball player with a 6-month history of anterior knee pain in his right knee (dominant limb). He was diagnosed as having chronic patellar tendinopathy. He complained of acute pain (less than 24 h) in the inferior pole of the patella. He had intensive training about 24 h ago. He experienced acute pain immediately after the training.

Treatment Parameters
- 10-min treatment
- Wavelength 480–3400 nm
- 95% polarization
- 40 mW/cm^2; 2.4 J/cm^2
- 10-cm distance from the device
- Twice a day
- Five days a week
- Five-day intervention

Outcome measures were pain and function, using a VISA-P questionnaire. The patient's evaluation was conducted before and after treatment.

Outcome
VISA-P score was 19 at the initial evaluation. At the end of the treatment (session 10), the VISA-P score increased to 57 units.

Interpretation
Since pain relief and improvements in function were noted in the present case study on a short-term basis, it is proposed that PPNCL may potentially have promoted an anti-inflammatory effect in the soft tissues. No side effects were reported during or after the treatment period. Future well-designed trials are needed to confirm the findings of this case report and to establish the effectiveness of this treatment approach in managing PT (acute, chronic, and calcific).

6.7.3.5 Case Report 4: Chronic Patellar Tendinopathy [29]

Patient Profile
The subject was a 19-year-old male basketball player with an eight-month history of anterior knee pain in his right (dominant) knee. He was diagnosed by a specialist (orthopedic) as having CPT. He has played basketball for about 10 years. The site of pain was over the inferior pole of the patella (the most common site of patellar tendinopathy) without spreading down. He complained of pain during his

training and while walking downstairs. The pain subsided within 2 h after his training.

Treatment Parameters
Supervised exercise program consisting of isometric quadriceps exercise, slow progressive eccentric-concentric training of quadriceps, and simple lumbo-pelvic control exercises five times per week for 6 weeks + PPNCL

- 10-min treatment
- Wavelength 480–3400 nm
- 95% polarization
- 40 mW/cm^2; 2.4 J/cm^2
- 10-cm distance from the device
- Twice a day
- Five days a week
- Six weeks of intervention

The patient was evaluated using the VISA-P questionnaire, the pain pressure threshold (PPT), and the strength of the knee extensor at baseline, at the end of treatment (week 6), and 1 month after treatment (week 10).

Outcome
At week 0, the VISA-P score was 45, the PPT was 22 newtons, and the knee extensor torque was 80 kg. At week 10 (1 month after the end of the treatment), the VISA-P was 83, the PPTs were 33 kg, and the knee extensor torque was 119 kg.

Interpretation
Even though a supervised exercise program is an effective treatment approach, a supplement to the program should be identified to shorten the treatment period. PPNCL was associated with clinical improvement in this case; however, causal mechanisms cannot be established from single-case observations.

6.8 Clinical Applications in Wound Healing

The strongest body of evidence for light-based therapies, including noncoherent systems, relates to wound healing.

Several randomized and controlled studies investigating photobiomodulation in acute and chronic wounds have reported:

- Accelerated epithelialization
- Increased granulation tissue formation
- Improved microcirculation
- Reduced healing time

The clinical trials done with PPNCL have shown a positive clinical impact and enhancement of wound healing in:

- Acute and chronic wounds
- Pressure ulcers
- Venous ulcers
- Diabetic ulcers
- Postsurgical wounds
- Burns (superficial to partial thickness)
- Grafts

6.8.1 Chronic Wounds: Ulcers, Decubitus, Stasis Ulcers

Chronic wounds represent a substantial clinical and socioeconomic burden, characterized by persistent pain, impaired mobility, and a profound decline in patient quality of life, often resulting in prolonged hospitalization and high readmission rates.

To address these stagnant healing processes, PPNCL therapy is an adjuvant phototherapeutic intervention that modulates cellular mechanisms to promote tissue regeneration. The clinical efficacy of this technology is substantiated by several trials in chronic ulceration, in which it has consistently demonstrated statistically significant reductions in wound area and volume.

6.8.1.1 Clinical Trial 9: Diabetic Foot Ulcers [31]

Patients Profile

Patients with Wagner Grade 1 or 2 diabetic foot ulcers.

Treatment Parameters

1. The treated group, receiving PPNCL in conjunction with standard care:
   - 12-min treatment
   - Wavelength 480–3400 nm
   - 95% polarization
   - 40 mW/cm^2; 2.4 J/cm^2
   - 10-cm distance from the device
   - Three days a week
   - 2 months of intervention
2. Control group, receiving standard care

Outcomes

Group 1 exhibited a significantly greater reduction in ulcer size than the control group receiving standard care alone ($p < 0.001$) over a two-month period (Fig. 6.17). Furthermore, the therapy demonstrated a potent antimicrobial effect, with 60% of the treated group achieving negative microbial cultures after eight weeks, compared to only 15% in the control group ($p = 0.02$).

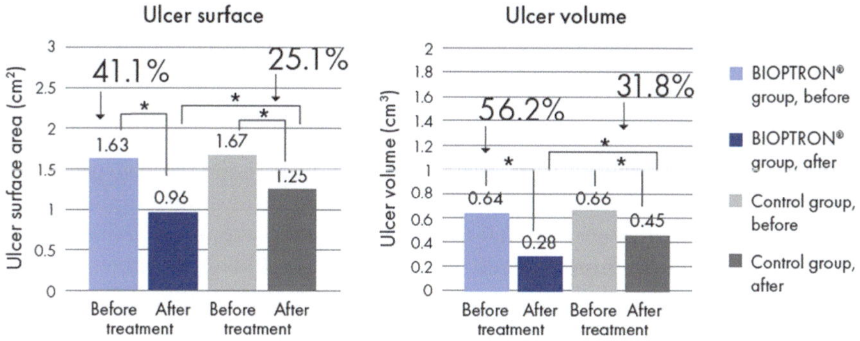

Fig. 6.17 Changes in ulcer parameters in patients treated ($n = 20$) and not treated ($n = 20$) with PPNCL (*$p < 0.001$ control vs. PPNCL group, and pre- vs. posttreatment within the same group). (Modified from Taha et al. [31])

Interpretation

These data suggest that integrating PPNCL therapy not only accelerates physical closure but also enhances the local immune environment in managing complex chronic wounds.

6.8.2 Burns

6.8.2.1 Clinical Trial 10: Burns [22]

Patients Profile

Forty patients with partial-thickness thermal burns affecting the foot, with the percentage of total body surface area (TBSA) ranging from 1% to 5%.

Treatment Parameters

1. Group 1, receiving PPNCL in conjunction with the traditional physical therapy routine and conservative treatment of the burn,
   - 10-min treatment
   - Wavelength 480–3400 nm
   - 95% polarization
   - 40 mW/cm^2; 2.4 J/cm^2
   - 10-cm distance from the device
   - Once daily
   - Three days a week
   - 1-month intervention
2. Group 2 was considered the control group, receiving LLLT in conjunction with the traditional physical therapy routine and conservative treatment of the burn
   - 90-second treatment
   - He-Ne laser
   - 1 mm distance from the device

- Once daily
- Three days a week
- 1-month intervention

Outcome
Comparative clinical trials evaluating the efficacy of nonpolarized polychromatic light against Low-Level Laser Therapy (LLLT) have shown improved outcomes in both antimicrobial activity and tissue regeneration. Following a four-week treatment regimen (three sessions weekly), PPNCL therapy achieved a 55.1% reduction in wound surface area and a 38.63% decrease in bacterial colony counts, yielding reductions of 37.92% and 15.6%, respectively ($p < 0.001$; Fig. 6.18).

Interpretation
These findings suggest that both techniques have a positive clinical impact on wound care management. Nevertheless, according to the results, the broad-spectrum, polarized technology was associated with greater improvements—including accelerated wound closure, reduced risk of secondary infection, and minimized cicatrization—compared with the control group in this study.

6.8.3 Postsurgery Scars

The management of postsurgical incisions remains a critical clinical challenge, as complications such as wound dehiscence, infection, and prolonged edema can severely impede patient recovery and increase the burden on healthcare systems. Beyond the acute phase, the formation of pathological fibrous scarring often leads to functional impairment, limited mobility, and long-term psychological distress.

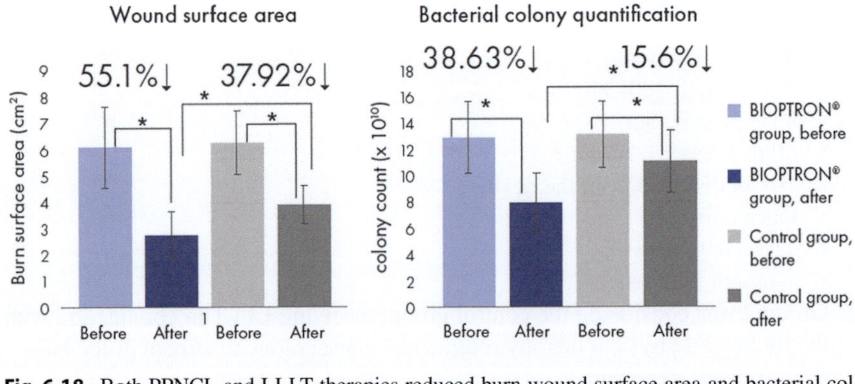

Fig. 6.18 Both PPNCL and LLLT therapies reduced burn wound surface area and bacterial colony counts. However, PPNCL significantly improved wound closure compared to LLLT (*$p < 0.001$), and demonstrated a double reduction in bacterial counts. (Modified from Mowafy et al. [22])

6.8.3.1 Clinical Trial 11: Postsurgery Mammoplasty [21]

Patients Profile

Thirty women with pain and fibrous scarring following mammoplasty, with ages ranging from 40 to 55 years.

Treatment Parameters

1. Group 1, receiving PPNCL in conjunction with the traditional physical therapy routine,
   - 10-min treatment
   - Wavelength 480–3400 nm
   - 95% polarization
   - 40 mW/cm^2; 2.4 J/cm^2
   - 10-cm distance from the device
   - Once daily
   - Seven days a week
   - Six-month intervention
2. Group 2 was considered the control group, receiving only the traditional physical therapy routine.

Outcome

Quantitative analysis revealed a 78% reduction in pain, as measured by the Visual Analog Scale (VAS), whereas the control group—receiving traditional physical therapy alone—showed no significant improvement. Furthermore, high-resolution ultrasonography confirmed an 84% reduction in scar tissue thickness (*$p < 0.05$) in the treated group (Fig. 6.19).

Interpretation

These findings suggest that the specific optical properties of PPNCL effectively modulate the inflammatory cascade and fibroblast activity, resulting in significant alleviation of postsurgical morbidity.

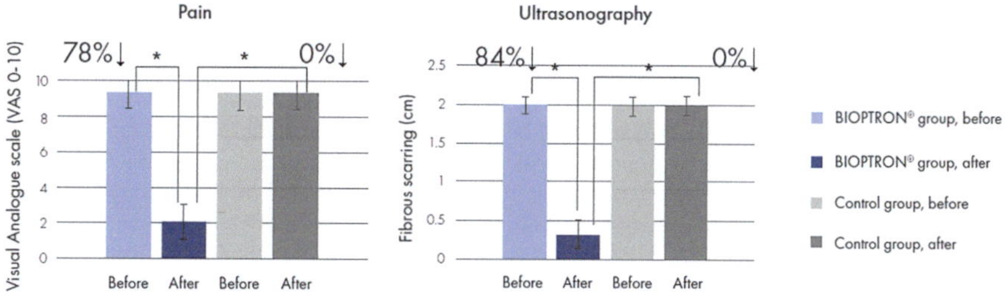

Fig. 6.19 VAS and ultrasonographic scarring changes in the group control and group treated with PPNCL (*$p < 0.05$). (Modified from Mowafy et al. [21])

6.9 Review Questions

1. Explain the difference between coherent and noncoherent light. Why is coherence not considered the primary determinant of biological response in photobiomodulation?
2. Describe the role of cytochrome c oxidase in the mechanism of action of polarized polychromatic noncoherent light.
3. How do wavelength and tissue optical properties influence penetration depth in light-based therapies?
4. Define irradiance and energy density.
5. Explain the biphasic dose–response (Arndt–Schulz principle) in the context of photobiomodulation.
6. Compare polarized polychromatic noncoherent light therapy with low-level laser therapy in terms of spectral characteristics, beam properties, and clinical implications.
7. Discuss the strength of current research evidence for wound healing applications. What are the main methodological limitations in existing studies?
8. Why should polarized polychromatic noncoherent light be considered an adjunct modality rather than a standalone treatment in rehabilitation?
9. In a patient with chronic tendinopathy, how would you integrate polarized light therapy into a comprehensive rehabilitation program? Provide clinical reasoning.

Declarations

Competing Interests The author(s) have no competing interests to declare that are relevant to the content of this manuscript.

References

1. Abramovich SG, Drobyshev VA, Koneva ES, Makhova AA. The efficacy of the comprehensive use of Naphthalan and non-selective chromotherapy in the treatment of patients with Gonarthrosis. Drug Res. 2020;70(04):170–3. https://doi.org/10.1055/a-1113-7062.
2. Akilbekova D, Boddupalli A, Bratlie KM. The effect of polarized light on the organization of collagen secreted by fibroblasts. Lasers Med Sci. 2017;33:539–47. https://doi.org/10.1007/s10103-017-2398-0.
3. Bahrami H, Moharrami A, Mirghaderi P, Mortazavi SMJ. Low-level laser and light therapy after Total knee arthroplasty improves postoperative pain and functional outcomes: a three-arm randomized clinical trial. Arthroplast Today. 2023;19:101066. https://doi.org/10.1016/j.artd.2022.10.016.
4. Chumak AG, Chichkan DN, Ulashchik VS, Soltanov VV, Kul'chitskii, V.A. Role of nitric oxide in modulation of afferent impulses in cutaneous branches of somatic nerves by polarized light. Bull Exp Biol Med. 2000;130(2):734–6. https://doi.org/10.1007/bf02681930.
5. de Melo CAV, Alves AN, Terena SML, Fernandes KPS, Nunes FD, da Silva Dd FT, Bussadori SK, Deana AM, Mesquita-Ferrari RA. Light-emitting diode therapy increases collagen deposition during the repair process of skeletal muscle. Lasers Med Sci. 2016;31(3):531–8. https://doi.org/10.1007/s10103-016-1888-9.

6. Feehan J, Burrows SP, Cornelius L, Cook AM, Mikkelsen K, Apostolopoulos V, Husaric M, Kiatos D. Therapeutic applications of polarized light: tissue healing and immunomodulatory effects. Maturitas. 2018;116:11–7. https://doi.org/10.1016/j.maturitas.2018.07.009.
7. Fenyö M, Mandl J, Falus A. Opposite effect of linearly polarized light on biosynthesis of interleukin-6 in a human B lymphoid cell line and peripheral human monocytes. Cell Biol Int. 2002;26(3):265–9. https://doi.org/10.1006/cbir.2001.0841.
8. Gasparyan LV, Brill G, Makela AM. Activation of angiogenesis under influence of red low level laser radiation. SPIE Proc. 2005;5968:596806. https://doi.org/10.1117/12.660039.
9. Gulyar SA, Tamarova ZA. Analgesic and sedative effects of blue LED light in combination with infrared LED irradiation. J US-China Med Sci. 2017;14:143–56. https://doi.org/10.17265/1548-6648/2017.04.001.
10. Gulyar SA, Tamarova ZA. Analgesic effects of the polarized red+infrared LED light. J US-China Med Sci. 2017;14:47–57. https://doi.org/10.17265/1548-6648/2017.02.001.
11. Gulyar S, Strelchenko YI, Jelskyj M. Physiological mechanisms of polychromatic polarized light influence at skin injuris by high temperature. 2016. Tdmu.edu.ua. [Online]. https://ojs.tdmu.edu.ua/index.php/here/article/view/5906.
12. Karu TI, Pyatibrat LV, Afanasyeva NI. Cellular effects of low power laser therapy can be mediated by nitric oxide. Lasers Surg Med. 2005;36(4):307–14. https://doi.org/10.1002/lsm.20148.
13. Karu TI, Pyatibrat LV, Afanasyeva NI. A novel mitochondrial signaling pathway activated by visible-to-near infrared radiation. Photochem Photobiol. 2007;80(2). https://doi.org/10.1111/j.1751-1097.2004.tb00097.x.
14. Lavi R, Shainberg A, Friedmann H, Shneyvays V, Rickover O, Eichler M, Kaplan D, Lubart R. Low energy visible light induces reactive oxygen species generation and stimulates an increase of intracellular calcium concentration in cardiac cells. J Biol Chem. 2003;278(42):40917–22. https://doi.org/10.1074/jbc.m303034200.
15. Lazovic J, Zopf LM, Hren J, Gajdoš M, Slavkovic M, Jovic Z, Stankovic I, Matovic V, Koruga D. Fullerene-filtered light spectrum and fullerenes modulate emotional and pain processing in mice. Symmetry. 2021;13(11):2004. https://doi.org/10.3390/sym13112004.
16. Leonard DR, Farooqi MH, Myers S. Restoration of sensation, reduced pain, and improved balance in subjects with diabetic peripheral neuropathy: a double-blind, randomized, placebo-controlled study with monochromatic near-infrared treatment. Diabetes Care. 2003;27(1):168–72. https://doi.org/10.2337/diacare.27.1.168.
17. Limansky YP, Tamarova ZA, Gulyar SA. Suppression of pain by exposure of acupuncture points to polarized light. Pain Res Manag. 2006;11(1):49–57. https://doi.org/10.1155/2006/784968.
18. Lubart R, Friedmann H, Peled I, Grossman N. Light effect on fibroblast proliferaton. Laser Ther. 1993;5(2):55–7. https://doi.org/10.5978/islsm.93-or-05.
19. Mihaylova M, Ruseva Z, Filkova S. The effect of polarized polychromatic non-coherent light (Bioptron) therapy on patients with lower back pain. Scripta Scientifica Salutis Publicae. 2017;3(1):23. https://doi.org/10.14748/sssp.v3i1.2165.
20. Mohamed MH, Selem MN, Mohamed MS, EL-Ghaffaar HAA. Interleukin-6 response to shock wave therapy versus polarized light therapy in the treatment of chronic diabetic foot ulcers. 2019. [Online] jprsolutions.info. Available at: https://www.researchgate.net/profile/Mohamed-Naeem-6/publication/338513938_Interleukin-6_response_to_shock_wave_therapy_versus_polarized_light_therapy_in_the_treatment_of_chronic_diabetic_foot_ulcers/links/5e1885cb4585159aa4c367e3/Interleukin-6-response-to-shock-wave-therapy-versus-polarized-light-therapy-in-the-treatment-of-chronic-diabetic-foot-ulcers.pdf.
21. Mowafy ZMET, Mohamedy TM, Khowailed KA-E, Mahmoud Saif S. Pain and fibrous scarring response to polarized light therapy following mammoplasty. Int J Pharm Tech Res. 2016;9(5):144–50.
22. Mowafy ZME, Abdelrahman SME, Ali KM, Ali AMA. Low level laser therapy versus polarized light therapy on healing of foot burn. Int J Health Sci. 2022;6:13053–63. https://doi.org/10.53730/ijhs.v6ns2.8444.

23. Petrovic D, Zlatkovic-Svenda M, Lazovic B. Could the complex regional pain syndrome (Sudeck atrophy), emerged as a distal radius at the typical site fracture complication, be prevented by physical therapy? Ann Phys Rehabil Med. 2018;61:e114. https://doi.org/10.1016/j.rehab.2018.05.246.
24. Safaa MMI, Botla AMM, El Kamel HE-DH. Effect of bioptron light therapy on pregnancy related carpal tunnel syndrome. Med J Cairo Univ. 2024;92(12):1151–6. https://doi.org/10.21608/mjcu.2024.411622.
25. Samoilova KA, Bogacheva ON, Obolenskaya KD, Blinova MI, Kalmykova NV, Kuzminikh EV. Enhancement of the blood growth promoting activity after exposure of volunteers to visible and infrared polarized light. Part I: stimulation of human keratinocyte proliferation in vitro. Photchem Photobiol Sci. 2004;3:96–101.
26. Samoilova KA, Zhevago NA, Petrishchev N, Zimin AP. Role of nitric oxide in the visible light-induced rapid increase of human skin microcirculation at the local and systemic levels: II. Healthy volunteers. Photomed Laser Surg. 2008;26(5):443–9. https://doi.org/10.1089/pho.2007.2205.
27. Stasinopoulos D, Papadopoulos K, Lamnisos D and Stasinopoulos I. (2017) The use of Bioptron(polarized, polychromatic, non-coherent) light therapy for the treatment of acute ankle sprains. Disability and Rehabilitation 39(5):450–457.
28. Dimitrios S, Stasinopoulos L. (2017) Treatment of Carpal Tunnel Syndrome in pregnancy with Polarized Polychromatic Non-coherent Light (Bioptron Light): A Preliminary, Prospective, Open Clinical Trial. Laser Therapy 26(4), 289–295.
29. Stasinopoulos D (2024) The Effectiveness of polarized polychromatic noncoherent light (Bioptron light) and a supervised exercise program on Pain and Disability in Chronic Patellar Tendinopathy: A Case Report. J Clin Cases Rep | July-2024.
30. Stasinopoulos D, Constantinou A, Lamnisos D. The effectiveness of polarized polychromatic noncoherent light (Bioptron light) in patients with chronic rotator cuff tendinopathy. A clinical trial. J Phys Fit Med Treat Sports. 2020;7(5). https://doi.org/10.19080/JPFMTS.2020.07.555724.
31. Taha MM, El-Nagar MM, Elrefaey BH, Elkholy RM, Ali OI, Alkhamees N, Felaya E-SEE-S. Effect of polarized light therapy (Bioptron) on wound healing and microbiota in diabetic foot ulcer: a randomized controlled trial. Photobiomodul Photomed Laser Surg. 2022;40(12):792–9. https://doi.org/10.1089/photob.2021.0175.
32. Tripodi N, Sidiroglou F, Fraser S, Husaric M, Kiatos D, Apostolopoulos V, Feehan J. The effects of polarized photobiomodulation on cellular viability, proliferation, mitochondrial membrane potential and apoptosis in human fibroblasts: potential applications to wound healing. J Photochem Photobiol B Biol. 2022;236:112574. https://doi.org/10.1016/j.jphotobiol.2022.112574.
33. Vacca RA, Marra E, Quagliariello E, Greco M. Activation of mitochondrial DNA replication by he-ne laser irradiation. Biochem Biophys Res Commun. 2002;195(2):704–9. https://doi.org/10.1006/bbrc.1993.2102.
34. Yoshida A, Shiotsu-Ogura Y, Wada-Takahashi S, Takahashi S, Toyama T, Yoshino F. Blue light irradiation-induced oxidative stress in vivo via ROS generation in rat gingival tissue. J Photochem Photobiol B Biol. 2015;151:48–53. https://doi.org/10.1016/j.jphotobiol.2015.07.001.
35. Yu W, Naim JO, McGowan M, Ippolito K, Lanzafame RJ. Photomodulation of oxidative metabolism and electron chain enzymes in rat liver mitochondria. Photochem Photobiol. 1997;66(6):866–71. https://doi.org/10.1111/j.1751-1097.1997.tb03239.x.
36. Zhevago NA, Samoilova KA, Calderhead RG. Polychromatic light similar to the terrestrial solar spectrum without its UV component stimulates DNA synthesis in human peripheral blood lymphocytes in vivo and in vitro. Photochem Photobiol. 2006;82(5):1301–8. https://doi.org/10.1562/2005-04-01-RA-473.

Magnetotherapy

7

Ivan Beljan

7.1 Introduction

Among the various forms of physical therapy, PEMF therapy has gained prominence in recent years and has become an indispensable component of therapeutic procedures in musculoskeletal rehabilitation. A magnetic field is a physical phenomenon generated by moving electric charges or by permanent magnets. It is characterized by field lines that conventionally extend from the north pole to the south pole, with field line density reflecting the strength of the magnetic field [1]. A magnetic field may be static, meaning constant and permanent, or it may be pulsed. Magnetic fields generated by modern therapeutic devices are predominantly pulsed; therefore, the term pulsed electromagnetic fields (PEMF) is commonly used. A fundamental property of magnetic fields is their ability to penetrate matter with relatively low energy loss. Consequently, therapeutically applied magnetic fields can pass through clothing and can penetrate deeply into biological tissues with minimal attenuation. This characteristic distinguishes PEMF therapy from many other physiotherapeutic modalities with limited tissue penetration, which therefore primarily have superficial effects. Magnetic field strength, or magnetic flux density, is expressed in Tesla (T) or Gauss (G), where 1 T corresponds to 10,000 G [2]. The strength of the magnetic field is determined by the properties of the coil system and the magnitude of the electric current. In addition to field strength, pulse frequency and polarity play an important role in determining therapeutic effects. Based on the assumption that different structures in the human body exhibit polarity preferences, specific organs may be treated accordingly. Although some earlier theoretical frameworks suggested polarity-specific biological effects (e.g., differential effects of north and south magnetic poles), such distinctions are not consistently supported by contemporary scientific evidence. Current understanding of PEMF therapy

I. Beljan (✉)
University of Mostar Faculty of Health Studies, Mostar, Bosnia and Herzegovina

D. Stasinopoulos (ed.), *Application of Electrophysical Agents in Physiotherapy*,
https://doi.org/10.1007/978-3-032-32144-2_7

focuses primarily on field characteristics such as frequency, intensity, and waveform rather than polarity-based therapeutic targeting. PEMF therapy refers to the therapeutic use of static or pulsed magnetic fields. Only a small percentage of individuals (approximately 15%) can perceive magnetic fields directly. Magnetic fields cannot be sensed by hearing, vision, smell, or taste, although some patients may experience a sensation of warmth during therapy. Electromagnetic interaction implies the combined influence of magnetic fields and electric currents. Magnetic fields can be generated by electric currents flowing through coils. Conversely, magnetic fields can induce electric currents in the conductive tissues of the human body, which is the basic principle underlying magnetic field interaction with biological tissues [1].

7.2 History of PEMF Therapy

According to historical records, magnetic fields have been used to treat various health conditions for more than 3500 years [1]. In ancient Greece and the Roman Empire, the use of magnetic fields was frequently mentioned by scholars and physicians, including Aristotle and Hippocrates, for the treatment of a wide range of diseases [1, 3]. Historical sources also indicate that Cleopatra wore a magnetic headband, reportedly to alleviate persistent migraine headaches. The first scientific works related to magnetism were published by Simon (1835) and Gauss (1838). In 1965, Linus Pauling, a two-time Nobel Prize laureate, described biomagnetic effects on the circulatory system. Professor C. A. Bassett demonstrated, through clinical studies, the effectiveness of PEMF therapy in treating bone fractures and accelerating bone healing (1982) [1, 4]. Since then, research interest in PEMF therapy has increased significantly, with results published in numerous scientific journals worldwide. Since 1996, the International Society for Energy Medicine has been active in organizing professional and scientific meetings and publishing books and journals addressing this increasingly relevant medical topic [1].

7.3 Biophysics of PEMF Therapy

PEMF therapy refers to the therapeutic use of pulsed electromagnetic fields, while the broader term magnetotherapy may also include static magnetic field applications. Understanding the biophysics of PEMF is essential for rational clinical use, appropriate parameter selection, and interpretation of therapeutic effects. In contemporary physiotherapy literature, the terms magnetotherapy and PEMF are sometimes used interchangeably; however, in clinical practice, PEMF represents the most commonly applied and scientifically investigated form of magnetotherapy.

Electromagnetic fields consist of two interrelated components: an electric field and a magnetic field. In PEMF devices, a time-varying magnetic field is generated externally and penetrates biological tissues without significant attenuation. Unlike thermal modalities, PEMF is considered a nonthermal modality, as it does not rely on tissue heating to produce physiological effects.

According to Faraday's law of electromagnetic induction, a changing magnetic field induces weak electric currents within conductive biological tissues such as blood, muscle, and interstitial fluid. These induced currents are thought to interact with cell membranes, ion channels, and intracellular signaling pathways rather than producing direct mechanical or thermal effects.

The depth of field penetration in PEMF is largely independent of tissue composition, in contrast to thermal modalities such as diathermy or ultrasound. This allows PEMF to influence deep structures, including bone and cartilage, without significant surface heating. The distribution of induced currents depends on the frequency, waveform, and intensity of the applied magnetic field, as well as tissue conductivity.

Frequency plays a central role in PEMF biophysics. Low-frequency fields (typically 5–100 Hz) are most commonly used in musculoskeletal rehabilitation, as they generate biologically relevant current densities without stimulating muscle contraction or causing discomfort. Higher frequencies tend to reduce biological responsiveness and may increase energy absorption without added clinical benefit.

Field intensity is usually measured in millitesla (mT) or gauss (G). Clinical devices typically operate at low to moderate field strengths that remain well within established safety limits. The therapeutic effect is not simply dose-dependent; rather, specific combinations of frequency, intensity, and waveform appear to be more important than maximal field strength alone.

At the cellular level, PEMF is proposed to influence membrane potential, calcium ion transport, nitric oxide production, and gene expression related to tissue repair. In bone, the piezoelectric properties of collagen and hydroxyapatite may interact with electromagnetic stimulation, potentially enhancing osteoblastic activity and callus formation.

From a tissue perspective, PEMF does not create temperature gradients or thermal stresses. Instead, its primary action is thought to be bioelectrical modulation, making it fundamentally different from diathermy or thermotherapy.

Overall, the biophysical foundation of PEMF therapy is based on electromagnetic induction, tissue conductivity, and frequency-dependent cellular responsiveness rather than heat transfer or mechanical vibration.

Based on these biophysical principles, several physiological mechanisms have been proposed to explain the therapeutic effects of PEMF.

7.4 Mechanisms and Principles of PEMF Therapy

Pulsed electromagnetic fields can influence multiple cell types within exposed tissues. The primary site of action is the cell membrane, which, through induced electrical currents, influences ion exchange. The biological effects of PEMF are primarily attributed to modulation of cellular activity rather than nonspecific "vitalizing" influences. These effects include alterations in membrane potential, ion transport, and intracellular signaling pathways that may contribute to tissue repair and functional recovery. These biological effects may be associated with improved cellular metabolism and enhanced regulation of local microenvironmental conditions that support tissue repair processes. This mechanism partly explains the effectiveness of PEMF therapy in the prevention and treatment of functional disorders.

The following cellular and subcellular mechanisms form the basis of the therapeutic effects of PEMF therapy:

- Cellular mechanism: Calcium signaling, a key physiological pathway of PEMF, is the modulation of calcium (Ca^{2+}) binding to calmodulin. This interaction accelerates the signaling cascades involved in tissue repair and anti-inflammatory responses. By influencing Ca^{2+}/Calmodulin-dependent nitric oxide (NO) signaling, PEMF can promote vasodilation and enhance the transition from the inflammatory to the proliferative phase of healing, providing a robust biological explanation for its clinical effects on tissue regeneration.
- Effects of the Lorentz force and Hall effect at the level of the cell membrane and piezoelectric effects [1].

At the molecular level, PEMF therapy is increasingly associated with modulation of intracellular signaling pathways rather than nonspecific biological stimulation. One of the most consistently proposed mechanisms involves calcium (Ca^{2+})-dependent signaling through calmodulin, which activates nitric oxide (NO) synthesis. This pathway may contribute to vasodilation, improved microcirculation, and regulation of inflammatory processes. In addition, PEMF exposure has been linked to modulation of adenosine receptor activity (particularly A2A and A3 receptors), which may influence anti-inflammatory responses and tissue repair. In bone tissue, electromagnetic stimulation appears to enhance osteoblastic activity and matrix-related gene expression, supporting its clinical application in delayed-union and nonunion fractures. However, despite increasing mechanistic understanding, most of these pathways remain biologically plausible rather than definitively confirmed in clinical populations.

7.5 Indications, Contraindications, Precautions, and Side Effects (Tables 7.1, 7.2, and 7.3)

Safety and Metal Implants: Regarding surgical implants, it is important to clarify that, unlike thermal modalities (e.g., Diathermy), PEMF typically does not cause significant heating of non-ferromagnetic metal implants such as titanium plates, screws, or intramedullary nails. In most clinical PEMF applications, the presence of such internal fixation is considered a precaution rather than an absolute contraindication, making it a safe and effective option for post-surgical bone healing and fracture management.

Table 7.1 Indications for PEMF therapy

Indications
Functional disorders caused by exogenous, endogenous, or iatrogenic harmful factors
Rehabilitation and mobilization following injuries, severe trauma, or diseases (e.g., stroke)
Preventive use in general preventive and prophylactic medicine
Broad applicability across multiple clinical indications with relatively few side effects
Improvement of tissue oxygenation and enhancement of local and systemic circulation
Psychological stabilization and improvement of stress-related functional disorders
Stimulation of metabolic processes
Acceleration of regenerative and reparative processes
Enhancement of immune system activity

It should be noted that the indications listed above represent broad clinical applications reported in the literature. In evidence-based clinical practice, PEMF therapy is most strongly supported for specific indications, particularly delayed bone healing and selected musculoskeletal conditions. Clinicians should critically evaluate the relevance of each indication based on current research evidence and individual patient presentation

Table 7.2 Absolute contraindications for PEMF therapy

Absolute contraindications
Implanted electronic medical devices (e.g., pacemakers, ICDs, neurostimulators)
Pregnancy (especially application to the abdominal or lumbar region)
Active malignant diseases
Acute bleeding or bleeding disorders
Severe cardiac arrhythmias
Acute infectious diseases accompanied by fever
Severe hypotension or unstable cardiovascular conditions

Table 7.3 Relative contraindications for PEMF therapy

Relative contraindications
Pediatric patients (depending on age and treatment area)
Menstruation (especially abdominal application)
Epilepsy
Endocrine disorders (e.g., uncontrolled hyperthyroidism)
Metallic implants without electronic components
Chronic diseases in an exacerbation phase
Hypersensitivity or discomfort during previous PEMF therapy sessions

Indications adapted from Kapetanović and Pecar [1]. Contraindications adapted from Jajić and Jajić [5]

7.6 Effects of PEMF Therapy on the Human Body

The effects of PEMF therapy on the human body are primarily related to the modulation of cellular and tissue-level processes rather than broad systemic effects. Experimental and clinical studies suggest that PEMF may influence pain perception, inflammatory responses, and tissue repair mechanisms. Reported effects include modulation of nociceptive signaling, potential enhancement of microcirculation, and support of cellular processes involved in tissue healing. However, many proposed systemic effects, such as hormonal regulation or generalized immune enhancement, remain insufficiently supported by high-quality clinical evidence and should therefore be interpreted with caution.

7.7 Dosology/Parameters

PEMF therapy is applied using devices that allow adjustment of intensity, polarity, waveform, frequency, and pulse duration. Both constant and variable magnetic fields can be generated. In medical practice, variable magnetic field generators are predominantly used. These devices can produce sinusoidal waves, series of sinusoidal waves, half-waves, trapezoidal impulses (monophasic or biphasic), and triangular impulses. Frequency ranges include low frequencies (1–5 Hz and 5–50 Hz), medium frequencies (50–100 Hz), and high frequencies exceeding 100 Hz, reaching up to 1–20 MHz for specific device categories. Most therapeutic devices generate magnetic fields between 5 and 100 gauss (0.5–10 mT). Treatment duration depends on frequency and clinical indication [6] (Table 7.4).

When selecting parameters, clinicians should consider the concept of "biological windows" (Adey windows). This principle suggests that biological tissues respond optimally only to specific combinations of frequency, intensity, and waveform. Most clinical evidence supports the use of extremely low frequencies (ELF), typically between 1 and 100 Hz, emphasizing that adherence to these "effective windows" is often more critical for therapeutic success than simply increasing the field intensity.

A key concept in PEMF application is the existence of so-called "biological windows" (Adey windows), which suggest that biological tissues respond optimally only to specific combinations of frequency, intensity, and waveform. Increasing the magnetic field strength beyond these effective ranges does not necessarily enhance therapeutic outcomes and may even reduce biological responsiveness. This phenomenon highlights that PEMF therapy is not purely dose-dependent in a linear sense, but rather parameter-specific. Consequently, clinical effectiveness depends less on maximal intensity and more on the selection of appropriate frequency ranges (commonly 1–100 Hz), waveform characteristics, and treatment duration. This principle partly explains the variability in clinical outcomes across studies using different devices and protocols.

Table 7.4 Examples of pulsed electromagnetic field (PEMF) dosing parameters reported in clinical studies

Condition	PEMF characteristics	Session duration	Treatment frequency	Total treatment period	Main outcome	Study
Delayed union/ nonunion fractures	Low-frequency PEMF; device-specific waveform and magnetic flux density	Several hours per day	Daily	Mean 4–5 months	Increased fracture union rates	[4]
Delayed union of tibial fractures	PEMF via coil applicators; preset device parameters	Several hours per day	Daily	Until radiological union	Superior to the placebo	[7]
Knee osteoarthritis	Low-frequency PEMF; parameters varied between devices	30–60 min	3–5 times/ week	4–6 weeks	Pain reduction and functional improvement	[8]
Knee osteoarthritis	Wearable PEMF system; low-frequency exposure	2 h per day	5 days/week	6 weeks	No clinically relevant difference vs placebo	[9]
Knee osteoarthritis	Wearable PEMF device; manufacturer-defined parameters	Up to 12 h per day	Daily	1 month	Significant pain and functional improvement	[10]
Bone healing (review of clinical protocols)	Heterogeneous PEMF protocols across studies	~8 h per day (typical)	Daily	~4–5 months	Supportive evidence for enhanced bone healing	[11]
Knee osteoarthritis (meta-analysis)	Wide variability in PEMF parameters	Variable	Variable	Variable	Mixed evidence due to protocol heterogeneity	[12]

PEMF dosing parameters vary considerably between studies due to differences in devices, waveforms, and clinical protocols. Therefore, reported values should be interpreted within the methodological context of each study

7.8 Devices for PEMF Therapy

PEMF applicators can be designed to target joints or soft tissues, such as the knee, shoulder, or spine. They are often used in outpatient physical therapy clinics and can be integrated with other modalities (e.g., exercise therapy, manual techniques). PEMF systems have been widely studied for conditions such as osteoarthritis, tendinopathy, and bone healing, with clinical evidence varying by condition and protocol [4, 13]. Devices in this category include tabletop units with interchangeable coils, hand-held applicators, and table-mounted configurations for treating larger body areas. Modern PEMF devices allow clinicians to set parameters such as frequency (typically in the low-Hz range), magnetic flux density, and treatment duration to tailor therapy to specific conditions [14].

Despite the availability of various device configurations, differences in technical specifications and treatment protocols may significantly influence clinical outcomes. Therefore, clinicians should not rely solely on device capabilities but should base their application on evidence-informed parameter selection and clinical reasoning.

Recent technological developments have introduced high-intensity pulsed electromagnetic field systems and electromagnetic transduction therapies (EMTT), which operate at higher frequencies and energy levels compared to conventional PEMF devices. While these approaches aim to enhance tissue penetration and biological responsiveness, current clinical evidence remains limited, and their superiority over traditional PEMF protocols has not been clearly established. As such, clinicians should interpret claims about newer technologies with caution and rely on evidence-informed parameter selection rather than on device-specific marketing (Figs. 7.1, 7.2, 7.3, 7.4, 7.5, 7.6 and 7.7).

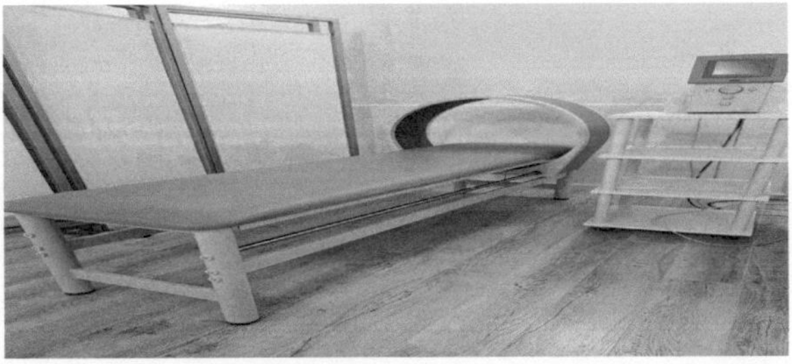

Fig. 7.1 Device for PEMF therapy with an intensity of 128 mT and a frequency of 0–166 Hz

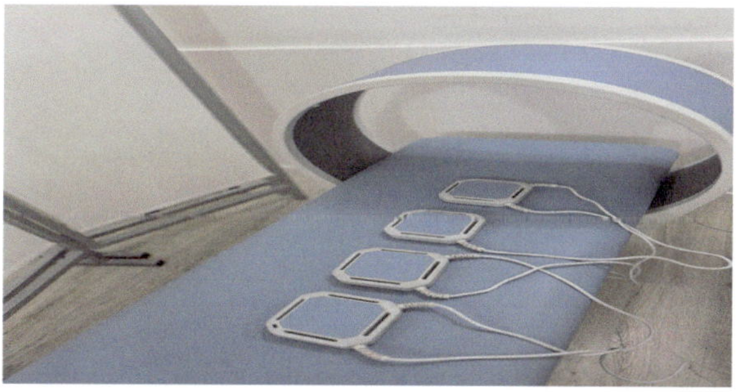

Fig. 7.2 Magnetic therapy bed with a large solenoid and multidisk PEMF applicators

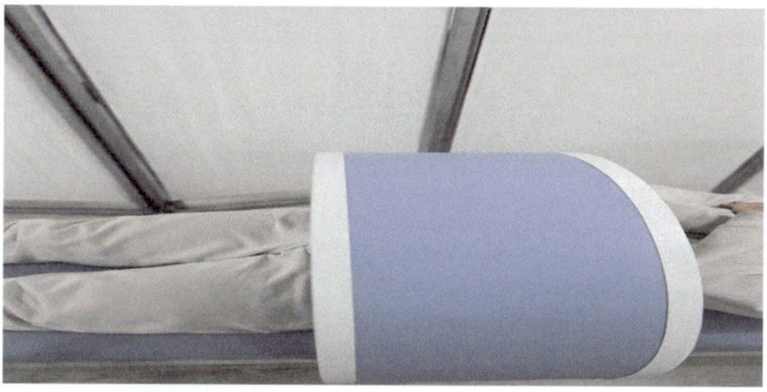

Fig. 7.3 Illustration of the application of PEMF therapy to the pelvic and hip area

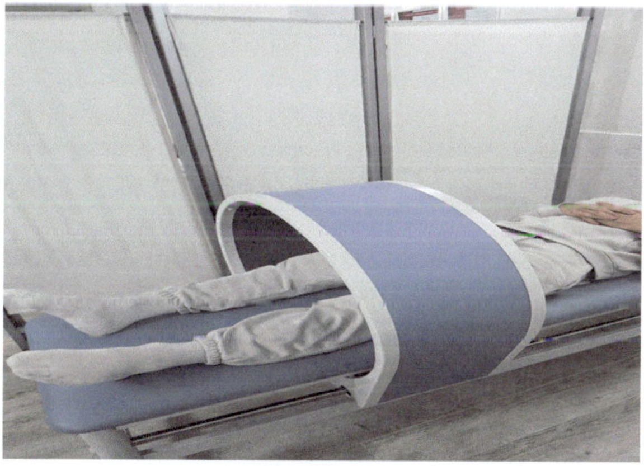

Fig. 7.4 Illustration of the application of PEMF therapy to the knee area

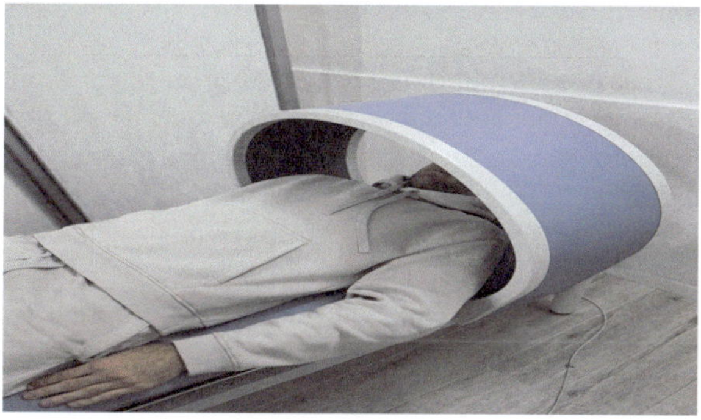

Fig. 7.5 Illustration of the application of PEMF therapy to the cervical spine and shoulder area

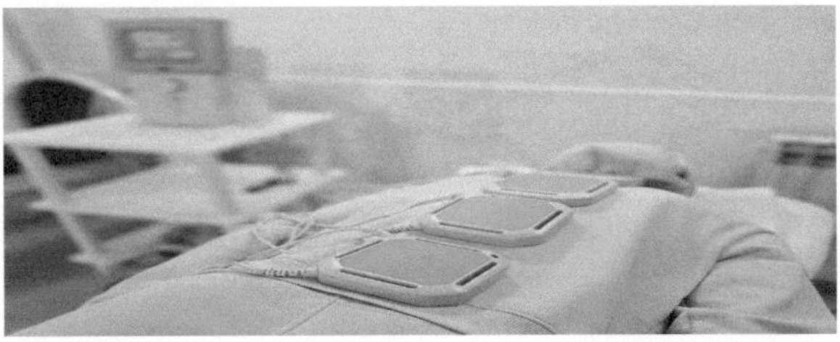

Fig. 7.6 Illustration of the application of a multidisk applicator to the spine area

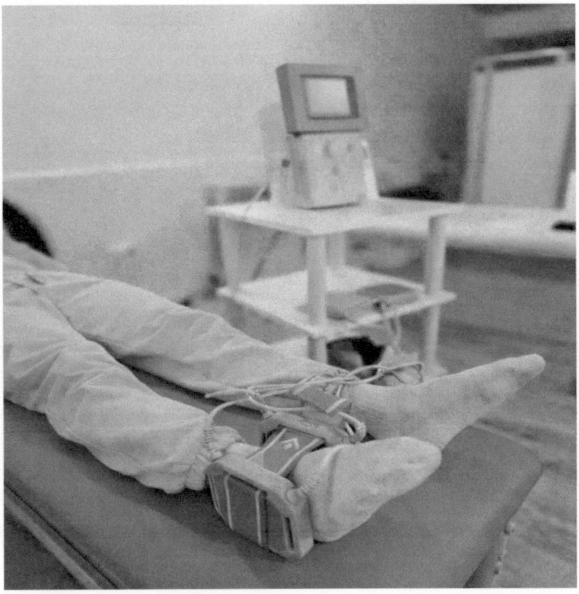

Fig. 7.7 Illustration of the application of the multidisk applicator to the area of the ankle joint

7.9 Evidence from Clinical Studies

Bone Healing

Clinical evidence for PEMF therapy indicates condition-specific efficacy with the strongest support for use in bone healing. Randomized controlled trials and long-term clinical use show that PEMF can improve fracture healing and increase the rate of healing in delayed-union and nonunion fractures [4, 7].

Osteoarthritis and Soft Tissues

These findings are supported by experimental evidence showing that electromagnetic stimulation affects cellular behavior in calcified tissues [4]. In musculoskeletal disorders, particularly knee osteoarthritis, multiple randomized controlled trials have investigated the effects of PEMF on pain and function. Several studies report significant improvements in pain intensity and functional outcomes after PEMF therapy [8, 10, 15], while other well-designed trials report no clinically significant difference compared to placebo interventions [9]. Systematic reviews and meta-analyses conclude that PEMF may provide functional benefits in selected patient populations, but highlight significant heterogeneity in treatment parameters and outcome measures, which limits definitive clinical recommendations [12]. New evidence suggests a potential role for PEMF therapy in the treatment of tendinopathies and soft tissue disorders. Recent randomized trials show that PEMF, especially when combined with exercise-based rehabilitation, can lead to short-term improvements in pain and function [16].

Overall Interpretation

However, the available evidence remains limited in scope and sample size. Overall, current evidence supports the use of PEMF therapy as an adjunctive electrophysical agent in specific clinical contexts, particularly bone healing. For other musculoskeletal conditions, the effectiveness of PEMF appears to be variable and depends on treatment parameters, patient selection, and combination with active rehabilitation. Future research should focus on standardized dosimetry, high-quality randomized controlled trials, and long-term outcomes to better define the clinical role of PEMF therapy [12]. PEMF should be used as an adjunct, and heterogeneity of protocols limits firm conclusions.

From a clinical perspective, PEMF therapy may be considered in selected cases, particularly in bone healing and specific musculoskeletal conditions. Still, it should always be integrated within a comprehensive rehabilitation program rather than used as a stand-alone intervention.

From a clinical perspective, PEMF therapy should not be selected based solely on diagnosis but on clearly defined treatment objectives. For example, in cases of delayed bone healing, the goal may be to support osteogenesis and enhance callus formation. In contrast, in osteoarthritis, the primary aim may be pain modulation and improvement of functional tolerance. Clinicians should therefore determine whether PEMF provides added value beyond active rehabilitation strategies such as exercise and loading. In many cases, its role is best understood as facilitating a therapeutic environment that supports tissue adaptation rather than directly producing structural change. The decision to apply PEMF should be continuously re-evaluated based on patient response and overall rehabilitation progress.

7.10 Summary/Conclusion

PEMF therapy is a widely used electrophysical tool in physiotherapy practice. Available scientific evidence indicates that PEMF can influence biological processes relevant to tissue repair and pain modulation, which supports its clinical use in selected indications. The strongest and most consistent clinical evidence supports the use of PEMF for bone healing, particularly in delayed and nonunion fractures, with randomized controlled trials and systematic reviews reporting improved healing outcomes. In musculoskeletal conditions such as knee osteoarthritis, clinical results are mixed: some randomized trials show improvements in pain and function, while others show no significant benefit compared with placebo. These inconsistencies are mainly attributed to the heterogeneity of treatment parameters, devices, and study designs. Emerging evidence suggests a potential role for PEMF therapy in the treatment of tendinopathies and other soft tissue disorders, particularly when used as an adjunct to exercise-based rehabilitation. However, the current body of evidence in these conditions remains limited and requires further confirmation through high-quality randomized controlled trials. Overall, PEMF therapy should be considered an additional method rather than an independent treatment in physiotherapy. Clinical decision-making should be guided by the specific condition, available evidence, patient response, and integration with active rehabilitation strategies. Future research should prioritize standardized dosing protocols, transparent reporting of treatment parameters, and long-term clinical outcomes to better define the role of PEMF therapy in modern physiotherapy practice.

7.11 Case Studies

7.11.1 Case Study 1—PEMF in Delayed Union Tibial Fracture

Patient:
A 52-year-old male presents with delayed union of a tibial shaft fracture 16 weeks postsurgery. Radiographs show incomplete callus formation. The patient reports persistent pain during weight bearing, but no signs of infection.

Clinical Reasoning:
The primary goal is to stimulate osteogenesis and improve bone healing in a delayed union while maintaining safe, progressive loading. PEMF is selected as an adjunct to standard orthopedic management rather than a replacement for surgical or mechanical stability.

Intervention:
- Low-frequency PEMF therapy
- Frequency: 15–30 Hz
- Duration: 30–60 min daily for 8–12 weeks
- Continued gradual weight-bearing as tolerated

Rationale:
PEMF is proposed to enhance osteoblastic activity, modulate calcium signaling, and improve local circulation within the fracture site.

Outcome:
After 10 weeks, radiographs show improved callus formation and the patient reports reduced pain and improved function.

7.11.2 Case Study 2—PEMF in Knee Osteoarthritis

Patient:
A 68-year-old female with symptomatic knee osteoarthritis reports pain, stiffness, and reduced walking tolerance. She is already in an exercise program.

Intervention:
- Low-frequency PEMF to the knee
- Frequency: 20–40 Hz
- 20–30 min, 3–5 times per week for 6–8 weeks
- Continued strengthening and mobility training

Outcome:
After 8 weeks, the patient reports reduced pain and improved exercise tolerance.

7.12 Review Questions

1. What is PEMF therapy, and how is it classified among electrophysical agents in physiotherapy?
2. What are the main physical characteristics of PEMF therapy?
3. How do PEMFs interact with biological tissues at the cellular level?
4. What are the proposed mechanisms of action of PEMF therapy on the human body?
5. Which clinical indications have the strongest scientific support for PEMF therapy?
6. What evidence supports the use of PEMF therapy in bone healing and fracture nonunion?
7. What are the reported clinical effects of PEMF therapy in knee osteoarthritis?
8. Which parameters are relevant when determining the dosage of PEMF therapy?
9. What types of PEMF therapy devices are used in clinical practice?
10. What are the main contraindications and safety considerations for PEMF therapy?
11. How do randomized controlled trials and systematic reviews contribute to the evidence base for PEMF therapy?
12. Why should PEMF therapy be considered an adjunctive rather than a stand-alone intervention in physiotherapy practice?

Declarations

Competing Interests The author(s) have no competing interests to declare that are relevant to the content of this manuscript.

References

1. Kapetanović H, Pecar D. Vodič u rehabilitaciju. Sarajevo; 2005.
2. Beljan I, Švraka E. Effectiveness of magnetotherapy in the treatment of patients with lumbar syndrome. Health Bull. 2023;9(1):74–85.
3. Basford JR. A historical perspective of the popular use of electric and magnetic therapy. Arch Phys Med Rehabil. 2001;82:1261–9.
4. Bassett CA. Pulsing electromagnetic fields: a new method to modify cell behavior in calcified and noncalcified tissues. Calcif Tissue Int. 1982;34(1):1–8.
5. Jajić I, Jajić Z. i suradnici. Fizikalna i rehabilitacijska medicina: osnove i liječenje. Zagreb; 2008.
6. Andrade R, Duarte H, Pereira R, Lopes I, Pereira H, Rocha R, et al. Pulsed electromagnetic field therapy effectiveness in low back pain: a systematic review of randomized controlled trials. Porto Biomed J. 2016;1(5):156–63.
7. Sharrard WJW. A double-blind trial of pulsed electromagnetic fields for delayed union of tibial fractures. J Bone Joint Surg Br. 1990;72-B(3):347–55.
8. Trock DH, Bollet AJ, Markoll R. Pulsed electromagnetic fields for treatment of osteoarthritis of the knee and cervical spine. J Rheumatol. 1994;21(10):1903–11.
9. Thamsborg G, Florescu A, Oturai P, Fallentin E, Tritsaris K, Dissing S. Effect of pulsed electromagnetic fields on knee osteoarthritis: a randomized, double-blind, placebo-controlled study. Osteoarthr Cartil. 2005;13(7):575–81.
10. Bagnato GL, Miceli G, Marino N, Sciortino D, Bagnato GF. Pulsed electromagnetic fields in knee osteoarthritis: a randomized, double-blind, placebo-controlled trial. Rheumatology. 2015;54(1):1–8.
11. Caruso G, et al. Pulsed electromagnetic field stimulation in bone healing: clinical evidence and dosing considerations. Appl Sci. 2024;14(5):1789.
12. Vavken P, Arrich F, Schuhfried O, Dorotka R. Effectiveness of pulsed electromagnetic field therapy in the management of knee osteoarthritis: a meta-analysis. J Rehabil Med. 2009;41(6):406–11.
13. McCarthy CJ, Oldham JA. Effectiveness of pulsed electromagnetic fields in knee osteoarthritis: a randomized controlled trial. Rheumatology. 2006;45(3):320–7.
14. Markov MS. Pulsed electromagnetic field therapy: history, state of the art and future. Environmentalist. 2007;27(4):465–75.
15. Pipitone N, Scott DL. Magnetic pulse treatment for knee osteoarthritis. Curr Med Res Opin. 2001;17(3):190–6.
16. Ko VMC, et al. Pulsed electromagnetic field therapy combined with exercise for Achilles tendinopathy: randomized controlled trial. 2024.

8 Extracorporeal Shockwave Therapy (ESWT)

Knobloch Karsten

8.1 Introduction

Extracorporeal shockwave therapy (ESWT) represents a clinically established energy-based modality within contemporary musculoskeletal rehabilitation, integrating biophysical stimulation with modern load-based therapeutic strategies. Initially introduced during the 1980s for lithotripsy in urology, shockwave technology was later adapted for musculoskeletal applications following observations that mechanical acoustic impulses could stimulate tissue healing and modulate pain [1, 2].

The transition of ESWT from urology to orthopedics and subsequently to rehabilitation represents an important conceptual evolution [3]. Early applications focused mainly on mechanical fragmentation of calcifications and stimulation of bone healing. Over time, the understanding of ESWT shifted toward its biological and regenerative potential with much lower energy levels applied, emphasizing cellular signaling and tissue adaptation rather than purely mechanical disruption [4].

In physiotherapy practice, ESWT is primarily used for chronic musculoskeletal conditions in which tissue healing has plateaued despite conservative management. These conditions are often characterized by degenerative changes rather than acute inflammatory pathology, reduced vascularity, and altered mechanical properties. In this context, ESWT is used to facilitate biological activity and restore tissue adaptability.

The modality is rarely used as a standalone intervention. Contemporary rehabilitation models position ESWT as an adjunct or congenial partner that facilitates progression of active treatment strategies such as progressive loading, neuromuscular control training, and functional rehabilitation.

K. Karsten (✉)
SportPraxis Professor Knobloch, Hannover, Germany

D. Stasinopoulos (ed.), *Application of Electrophysical Agents in Physiotherapy*, https://doi.org/10.1007/978-3-032-32144-2_8

Extracorporeal shockwave therapy is an energy-based therapy, alongside magnetic field therapy [5], low-level laser therapy (LLLT) [6, 7], and vibration therapy (Fig. 8.1).

All of the aforementioned energy-based therapies share the noninvasive feature, a paramount consideration in daily patient and athlete care.

Ludger Gerdesmeyer from Kiel, Germany, has proposed the term "soft tissue engineering" to describe the combination of the aforementioned tools from the regenerative toolbox. In 2024, I introduced the concept of the "regenerative clockwork" at the D.A.F. foot conference in Vienna, Austria, adding precision, timing, and a distinct, consecutive order to this framework, highlighting the need for optimal dosages and performance of each component of this holistic regenerative approach (Fig. 8.2).

Two principal shockwave technologies are used clinically:

Focused extracorporeal shockwave therapy (fESWT)
Radial pressure wave therapy (RPWT or rESWT)

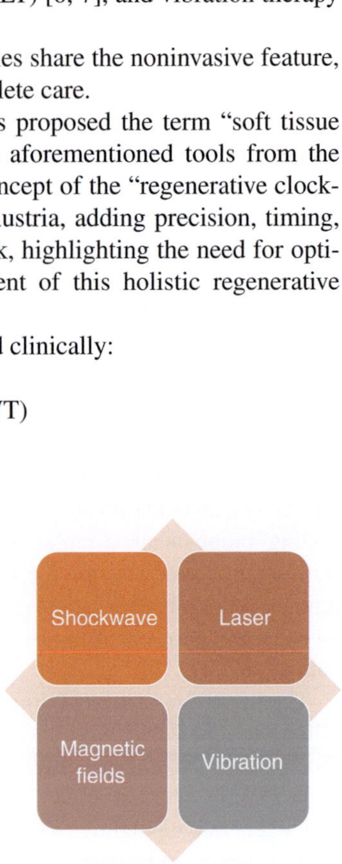

Fig. 8.1 Energy-based therapies include extracorporeal shockwave therapy (ESWT), low-level laser therapy (LLLT), oscillating magnetic field therapy with pulsed electric field therapy (PEMF), extracorporeal magnetotransduction therapy (EMTT), and vibration therapy

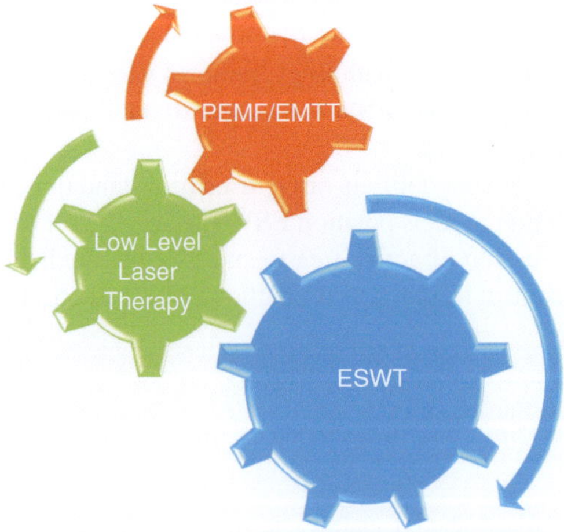

Fig. 8.2 Regenerative clockwork combining ESWT, magnetic field therapy, and low-level laser therapy (LLLT) to have even faster and more pronounced regenerative responses

Although often grouped, these technologies differ significantly in physical characteristics, energy distribution, penetration depth, and clinical applications. Understanding these differences is essential for safe and effective use.

Although radial systems are commonly included under the ESWT umbrella in clinical practice, radial devices generate pressure waves rather than true shockwaves in the strict physical sense; the shared terminology reflects historical development and therapeutic overlap rather than identical physical properties.

From a broader clinical perspective, ESWT occupies an intermediate position between passive modalities and active rehabilitation. Its primary role is not to replace exercise therapy but to enhance tissue readiness, reduce pain, and improve tolerance to mechanical loading. Clinically, ESWT is increasingly viewed as a means of creating a "window of opportunity" in which pain reduction and altered tissue sensitivity enable more effective loading interventions.

In addition, clinicians should recognize that treatment goals may differ between patients. In some cases, the intent is primarily analgesic, whereas in others the focus is on longer-term tissue adaptation. This distinction influences parameter selection, patient education, and expectations regarding the timeline of improvement.

The terminology used in clinical practice is often inconsistent. The term ESWT traditionally refers to true shockwaves generated by focused devices. Radial systems produce ballistic pressure waves and may be described as radial pressure wave therapy (RPWT or rESWT). Commercial terms such as "acoustic wave therapy" are frequently used in marketing but do not represent a distinct physical technology. Understanding these distinctions is essential for interpreting research and device specifications.

8.2 Biophysics of ESWT

8.2.1 Definition of Shockwaves

From a physical point of view, a shock wave is defined by an abrupt, nearly discontinuous change in pressure and by a velocity greater than the speed of sound in the medium through which it propagates [8]. Generally, a shock wave can be described as a single pulse with a wide frequency range (from approx. 150 kHz up to 100 MHz), high pressure amplitude (up to 150 MPa), low tensile wave (up to −25 MPa), small pulse width, and a short rise time of up to a few hundred nanoseconds.

Unlike sinusoidal waves used in ultrasound therapy, shockwaves deliver energy in isolated high-amplitude pulses.

A typical shockwave consists of a rapid positive-pressure phase (Fig. 8.3), followed by a negative-pressure phase, with a short total duration measured in microseconds. This rapid pressure change produces unique mechanical effects that distinguish ESWT from other electrophysical agents.

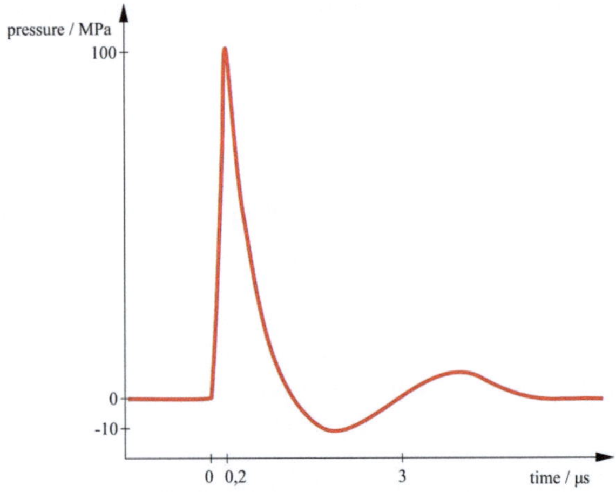

Fig. 8.3 Schematic pressure profile of a focused shockwave

8.2.2 Shockwave Pressure Profile and Wave Characteristics

The physical profile of a shockwave is central to understanding its therapeutic effects. The positive-pressure phase compresses tissues, while the subsequent negative phase may induce tensile stress and cavitation.

Rise Time

The rise time of a shockwave typically occurs in the nanosecond range, depending on the generator technology, producing steep pressure gradients that can mechanically stimulate cells and extracellular structures. Focused electrohydraulic (EH) devices have the fastest rise time, followed by electromagnetic (EM) and piezoelectric (PE) focused generators.

Peak Pressure

Peak pressures may reach tens of 150 Mega Pascal (MPa), far exceeding those produced by conventional therapeutic ultrasound.

Negative Phase and Cavitation

The negative-pressure phase up to −25 MPa may induce cavitation [9], particularly in fluid environments. The collapse of microscopic gas bubbles may generate localized mechanical forces; however, the extent and clinical relevance of cavitation effects in vivo remain under investigation.

These characteristics help explain why ESWT can induce mechanotransduction even without significant thermal effects. It is important to note that the biological response depends not only on the magnitude of the pressure but also on the repetition rate and the energy distribution within tissues.

8.2.3 Fundamental Physical Principles Relevant to ESWT

Several physical principles govern the behavior of ESWT energy in biological tissues.

Acoustic Impedance
When shockwaves encounter tissue boundaries with different impedances, some energy is reflected and some is transmitted, creating localized stress concentrations [10].

Energy Attenuation
As waves travel through tissue, energy decreases due to absorption and scattering, influencing treatment depth and parameter selection.

Focal Zone Concept
Focused ESWT devices converge acoustic energy into a specific focal area, enabling precise targeting of deep structures while reducing exposure to superficial tissues [11]. Depending on the device in focus, the focus varies tremendously (Fig. 8.4).

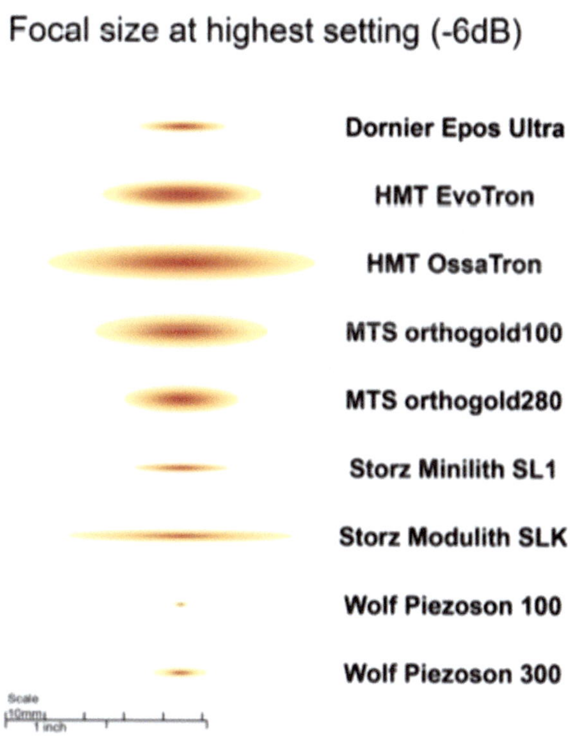

Fig. 8.4 Focus sizes of different focused electrohydraulic (HMT), electromagnetic (Storz), and piezoelectric (Wolf) generators

Electrohydraulic focused ESWT devices have the largest focus zone, followed by electromagnetic focused devices. The piezoelectric focus size is the smallest among the focused generators.

Energy Dispersion in Radial Systems
Radial pressure waves propagate outward from the applicator, producing maximal energy at the skin interface and gradually decreasing with depth.

Understanding these principles helps clinicians match device type to the location of pathology. Tissue composition, hydration, and anatomical interfaces may also influence energy transmission, emphasizing the importance of coupling medium and applicator positioning during treatment.

8.2.4 Generation Technologies

Three primary technologies can produce focused shockwaves:

- Electrohydraulic: spark discharge creates pressure waves reflected into a focal zone
- Electromagnetic: magnetic forces accelerate a membrane, generating acoustic waves
- Piezoelectric: multiple piezo crystals expand rapidly to create focused energy

Each system produces slightly different focal characteristics and energy distributions. While clinical differences may be subtle, understanding generation mechanisms helps interpret device specifications. Based on the aforementioned differences in rise time and focus size, the same energy flux densities across different focused devices may exert different effects, which is paramount when interpreting clinical studies and devices.

Radial devices use a ballistic projectile accelerated by compressed air to transfer kinetic energy to an applicator that transmits pressure waves into tissues. The design of applicator heads and interfaces may further influence surface pressure distribution and patient comfort.

8.2.5 Radial Versus Focused Shockwaves

Feature	Focused ESWT	Radial pressure waves
Energy profile	Convergent focus at depth	Maximal at the skin interface
Penetration depth	Up to ~8 cm	Superficial to moderate
Energy descriptor	Energy flux density (mJ/mm^2)	Pressure (bar)
Typical targets	Bone, deep tendons	Fascia, superficial tendons

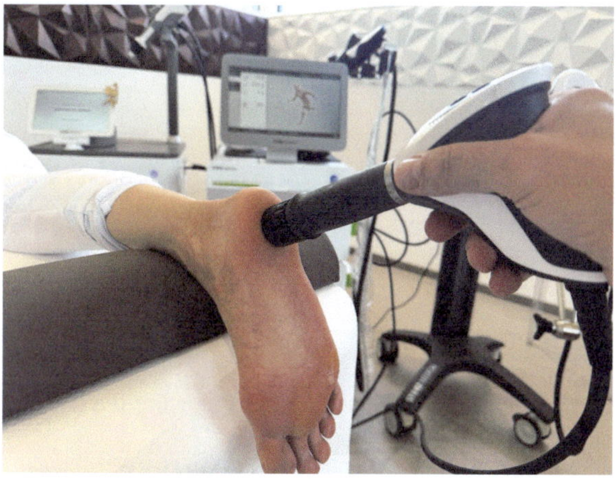

Fig. 8.5 Radial pressure wave therapy for plantar fasciitis

While both technologies provide mechanical stimulation and may yield similar clinical outcomes in certain indications, their underlying generation mechanisms and energy distributions differ substantially. Clinical selection, therefore, depends not only on diagnosis but also on anatomical depth, tissue type, and treatment intent. Radial devices do not generate a true shock front with an abrupt pressure discontinuity and are therefore physically classified as ballistic pressure waves rather than true shockwaves.

From a strict physical perspective, radial devices do not generate a classical shockwave characterized by a discontinuous pressure front and ultrafast rise time. They are therefore more accurately described as ballistic pressure-wave systems, as introduced in the PhD thesis of German urologist Gerald Haupt in 1997 (Fig. 8.5).

The continued use of the term rESWT also known as radial pressure waves (RPW) reflects historical clinical terminology rather than physical equivalence with focused shockwaves.

8.2.6 Mechanotransduction

Mechanotransduction describes the conversion of mechanical stimuli into cellular biochemical signaling, providing the theoretical framework by which ESWT is believed to influence tissue adaptation and repair [12]. Mechanical stress is thought to deform cell membranes and cytoskeletal structures, activating mechanosensitive pathways such as integrins and PIEZO1 and PIEZO2 receptors, which may contribute to intracellular signaling cascades that influence gene expression, protein synthesis, cellular proliferation, and extracellular matrix remodeling.

Mechanotransduction is considered a central biological mechanism through which ESWT may promote tissue healing. Emerging experimental evidence suggests that repeated mechanical stimulation may influence cell-signaling thresholds

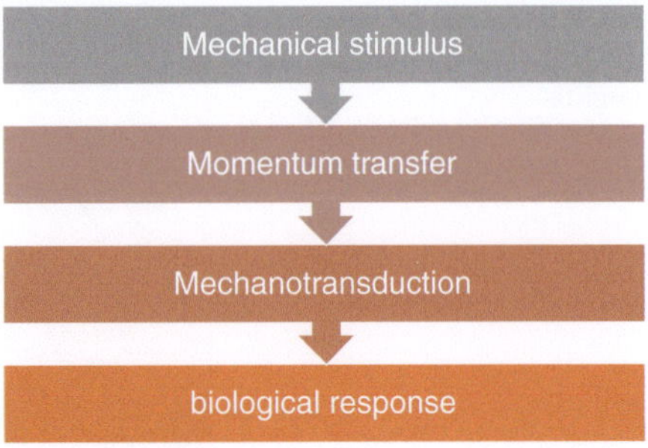

Fig. 8.6 A mechanical stimulus by focused shockwaves and radial pressure waves exerts a momentum transfer, eliciting mechanotransduction and a subsequent biological response

and tissue adaptation over time, supporting the use of repeated sessions rather than single applications.

Extracorporeal shockwave therapy (ESWT) uses acoustic waves characterized by a rapid, steep rise to elicit a biological response via mechanotransduction. Momentum transfer underlies mechanotransduction at interfaces between tissue layers with different acoustic impedances. Mechanical energy induces changes in the cellular skeleton, which trigger a response in the cell core (e.g., the release of mRNA) that influences various cellular structures, such as mitochondria, endoplasmic reticulum, and intracellular vesicles, thereby improving the healing process (Fig. 8.6).

Compared with therapeutic ultrasound, ESWT delivers single high-amplitude pulses with predominantly mechanical effects, whereas ultrasound applies sinusoidal waves that produce combined thermal and mechanical effects.

8.3 Dosology and Treatment Parameters

ESWT dosology remains one of the most debated aspects of clinical practice, requiring integration of physical parameters, device characteristics, tissue properties, and clinical presentation rather than reliance on fixed protocols. Effective dosing requires integration of device characteristics, tissue depth, pathology stage, and patient tolerance.

Energy descriptors and output values are device-specific and not always directly comparable between manufacturers. Clinical dosing should therefore be interpreted within the context of each system's calibration and clinical guidelines.

Clinicians should also consider tissue irritability and symptom behavior when selecting initial dosage, adjusting parameters progressively as tolerance improves.

8.3.1 Core Parameters

Radial ESWT (Radial Pressure Waves)

- Pressure (0.1–5 bar)
- Frequency (1–27 Hz)
- Number of impulses (usually 2000–4000/session)
- Sessions (3–6 on a weekly basis)
- Applicator size and material

Focused ESWT (Figs. 8.7 and 8.8)

- Energy flux density (mJ/mm^2)
- Frequency (Hz)
- Number of impulses
- Generator type
- Focus depth

In addition to individual parameters, total energy delivered per session (energy flux density multiplied by the number of impulses) represents an important dosing concept, as similar energy levels combined with different impulse numbers may produce substantially different biological stimulation.

Direct comparisons of dosage between devices should be made with caution, as calibration methods and energy reporting are not fully standardized across manufacturers.

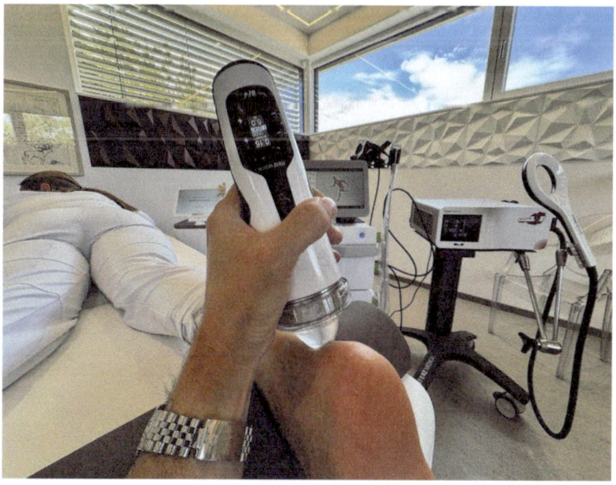

Fig. 8.7 Focused electromagnetic ESWT for midportion Achilles tendinopathy

Fig. 8.8 Focused electromagnetic ESWT in sesamoid nonunion

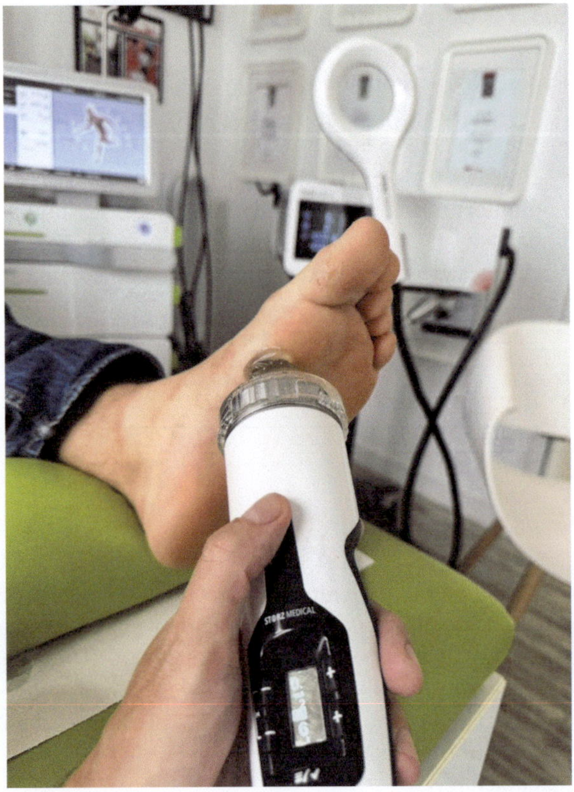

8.3.2 Energy Levels (Focused ESWT)

Very low (nano-energetic): 0.01–0.05 mJ/mm^2
Low: 0.07–0.10 mJ/mm^2
Medium: 0.12–0.25 mJ/mm^2
High: >0.25 mJ/mm^2

Energy level classifications vary across publications and manufacturers and should therefore be interpreted relative to device-specific calibration and reporting standards. Of note: in urology-based papers, everything below 0.5 mJ/mm^2 is called "low energetic," whereas in the MSK world, the aforementioned energy threshold is much lower.

Proposed energy classifications vary considerably across studies and device manufacturers. Consequently, energy categories should be interpreted as approximate clinical ranges rather than universally accepted thresholds.

8.3.3 Dose–Response Relationships

Clinical effects appear to follow a nonlinear dose–response relationship. Very low doses may fail to stimulate adaptation, while excessive doses can increase discomfort without improving outcomes. Furthermore, the target tissue is important in this regard: while nerves and lymphatics respond well to very low (nano-energetic; Fig. 8.9) and low energies, bone ESWT indications require high energy.

Lower energy levels are often associated with analgesic intent, whereas moderate to higher energy levels are thought to promote regenerative cellular responses, although clear thresholds remain debated.

Current clinical practice often uses gradual titration of energy according to patient tolerance. Typically, VAS scores <5/10 are recommended during ESWT treatment with local anesthesia. However, pain-guided dosing remains debated, as pain perception does not always correlate with biological stimulation. Excessive discomfort is not necessarily associated with improved outcomes, and patient-centered biofeedback communication is paramount for balancing ESWT efficacy and tolerability.

8.3.4 Treatment Frequency and Session Timing

Biological responses to ESWT unfold over days to weeks. Sessions are typically spaced 5–10 days apart; excessive treatment frequency may not allow tissue adaptation, and cumulative effects should be considered in treatment planning. Furthermore, tissue biologics are important: while a muscle cell divides in a week, a tendon cell has a much slower turnover of 8 weeks.

A proposed biological timeline suggests immediate neurophysiological effects within hours to days, followed by vascular and cellular responses over subsequent weeks, and structural remodeling over longer periods. This delayed timeline should be explained clearly to patients.

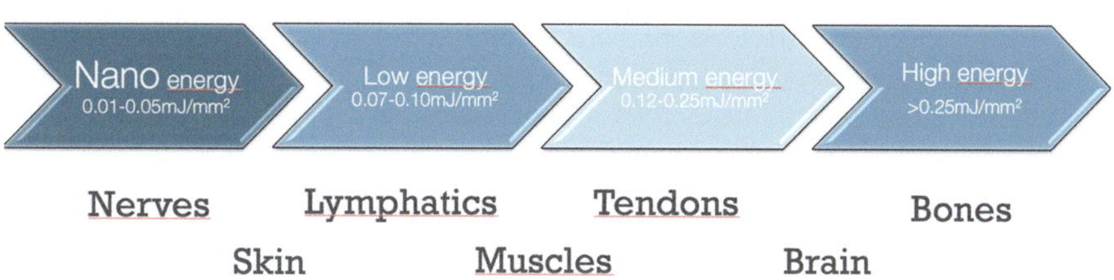

Fig. 8.9 Energy levels with an electromagnetic device in relation to the target tissue

8.3.5 Clinical Dosology by Condition (Example Ranges Reported in Clinical Studies)

Condition	Radial pressure wave	Focused ESWT (mJ/mm^2)
Achilles tendinopathy	0.5–2.0 bar, 8 Hz, ~2000 shots	0.07–0.25
Patellar tendinopathy	0.5–2.0 bar	0.07–0.25
Lateral epicondylitis	0.5–1.5 bar	0.03–0.12
Trigger finger	0.3–1.5 bar	0.03–0.10
Carpal tunnel syndrome	0.3–1.2 bar	0.03–0.10
Myofascial trigger points	0.7–2.5 bar	0.07–0.25

8.4 Mechanism of Action (Physiological and Therapeutic Effects)

Box 8.1 Clinical Decision-Making Considerations in ESWT

- Chronicity of symptoms (>3 months)
  Since the majority of clinical ESWT tendinopathy trials have included at least 3 months of symptom duration, the evidence for ESWT in chronic tendinopathies is strong. Basic science studies have shown beneficial effects on tendon properties regardless of duration. Therefore, even acute tendinopathies may respond positively to ESWT.
- Tissue depth and pathology type
  As mentioned before, the radial pressure wave interacts only superficially with the energy maximum at the skin-applicator interface. Then, by the square of the radius, the energy in the radial pressure wave diminishes. In focused ESWT, deeper tissues, such as the piriformis muscle or the hip joint, are targeted and are not accessible with radial pressure wave devices at sufficient energy. Advancements in technology, such as the deep radial pressure wave concept with a repetitive burst mode of 50 Hz, allow, for example, frozen shoulder to reach the shoulder capsular region, especially from an axillary inferior approach.
- Goal: analgesia versus regeneration
  Both radial and focused ESWT are strong pain-reducing devices. In addition, regenerative effects have been shown for both techniques. Focused ESWT induces toll-like receptor 3 (TLR3), revealing its central role in the innate immune system [13]. In addition, focused ESWT increases nitric oxide, leading to anti-inflammatory effects; stimulates exosomal release; increases VEGF-C, the lymphogenic growth factor; enhances DNA accessibility via TLR-3 activation; and facilitates the transdifferentiation of fibroblasts toward endothelial cells in ischemic myocardium [14].
- Previous response to loading programs

In tendinopathies, especially of the Achilles tendon, numerous clinical trials have demonstrated beneficial effects of collagen stimulation, including reductions in pathological neovascularization [15]. The combination of ESWT and eccentric training in Achilles tendinopathy is superior to eccentric training alone [16–19]. Home-based eccentric training should be performed with at least 6 × 15 repetitions per day for at least 12 weeks to achieve a response. Concomitantly, the combined ESWT should be applied over three to five sessions weekly initially.

- Integration with rehabilitation plan
  ESWT does not replace proper rehabilitation. Together, ESWT biostimulation and rehabilitation will improve clinical outcomes for tendinopathies and muscle injuries.
- Patient tolerance and risk profile
  Both radial and focused ESWT should be applied with pain <5/10 on the VAS during treatment, without local anesthesia. It is recommended to start at low energy levels and then titrate them up based on continuous patient feedback.
- Tissue irritability and sensitivity during assessment

  Both radial and focused ESWT are not harmful to the tissue. Even in chronic wounds, the application of ESWT has been found both feasible and successful. Different tissue types necessitate different energy levels: while nerves and lymphatics react to very low, aka nano energies, bones need high energies.

Current evidence suggests that the clinical effects of ESWT arise from the interaction of mechanical, neurophysiological, vascular, and cellular mechanisms rather than from a single dominant pathway. In other words, ESWT can stimulate a plethora of biological effects, depending on the energy levels applied, the target tissue, and the disease.

8.4.1 Mechanical Effects

Mechanical stimulation induces controlled microstress within tissues, initiating reparative responses. These effects may alter tissue stiffness and local mechanical signaling without causing clinically relevant structural damage when appropriate parameters are used. In bone, ESWT activates osteogenesis by promoting osteoblast differentiation and subsequent proliferation, as demonstrated in both in vivo and in vitro studies [20].

8.4.2 Cellular Responses

Activation of mechanotransduction pathways may stimulate the release of growth factors, including VEGF and BMP-related signaling molecules, influence tenocyte and osteoblast activity, and enhance collagen remodeling. Experimental studies also suggest the involvement of nitric oxide signaling and intracellular pathways such as the ERK/MAPK pathway, supporting the concept that mechanical stimulation may trigger broader biochemical cascades associated with tissue adaptation.

It should be emphasized that much of the mechanistic evidence regarding molecular signaling pathways derives from in vitro and animal studies. Direct confirmation of these mechanisms in human clinical populations remains limited, and current interpretations should therefore be considered biologically plausible rather than definitively proven. Consequently, mechanistic explanations should be interpreted as proposed biological models rather than fully established clinical mechanisms.

8.4.3 Inflammatory Modulation

ESWT may modulate chronic low-grade inflammatory activity and promote a shift toward a more regenerative tissue environment. ESWT reduces the proinflammatory M1 action, while the anti-inflammatory M2 response is enhanced [21, 22].

8.4.4 Vascular Effects

Angiogenesis and improved microcirculation may enhance nutrient delivery and metabolic activity, particularly in poorly vascularized tendons [23, 24].

8.4.5 Analgetic Mechanisms

Pain reduction may involve modulation of nociceptors, hyperstimulation analgesia, reduced substance P, and altered peripheral pain signaling. Central modulation and changes in pain expectation may also contribute to clinical outcomes. Burn scar pain can be reduced by ESWT via modulation of neuropeptides like substance P and calcitonin gene-related peptide CGRP [25].

8.4.6 Temporal Dynamics of Response

Clinical improvement often appears gradually after 6–8 weeks. Biological changes may begin immediately, while functional outcomes typically emerge over several weeks. Pain reduction should therefore not be interpreted as immediate structural healing via substance P modulation but rather as part of a broader adaptive process.

8.4.7 Clinical Effects of ESWT

Extracorporeal shockwave therapy is associated with several clinically relevant effects, including pain reduction, improvement in tissue loading capacity, and facilitation of functional recovery. Analgesic effects are thought to result from modulation of nociceptive activity and altered peripheral and central pain processing. In addition, ESWT may enhance tissue adaptability by promoting cellular and vascular responses that support long-term structural and functional improvement.

Clinically, these effects contribute to improved tolerance to mechanical loading, which is essential for successful rehabilitation outcomes.

8.5 Indications, Contraindications, Precautions, and Side Effects

8.5.1 Clinical Indications

The International Society for Medical Shockwave Therapy (www.ISMST.com), established in 1997, has proposed and continues to evaluate ESWT indications and contraindications based on available evidence and the long-term shockwave expertise of its board members.

As such, the ISMST categorized four indication levels: beginner, advanced, expert, and experimental (Fig. 8.10). The indication list is updated annually at the respective ISMST world conference.

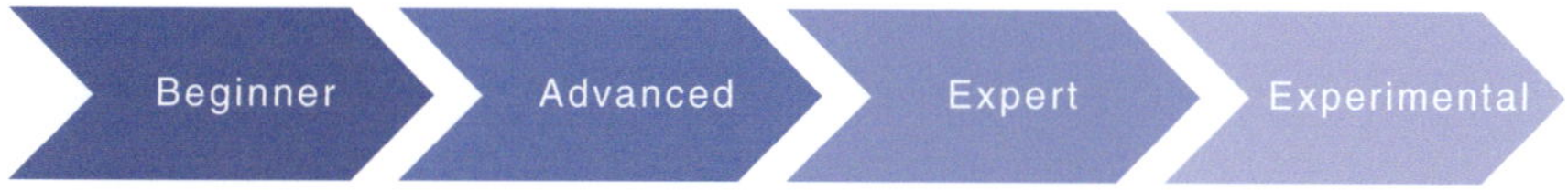

Fig. 8.10 ISMST shockwave indication levels for beginner, advanced, and expert shockwave are provided, as well as current experimental indications

1. **Approved standard indications**

1.1. Chronic Tendinopathies

1.1.1. Calcifying tendinopathy of the shoulder

1.1.2. Lateral epicondylopathy of the elbow (tennis elbow)

1.1.3. Greater trochanter pain syndrome (GTPS)

1.1.4. Patellar tendinopathy

1.1.5. Achilles tendinopathy

1.1.6. Plantar fasciitis, with or without heel spur

1.1.7 Trigger finger

1.2. Bone Pathologies

1.2.1. Delayed bone healing

1.2.2. Bone Non-Union (pseudarthroses)

1.2.3. Stress fracture

1.2.4. Avascular bone necrosis without articular derangement

1.2.5. Osteochondritis Dissecans (OCD) without articular derangement

1.3. Skin Pathologies

1.3.1. Delayed or non-healing wounds

1.3.2. Skin ulcers

1.3.3. Non-circumferential burn wounds

1.3.4. Cellulite

1.4 Spasticity

2. Common empirically-tested clinical uses

2.1. Tendinopathies

2.1.1. Rotator cuff tendinopathy without calcification

2.1.2. Medial epicondylopathy of the elbow

2.1.3. Adductor tendinopathy syndrome

2.1.4. Pes-Anserinus tendinopathy syndrome

2.1.5. Peroneal tendinopathy

2.1.6. Foot and ankle tendinopathies

2.2. Bone Pathologies

2.2.1. Bone marrow edema

2.2.2. Osgood Schlatter disease: Apophysitis of the anterior tibial tubercle

2.2.3. Tibial stress syndrome (shin splint)

2.2.4. Knee Osteoarthritis

2.3. Muscle Pathologies

2.3.1. Myofascial Syndrome

2.3.2. Muscle sprain without discontinuity

2.4. Neurological Pathologies

2.4.1. Mild to moderate carpal tunnel syndrome

2.5 Lymphedema

3. Exceptional indications – expert indications

3.1. Musculoskeletal pathologies

3.1.1. Osteoarthritis

3.1.2. Dupuytren disease

3.1.3. Plantar fibromatosis (Ledderhose disease)

3.1.4. De Quervain disease

3.1.5. Facet join syndrome

3.2. Neurological pathologies

3.2.1. Morton's neuroma

3.2.2. Polyneuropathy

3.3. Urologic pathologies

3.3.1. Pelvic chronic pain syndrome (abacterial prostatitis)

3.3.2. Erectile dysfunction

3.3.3. Peyronie disease

3.4. Others

3.4.1. Painful Lipedema

3.4.2 Heart muscle failure

4. **Experimental Indications**
4.1. Peripheral nerve lesions
4.1.1 Alzheimer's disease
4.1.2 Parkinson's disease
4.1.3 Attention Deficit Hyperactivity syndrome ADHS
4.1.4 Concussion
4.1.5 Post-Covid syndrome
4.2. Spinal cord injury
4.3. Skin calcinosis
4.4. Periodontal disease
4.5. Jawbone pathologies
4.6. Complex Regional Pain Syndrome (CRPS)
4.7. Osteoporosis

Strongly supported indications include chronic Achilles tendinopathy, plantar fasciitis, calcific rotator cuff tendinopathy, patellar tendinopathy, and lateral elbow tendinopathy.

Bone-related applications include delayed union or nonunion fractures, bone stress injuries, and bone marrow edema syndromes. Evidence supporting these indications largely originates from orthopedic and specialized medical settings, and their routine use may extend beyond standard physiotherapy practice.

These indications are frequently managed in physician-led or specialized orthopedic settings and may fall outside the scope of routine physiotherapy, depending on local regulations and clinical training.

Emerging indications include myofascial trigger points, carpal tunnel syndrome, lymphedema, and selected scar-related conditions. These applications should be interpreted cautiously, as evidence remains heterogeneous and protocols are not yet standardized. Evidence for these emerging indications remains preliminary and heterogeneous, and they are not yet universally considered standard first-line indications.

Appropriate diagnosis and confirmation of load-related symptom behavior remain essential to optimize clinical outcomes.

8.5.2 Clinical Selection Principles

ESWT is typically considered when symptoms persist beyond 3–6 months, conservative exercise-based treatment has failed, imaging supports structural pathology, and patient tolerance allows mechanical stimulation.

Clinical reasoning should also include assessment of psychosocial factors, activity demands, and previous treatment responses to ensure realistic expectations.

ESWT is generally not considered a first-line intervention for acute reactive tendon presentations, where load modification and symptom management are prioritized.

8.5.3 Contraindications

The ISMST recommends the following contraindications:

Absolute contraindications: radial pressure waves (RPW) and/or focused shockwaves with low energy:

1.1. Malignant tumor in the treatment area (not as underlying disease)
1.2. Fetus in the treatment area

Relative contraindications:

1.3. Epiphyseal plate in the treatment area
1.4. Brain or Spine in the treatment area

Absolute contraindications with high energy focused waves:

1.5. Lung tissue in the treatment area
1.6. Malignant tumor in the treatment area (not as underlying disease)
1.7. Severe coagulopathy
1.8. Fetus in the treatment area

For radial technique and focused technique with low energy (focused and defocused):

1.9. Malignant tumor in the shockwave field (not the tumor disease itself)
1.10. Fetus in the shockwave field (not the pregnancy itself)
1.11. Pacemaker/defibrillator in the shockwave field

For focused sources with high energy, the following contraindications apply:

1.12. Brain tissue/CNS in the shockwave field (at high energy)
1.13. Vertebral bodies, skull bones and ribs
1.14. Lung tissue in the shockwave field
1.15. Malignant tumor in the shockwave field (not the tumor disease itself)
1.16. Significant coagulation disorder
1.17. Fetus in the shockwave field (not the pregnancy itself)
1.18. Pacemaker/defibrillator in the shockwave field

8.5.4 Precautions

Relative contraindications include anticoagulant medication, peripheral neuropathy or altered sensation, severe osteoporosis, pediatric growth plates, and recent corticosteroid injections.

Care should be taken when treating near neurovascular structures or highly sensitive periosteal regions.

8.5.5 Side Effects and Safety Considerations

Adverse effects are usually mild and transient, including localized soreness, erythema, bruising, and a temporary increase in symptoms during early sessions.

Proper patient education regarding temporary posttreatment discomfort can reduce anxiety and improve adherence to rehabilitation plans.

A temporary increase in symptoms during the first 24–72 hours after treatment is relatively common and should be explained to patients as a normal short-term response rather than treatment failure.

8.5.6 Role of Anesthesia

In the early 2000s, trials of high-energy shockwave protocols with large machines often employed local anesthesia to improve tolerance. Notably, in epicondylitis, trials using local anesthesia with focused ESWT failed to demonstrate a clinical effect, whereas those without local anesthesia did. As early as 2005, Labek, Auersperg, and Niki Böhler from Austria conducted a triple-arm RCT to study the effect of local anesthesia on plantar fasciitis [26]. At 6 weeks, success rates after low-energy ESWT (0.09 mJ/mm^2) with local anesthesia were significantly lower than after identical low-energy ESWT without local anesthesia. Higher energy levels (0.18 mJ/mm^2) could not offset the disadvantage of this effect. LA had a significant negative effect on clinical outcomes following low-energy ESWT.

Contemporary musculoskeletal practice generally avoids anesthesia, as reduced sensory feedback and altered neural responses may diminish therapeutic effectiveness.

Box 8.2 Common Clinical Errors in ESWT Application

- Using ESWT as a standalone intervention
- Selecting parameters solely based on pain tolerance, especially with local anesthesia
- Wrong or nonprecise diagnosis
- Over-treating acute or highly irritable tissues
- Ignoring progressive loading after treatment
- Assuming higher energy automatically leads to better outcomes

8.6 Research Evidence

8.6.1 Overview of Current Evidence

Over the past decades, several hundred evidence-based papers have been published on extracorporeal shockwave therapy (ESWT).

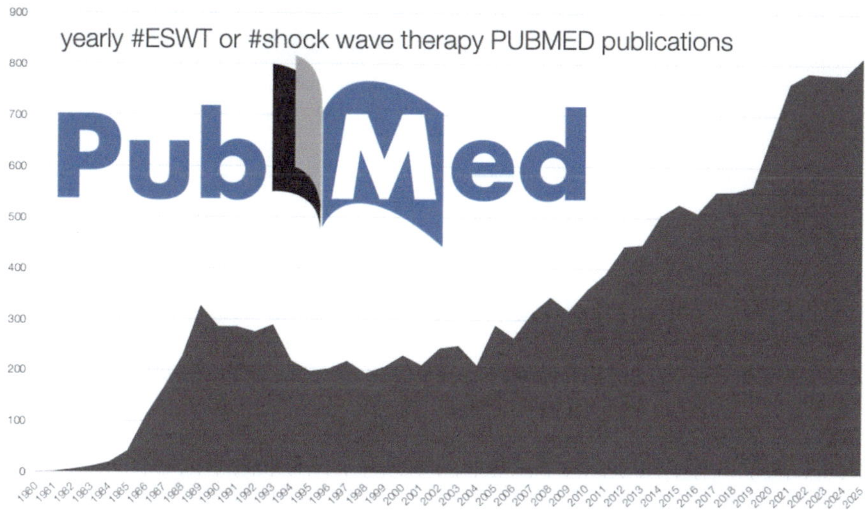

Fig. 8.11 Yearly PUBMED publication *#eswt* or *#shockwave therapy* culminating in 815 publications in 2025, the record year since the first ESWT publication in 1980

Randomized controlled trials and meta-analyses suggest moderate-to-strong evidence for several chronic tendinopathies, although variability in protocols remains a major methodological limitation. Differences in device technology, treatment parameters, and study design complicate the interpretation of findings. Differences in outcome measures, follow-up duration, and patient populations likely contribute to inconsistencies across trials.

Since the first clinical application of focused ESWT for lithotripsy in February 1980, numerous publications have reported on the experimental and clinical effects of ESWT on biological tissues. The number of PUBMED-listed publications peaked in 2025 at 815, a record year (Fig. 8.11). This underscores the still high scientific interest in a 45-year-old technology.

ESWT is a well-established modality for enhancing healing by stimulating osteogenesis, angiogenesis, and cellular regeneration [27]. Studies suggest that ESWT promotes the release of growth factors such as bone morphogenetic proteins (BMPs) and vascular endothelial growth factors (VEGFs) [28–30].

8.6.2 Evidence Table

Evidence strength categories reflect overall consistency of randomized controlled trials and meta-analyses rather than a formal grading system such as GRADE.

Condition	Evidence strength	Clinical outcome
Plantar fasciitis	Strong	Pain reduction and functional improvement
Calcific shoulder tendinopathy	Strong	Pain reduction and calcification resorption

Condition	Evidence strength	Clinical outcome
Achilles tendinopathy	Moderate–strong	Improved loading tolerance
Patellar tendinopathy	Moderate	Functional gains with combined exercise
Lateral epicondylitis	Moderate	Medium-term benefits
Bone nonunions	Strong (specialized)	Healing stimulation
Myofascial pain	Emerging	Variable outcomes

8.6.3 Interpretation of Evidence

Variability across studies may reflect differences in device technology, inconsistent energy dosing, heterogeneous patient populations, varying definitions of chronicity, and inconsistent combination with exercise therapy. Future trials may benefit from clearer reporting of dose parameters and integration with rehabilitation programs.

8.6.4 Placebo and Contextual Effects

Because ESWT produces strong sensory stimulation, placebo-controlled designs are challenging. The strong auditory and sensory characteristics of ESWT may enhance contextual and expectancy effects, making high-quality sham-controlled study designs particularly difficult to conduct. Therapeutic alliance and communication may therefore contribute meaningfully to treatment success.

8.6.5 Methodological Limitations and Future Directions

Future research should focus on standardized dosing protocols, comparative studies of radial versus focused devices, long-term outcomes, responder profiles, and integration with load-based rehabilitation frameworks.

8.7 Practical Integration of ESWT in Rehabilitation Programs

A key concept in modern physiotherapy is that ESWT should be integrated within a staged rehabilitation approach rather than applied as an isolated treatment.

8.7.1 Suggested Clinical Framework

Phase 1—Pain modulation and tissue stimulation
ESWT is applied to reduce pain and improve the tissue environment.
Phase 2—Progressive loading

Introduction or modification of tendon or muscle loading exercises.
Phase 3—Functional retraining
Restoration of movement patterns and neuromuscular control.
Phase 4—Return to activity
Sport or task-specific progression.

The timing of progression between phases should depend on symptom behavior, functional testing, and load tolerance rather than predetermined timelines.

8.7.2 Clinical Timing Considerations

ESWT sessions are often scheduled weekly. Loading intensity may be temporarily modified after treatment, and patient response guides progression rather than fixed protocols.

Box 8.3 Clinical Integration Pearls

- ESWT enhances tolerance to loading—it does not replace loading.
- Pain reduction following ESWT does not necessarily indicate structural recovery.
- Improvements often appear 4–8 weeks after treatment completion.
- Patient education is critical to prevent unrealistic expectations.
- ESWT should be embedded within a comprehensive rehabilitation strategy.

8.7.3 Current Controversies in ESWT

Despite growing evidence, important controversies remain, including the clinical equivalence of radial and focused technologies, the absence of universally accepted dosing standards, and the extent to which observed benefits reflect biological versus contextual mechanisms. Ongoing research is expected to refine patient selection and optimize treatment protocols.

8.7.4 ESWT Compared with Other EPAs

Compared with therapeutic ultrasound or laser, ESWT delivers high-amplitude, single mechanical pulses with minimal thermal contribution. Its primary therapeutic rationale focuses on mechanotransduction and load adaptation rather than thermal tissue effects.

Key Messages

- ESWT is an adjunctive modality that enhances, but does not replace, active rehabilitation.
- Mechanical stimulation via shockwaves induces biological responses through mechanotransduction.
- Treatment effects depend on appropriate dosing, tissue characteristics, and clinical context.
- Strongest evidence supports ESWT in chronic tendinopathies and selected bone conditions.
- Clinical outcomes are optimized when ESWT is combined with progressive loading strategies.
- Differences between radial and focused technologies are clinically relevant and should guide treatment selection.

8.8 Summary/Conclusion

ESWT should be viewed as a biologically active mechanostimulatory intervention rather than a purely symptomatic modality. Its clinical value appears greatest when applied within a broader rehabilitation framework that includes progressive loading, patient education, and functional restoration. Understanding differences between focused and radial technologies is essential for selecting appropriate treatment strategies.

Current evidence supports ESWT primarily in chronic tendinopathies and selected bone conditions. The strongest clinical outcomes occur when ESWT is integrated into multimodal rehabilitation programs emphasizing progressive mechanical loading and functional recovery.

Proper dosing, patient selection, and clinical reasoning remain fundamental to maximizing therapeutic outcomes.

Current evidence supports clinical improvements in pain and function; definitive structural regeneration in humans remains less clearly established.

8.9 Clinical Case Studies

8.9.1 Case 1—Chronic Achilles Tendinopathy

A 38-year-old recreational runner presented with persistent mid-portion Achilles pain lasting 8 months despite eccentric loading exercises. Assessment revealed pain during loading activities, reduced calf endurance, and ultrasound evidence of tendon thickening.

Clinical reasoning suggested a chronic tendinopathic presentation with reduced biological responsiveness. ESWT was selected to facilitate adaptation and improve tolerance to progressive loading.

Intervention included radial pressure waves, 2000 impulses at 1.2 bar, 8 Hz, weekly for five sessions, combined with monitored loading progression.

Outcome included pain reduction, improved running tolerance, and return to full activity within 8 weeks.

8.9.2 Case 2—Calcific Rotator Cuff Tendinopathy

A 52-year-old patient presented with chronic shoulder pain and imaging-confirmed calcific deposits. Assessment showed a painful arc and reduced abduction following failed conservative management.

Focused ESWT was selected due to the depth and density of calcification.

Intervention consisted of focused ESWT (0.18–0.25 mJ/mm^2), 2000 shots, three sessions combined with shoulder mobility and strengthening exercises.

Outcome included improved range of motion, reduced pain, and functional recovery at 3-month follow-up.

Review Questions

1. Differentiate radial and focused ESWT in terms of physical properties and clinical indications.
2. Explain the role of acoustic impedance in ESWT effectiveness.
3. Describe the concept of mechanotransduction and its therapeutic relevance.
4. How does energy dose influence clinical outcomes?
5. Why should ESWT be integrated with progressive loading programs?
6. Discuss common methodological limitations in ESWT research.
7. Identify major contraindications and precautions.
8. Describe a staged rehabilitation model incorporating ESWT.

Declarations

Competing Interests The author(s) have no competing interests to declare that are relevant to the content of this manuscript.

References

1. d'Agostino MC, et al. Shockwave therapy in musculoskeletal disorders: biological mechanisms and clinical evidence. Int J Surg. 2015.
2. Buarque de Gusmão CV, Batista NA, Lemes VTV, et al. Effects of extracorporeal shockwave therapy on musculoskeletal tissues. Ultrasound Med Biol. 2019.
3. Cheng JH, Jhan SW, Chen PC, et al. Effects of extracorporeal shockwave therapy in musculoskeletal conditions. Bone Joint Res. 2023.
4. Cho HK, Sung WJ, Lee YJ. Clinical outcomes following extracorporeal shockwave therapy in musculoskeletal disorders. J Int Med Res. 2021.
5. Duarte de Oliveira, et al. https://doi.org/10.1136/bmjopen-2025-104789.
6. de la Barra Ortiz, et al. https://doi.org/10.1007/s10103-026-04812-9.

7. Shivappa P, et al. https://doi.org/10.1186/s12967-025-07466-3.
8. ISMST ESWT guideline. www.ismst.com.
9. Csaszar NBM, et al. https://doi.org/10.1371/journal.pone.0140541.
10. Knemoku T, et al. https://doi.org/10.1016/j.jos.2020.07.009.
11. Auersperg V, et al. https://doi.org/10.1302/2058-5241.5.190067.
12. d'Agostino MC, et al. Mechanotransduction and regenerative effects of extracorporeal shockwave therapy. Int J Surg. 2015.
13. Holfeld J, Tepeköylü C, Reissig C, et al. https://doi.org/10.1186/s13578-020-00522-z.
14. Graber M, Gollmann-Tepeköylü C, Schweiger V, et al. https://doi.org/10.1093/ehjopen/oeaf011.
15. Knobloch K, et al. https://doi.org/10.1177/0363546505278705.
16. Rompe JD, et al. https://doi.org/10.1177/0363546508326983.
17. Rompe JD, et al. https://doi.org/10.2106/JBJS.F.01494.
18. Rompe JD, et al. https://doi.org/10.1177/0363546506295940.
19. Korakakis V, et al. https://doi.org/10.1136/bjsports-2016-097347.
20. Wang FS, Wang CJ, Chen YJ, et al. https://doi.org/10.1074/jbc.M308013200.
21. d'Agostino MC, et al. https://doi.org/10.1016/j.ijsu.2015.07.719.
22. d'Agostino MC, et al. https://doi.org/10.1016/j.ijsu.2015.11.030.
23. Wang CJ, et al. https://doi.org/10.1007/s00402-008-0663-1.
24. Wang CJ, et al. https://doi.org/10.1016/j.niox.2009.02.006.
25. Zhao M. https://doi.org/10.3389/fphys.2025.1627798.
26. Labek G, et al. https://doi.org/10.1055/s-2004-832379.
27. Lv F, Li Z, Jing Y, et al. https://doi.org/10.3389/fendo.2023.1188297.
28. Cheng JH, Jhan SW, Chen PC, et al. https://doi.org/10.1302/2046-3758.137.BJR-2023-0264.R2.
29. Buarque de Gusmao CV, Batista NA, Lemes VTV, et al. https://doi.org/10.1016/j.ultrasmedbio.2019.04.011.
30. Gerdesmeyer L, Zielhardt P, Klüter T, et al. https://doi.org/10.1080/15368378.2022.2079672.

The Use of Electrophysical Agents (EPAs) in the Healing Process, in the Management of Pain and Edema, and for Increasing Tissue Extensibility, Flexibility, and Range of Motion

9

Dimitrios Stasinopoulos

9.1 Introduction

Electrophysical agents (EPAs) can be valuable tools in rehabilitation when applied within a structured clinical reasoning framework. Their effectiveness does not depend solely on the modality itself but on the clinician's ability to select, dose, and integrate them appropriately based on the patient's presentation and stage of healing. Rather than following prescriptive protocols, clinicians should adopt a goal-oriented approach, tailoring EPA use to the specific needs of each clinical scenario [10].

EPAs are used to:

- Facilitate tissue healing
- Relieve pain
- Decrease edema
- Alter collagen extensibility

These core objectives are rarely pursued in isolation; rather, they overlap throughout the recovery period. For instance, facilitating tissue healing often concurrently modulates pain, while reducing edema is a prerequisite for restoring range of motion (ROM). Understanding these interdependencies allows the clinician to transition from a modality-centered approach to a goal-oriented strategy.

A summary of the above processes is presented below. A complete discussion of the physiological processes affected by EPAs is provided in Chaps. 2, 3, 4, 5, 6, 7, and 8. It is important to reiterate that in any rehabilitation program, EPAs should be used as adjuncts to manual therapy (assessment, exercise programs, and

D. Stasinopoulos (✉)
University of West Attica, Athens, Greece
e-mail: dstasinopoulos@uniwa.gr

D. Stasinopoulos (ed.), *Application of Electrophysical Agents in Physiotherapy*,
https://doi.org/10.1007/978-3-032-32144-2_9

mobilization/manipulation/soft-tissue techniques) and should certainly not be used to the exclusion of therapeutic exercises.

This chapter synthesizes the biophysical principles, physiological effects, and clinical applications discussed throughout this textbook. It translates them into practical clinical reasoning for the use of EPAs across the rehabilitation continuum.

9.2 Facilitating Tissue Healing

Facilitating tissue healing represents one of the fundamental clinical applications of electrophysical agents. Appropriate selection and timing of EPAs require integrating tissue pathology, the healing stage, and rehabilitation goals.

Inflammation is the first stage of healing, followed by proliferation and maturation. It must be stressed that although the phases of healing are presented as three separate entities, the healing process is a continuum [10]. The mechanisms of tissue healing are described in detail in many textbooks and are outside the scope of this chapter. Tissue healing is facilitated by selecting appropriate EPAs. Thus, the therapist must understand the healing process to effectively incorporate EPAs into rehabilitation.

Nonthermal modalities are applied during the inflammatory stage. When the symptoms of inflammation (swelling, pain, redness, heat, and loss of function) are reduced, the therapist can use thermal or nonthermal modalities. The choice between thermal and nonthermal modalities after the inflammatory stage depends on the therapy's goal. Many clinicians continue using nonthermal modalities for weeks after injury; in fact, some never switch to thermal EPAs [10]. This procedure is often a matter of personal preference, determined by experience. Pulsed shortwave diathermy (PSWD) with thermal effects (increased intensity) appears to be superior to US in reducing pain and improving function and strength during tissue healing [6].

Nonthermal modalities are applied differently (dosage) at different stages of tissue healing. For example, pulsed US can be used during the inflammatory period at a duty cycle of 20%, an intensity of 0.1–0.3 W/cm^2, and twice daily. Once the inflammatory stage is complete, pulsed US can be used once daily or every other day, with a higher duty cycle and intensity. Low-level laser therapy (LLLT), pulsed shortwave therapy (PSWT), and PEMF therapy can be applied similarly, with lower doses during the inflammatory stage and higher doses in subsequent healing stages.

Cryotherapy is primarily used during the inflammatory stage. Many people think the purpose of cryotherapy is to decrease inflammation. However, inflammation is necessary to prepare the body for healing. One purpose of cryotherapy is to minimize secondary tissue injury [6].

Extracorporeal shock wave therapy (ESWT) is generally avoided during the inflammatory stage. However, some trials, particularly for muscle injuries, recommend ESWT during the inflammatory stage [9]. ESWT appears to play an important role in soft-tissue repair and healing.

The strategic timing of these interventions is paramount. While the traditional view suggested a rigid progression from nonthermal to thermal agents, modern clinical reasoning advocates a more flexible approach based on the tissue's specific biological "readiness" and the patient's individual inflammatory profile.

Polarized polychromatic non-coherent light (PPNCL) can be used at all stages of healing, but appears to work best during the inflammatory stage [5].

A popular therapy for subacute and chronic conditions is applying thermal EPAs before practice or exercise, followed by cryotherapy afterward. However, evidence neither supports nor refutes this regimen. A pilot study does not support the use of cryotherapy in patients with lateral elbow tendinopathy (LET) after an exercise program [8].

Ultimately, the clinical value of EPAs in tissue healing lies not in selecting isolated parameters but in integrating them into staged rehabilitation programs, where they support biological repair while enabling progressive loading and functional restoration. The choice between thermal and nonthermal EPAs should be guided by tissue-healing status and therapeutic goals rather than by rigid, stage-based rules.

Clinical Implication The selection of EPAs for tissue healing should be guided by the biological stage of repair and the intended therapeutic goal, with emphasis on supporting tissue adaptation rather than attempting to accelerate healing through isolated interventions.

9.3 Management of Pain

Pain management is not only a symptomatic goal but also a prerequisite for functional recovery, movement restoration, and patient engagement in rehabilitation.

Pain is the main reason patients seek treatment [2]. Pain is an unpleasant sensory and emotional experience, and its management is challenging [4]. Pain is modulated through the gate control theory and the descending endogenous opioid system. Many textbooks explain pain physiology and offer evidence-based management recommendations. This textbook does not cover those details. Electrical stimulation may be used as one evidence-informed option for pain modulation within a broader rehabilitation program. Therapists should teach patients how to manage pain at home.

The question that arises is whether EPAs can be applied for pain management. Pain is a complex and multifactorial phenomenon. Applying appropriate EPAs to manage pain is not a simple process, as different EPAs have specific, often beneficial effects on tissues. However, they also have nonspecific sensory, cognitive, and emotional impacts on patients that should be considered [4].

From a contemporary biopsychosocial perspective, the effects of EPAs on pain should be understood not only through peripheral tissue mechanisms but also through central modulation, contextual factors, and patient expectations.

Cryotherapy is used to manage acute pain during the inflammatory stage (see Chap. 2). Moreover, cryotherapy applied during the proliferation and maturation phases should be used for pain control; therefore, only the skin temperature needs to be reduced sufficiently to modulate pain [6]. This is when clinicians should choose cryotherapy treatment settings that focus on cooling the patient's skin tissue rather than the underlying musculoskeletal tissue [6].

Although thermotherapy may reduce pain of any origin (by washing away chemical irritants that cause pain), it is contraindicated in acute pain.

The main clinical effect of nonthermal EPAs (PSWT, pulsed US, LLLT, and pulsed electromagnetic field therapy (PEMF) is the promotion of tissue repair processes. In cases where stimulation of repair mechanisms is the primary goal of treatment (for acute or chronic conditions), pain relief will occur concomitantly with repair progression; that is, the patient's pain will decrease as repair progresses. Therefore, clinicians should understand the healing process to select appropriate EPAs for managing pain.

ESWT may be used as a counterirritant; overstimulation of mechanoreceptors at the treated site can reduce the transmission of nociceptive signals to the brainstem [1].

Ultimately, pain management through EPAs serves as more than just symptomatic relief; it acts as a "neuromodulatory bridge" that reduces kinesiophobia and facilitates the transition to active, movement-based therapy. By altering nociceptive input, EPAs help patients regain confidence in their physical capabilities.

Clinical Implication EPAs should be viewed as neuromodulatory tools that facilitate patient engagement in active rehabilitation by reducing pain and fear of movement, rather than as stand-alone pain-relieving interventions.

9.4 Management of Edema

Effective management of edema is essential, as persistent swelling interferes with tissue repair, joint mobility, neuromuscular control, and functional recovery.

Edema, also known as fluid retention, swelling, dropsy, and hydropsy, is the accumulation of fluid in the body's tissues. Edema is one of the five primary signs of inflammation (see Sect. 9.2). One purpose of cryotherapy is to minimize edema (see Sect. 9.2). The less edema present, the faster the injury can heal. The clinician should use cryotherapy immediately after injury. Once edema has developed, cryotherapy cannot decrease it. Cryotherapy does not act as monotherapy to reduce edema. It should be combined with other therapeutic approaches (compression, elevation, protection) during the first 2–3 days (or 2–5 days, according to some sources) after injury.

EPAs with nonthermal effects may be used in the first days after injury to reduce swelling; however, evidence supporting this for some EPAs, such as pulsed US and PSWT, remains insufficient.

As edema and other inflammatory symptoms subside, the therapist can use thermal or nonthermal modalities within the scope of treatment (see Sect. 9.2 for more details). No patient with edema should be treated with any heat modality until the cause of the edema has been determined.

The therapist should use cryotherapy immediately after injury. However, if, 5 days after injury (when the inflammatory stage has ended), a small amount of swelling remains, the therapist may consider whether to continue cryotherapy or switch to thermotherapy. The recommendation is to continue cryotherapy and non-thermal modalities alongside a manual therapy program until the edema resolves. Cryotherapy is effective at preventing edema but not at removing it. Edema reduction occurs as free protein is removed from the area [6]. When the edema resolves, the patient can use thermal or nonthermal modalities alongside a manual therapy program, depending on the treatment goal.

If, on day 5 after injury, a large amount of edema is present due to the patient not receiving cryotherapy immediately, cryotherapy is unlikely to be effective. An appropriate manual therapy program will help reduce the edema. EPAs with thermal or nonthermal effects can also be used, in line with the goals of therapy.

Clinicians should therefore conceptualize edema management as a dynamic process that requires continuous reassessment and the coordinated application of EPAs, manual techniques, and movement-based interventions. It is essential to recognize that edema management is a time-sensitive intervention. The physiological transition from acute fluid accumulation to organized swelling dictates a change in EPA selection, shifting from vasoconstrictive cryotherapy to modalities that support lymphatic drainage and metabolic activity.

Clinical Implication Effective edema management requires early, coordinated intervention that combines EPAs with mechanical and functional strategies to optimize fluid dynamics and tissue recovery.

9.5 Increasing Tissue Extensibility, Flexibility, and Range of Motion

Restoration of tissue extensibility and joint range of motion is a central objective of rehabilitation and directly influences movement quality, functional capacity, and the risk of injury recurrence.

Range of motion (ROM) refers to how far and in what direction a joint or muscle can move. Loss or impairment of motion can result from pain, edema, joint stiffness, soft-tissue shortening, or altered muscle tone (e.g., spasticity). Decreased muscle strength can also limit ROM, as can pain. It is crucial to determine the cause of limited or impaired ROM to develop an appropriate management plan.

Pain can limit ROM. To manage acute pain or pain at rest that limits ROM, nonthermal EPAs can be used. Please refer to Sects. 9.1 and 9.2 for guidance on applying appropriate EPAs as pain subsides and ROM increases. To address chronic pain or pain with motion that is associated with decreased muscle strength and loss of ROM, thermal or nonthermal EPAs, as well as ESWT, can be used, depending on the rehabilitation goal. Muscle spasm is relieved more quickly with cold and stretching than with heat and stretching [6]. The patient must be able to tolerate cryotherapy.

Acute or chronic edema can lead to ROM impairment. Please refer to Sect. 9.4 for the management of edema using appropriate EPAs.

Joint stiffness is another cause of loss of mobility and ROM. Adhesive capsulitis, osteoarthritis, and rheumatoid arthritis are examples of conditions that can cause joint stiffness. When inflammatory signs are absent, thermal EPAs may be used to heat the affected restricted areas. Diathermy is recommended for capsular stiffness. Nonthermal EPAs may be used if tissues are inflamed. For example, a patient with adhesive capsulitis presenting with decreased ROM but without signs of inflammation may be managed with thermal EPAs. On the other hand, if the same patient presents with decreased ROM and signs of inflammation (acute pain or pain at rest), nonthermal EPAs may be used. As mentioned in the introduction to this chapter (Sect. 9.1), EPAs are not used as monotherapy. EPAs prepare tissues for manual therapy.

Soft-tissue shortening is another cause of loss of ROM and results from many injuries. Although soft-tissue shortening is outside the scope of this section, it is usually the result of disorganization of collagen fibers and structural changes within them [2]. Thermal EPAs are used to improve tissue extensibility before or during a manual therapy program (see Sect. 9.1), thereby enhancing the effectiveness of these interventions. Thermal EPAs cause collagen fibers to relax. Diathermy is usually recommended for muscle stiffness, whereas US is recommended for other causes of soft-tissue shortening.

Cryotherapy is known to increase stiffness. The question, therefore, arises whether nonthermal EPAs, such as cryotherapy, can be applied to muscle length. Research has shown that cryotherapy increases hamstring length when applied before stretching, compared with stretching alone or stretching with hot packs [3, 7]. Therefore, cryotherapy can be used to improve ROM limited by muscle inflexibility. Some clinicians recommend heat, followed by stretching, and then cryotherapy. Cryotherapy may enable collagen fibers to reattach in a lengthened position.

The synergy between thermal EPAs and mechanical loading is perhaps the clearest example of the integrative role of physical agents. By temporarily altering the viscoelastic properties of collagenous structures, EPAs create an optimal "biomechanical environment" for manual stretching and mobilization, thereby achieving permanent structural changes.

The application of EPAs in this context should be viewed as preparatory and supportive, facilitating manual therapy and active movement interventions rather than substituting for them.

Loss of ROM secondary to spasticity may also be observed. Thermal or nonthermal EPAs and ESWT can be used to manage this cause of ROM limitation.

Clinical Implication EPAs are most effective in improving range of motion when used as preparatory interventions that enhance the response to manual therapy and active movement.

9.6 Conclusion

This final chapter integrates the scientific principles and clinical applications presented throughout this textbook.

EPAs play a vital role in the rehabilitation process (tissue healing, pain management, edema control, and ROM restoration) when applied appropriately. Some EPAs can be used at home (e.g., cryotherapy and thermotherapy), whereas others can only be applied in a clinical setting (e.g., US, diathermy, LLLT, HILT, ESWT, and PEMF therapy). As mentioned in Sect. 9.3 (Pain), one of the critical roles of physical therapists is to educate patients throughout the rehabilitation process. Using EPAs in isolation is unlikely to result in meaningful improvements in rehabilitation. However, when administered in combination with other therapeutic approaches, the likelihood of facilitating healing by reducing pain and edema and improving ROM increases.

Future advances in technology, research methodology, and rehabilitation science will continue to refine the role of EPAs, reinforcing physiotherapists' responsibility to apply these interventions within evidence-informed, patient-centered, and ethically grounded frameworks.

Ultimately, the clinical effectiveness of EPAs depends less on the specific modality selected and more on the quality of clinical reasoning, appropriate dosing, and their integration within active, patient-centered rehabilitation strategies.

Declarations

Competing Interests The author(s) have no competing interests to declare that are relevant to the content of this manuscript.

References

1. Alsulaimani B, Perraton L, Vallance P, Powers T, Malliaras P. Does shockwave therapy lead to better pain and function than sham over 12 weeks in people with insertional Achilles tendinopathy? A randomised controlled trial. Clin Rehabil. 2025;39:174–86.
2. Bellew J, Nolan T. Michlovitz's modalities for therapeutic intervention. 7th ed. Philadelphia: FA Davis; 2022.
3. Brodowicz GR, Welsh R, Wallis J. Comparison of stretching with ice, stretching with heat, or stretching alone on hamstring flexibility. J Athl Train. 1996;31:324–7.
4. Cameron M. Physical agents in rehabilitation. An evidence – based approach to practice. 6th ed. St. Louis: Elsevier; 2023.
5. Dimitrios S. Recommendations of polarized polychromatic non-coherent light (Bioptron light) in the management of musculoskeletal conditions. Ann Physiother Occup Ther. 2021;4:000191.
6. Draper D, Juttle L, Knight K. Therapeutic modalities. The art and science. 3rd ed. Philadelphia: Wolters Kluwer; 2021.
7. Larsen CC, Troiano JM, Ramirez RJ, Miller MG, Holcomb WR. Effects of crushed ice and wetted ice on hamstring flexibility. J Strength Cond Res. 2015;29:483–8.
8. Manias P, Stasinopoulos D. A controlled clinical pilot trial to study the effectiveness of ice as a supplement to the exercise program for the management of lateral elbow tendinopathy. Br J Sports Med. 2006;40:81–5.

9. Morgan JPM, Hamm M, Schmitz C, Brem MH. Return to play after treating acute muscle injuries in elite football players with radial extracorporeal shock wave therapy. J Orthop Surg Res. 2021;16:708.
10. Prentice WE. Therapeutic modalities in rehabilitation. 6th ed. New York: McGraw-Hill Medical; 2021.

MIX
Papier aus verantwortungsvollen Quellen
Paper from responsible sources
FSC® C105338

If you have any concerns about our products,
you can contact us on
ProductSafety@springernature.com

In case Publisher is established outside the EU,
the EU authorized representative is:
Springer Nature Customer Service Center GmbH
Europaplatz 3, 69115 Heidelberg, Germany

Printed by Libri Plureos GmbH
in Hamburg, Germany